Medical Response to

Child Sexual

Abuse

A Resource for Professionals
Working with Children and Families

STM **Learning,** Inc.

Leading Publisher of Scientific, Technical, and Medical Educational Resources
Saint Louis
www.stmlearning.com

OUR MISSION

To become the world leader in publishing and

information services on child abuse,

maltreatment, diseases, and domestic violence.

We seek to heighten awareness of these issues,

and provide relevant information to

professionals and consumers.

*A portion of our profits is contributed to nonprofit organizations
dedicated to the prevention of child abuse and the care of victims
of abuse and other children and family charities.*

This book is dedicated to everyone who has been affected by child sexual abuse. It is our sincere hope that this will empower medical providers to give the most up-to-date and scientifically based care for victims. No one should undergo the trauma that these youngsters have undergone without high quality and responsive medical care in addition to other community interventions. It is our profound hope that this text makes a difference.

Rich Kaplan, MSW, MD, FAAP
Joyce A. Adams, MD
Suzanne P. Starling, MD, FAAP
Angelo P. Giardino, MD, PhD, MPH, FAAP

Medical Response to

Child Sexual

Abuse

A Resource for Professionals
Working with Children and Families

Rich Kaplan, MSW, MD, FAAP
Child Abuse Pediatrician
Children's Hospitals and Clinics of Minnesota
Associate Professor of Pediatrics
University of Minnesota Medical School
Medical Director
The Center for Safe and Healthy Children
University of Minnesota Amplatz
Children's Hospital
Associate Medical Director
Midwest Children's Resource Center
Children's Hospitals and Clinics of Minnesota
Minneapolis, Minnesota

Joyce A. Adams, MD
Professor of Clinical Pediatrics
Division of General Academic Pediatrics and
Adolescent Medicine
School of Medicine
University of California, San Diego
Specialist in Child Abuse Pediatrics
Rady Children's Hospital
San Diego, California

Suzanne P. Starling, MD, FAAP
Professor of Pediatrics
Eastern Virginia Medical School
Division Director, Child Abuse Pediatrics
Medical Director, Child Abuse Program
Children's Hospital of The King's Daughters
Norfolk, Virginia

Angelo P. Giardino, MD, PhD, MPH, FAAP
Medical Director
Texas Children's Health Plan
Clinical Professor of Pediatrics
Baylor College of Medicine
Attending Physician
Children's Assessment Center
Texas Children's Hospital
Houston, Texas

STM Learning, Inc.

Leading Publisher of Scientific, Technical, and Medical Educational Resources
Saint Louis
www.stmlearning.com

Publishers: Glenn E. Whaley and Marianne V. Whaley
Art Director: Glenn E. Whaley
Managing Editor: Sharifa N. Barakat
Associate Editor: Mallory C. Skinner
Book Design/Page Layout: G.W. Graphics
                              Heather N. Green
Print/Production Coordinator: Heather N. Green
Cover Design: G.W. Graphics
Color Prepress Specialist: Kevin Tucker
Acquisition Editor: Glenn E. Whaley
Developmental Editor: Laurie Sparks
                          Shawn Greene
Copy Editor: Sheri Kubasek
                Leigh Smith
Proofreader: Katie Sharp
Indexer: Donna M. Drialo

Printed in China.

Publisher:
STM Learning, Inc.
609 East Lockwood Avenue, Suite 203, Saint Louis, Missouri 63119-3287 USA
Phone: (314)993-2728 Fax: (314)993-2281 Toll Free: (800)600-0330
http://www.stmlearning.com

Library of Congress Cataloging-in-Publication Data

Medical response to child sexual abuse : a resource for professionals working with children and families / Rich Kaplan ... [et al.].
     p. ; cm.
  Includes bibliographical references and index.
  ISBN 978-1-878060-12-9
  1. Sexually abused children. 2. Child sexual abuse--Diagnosis. I. Kaplan, Rich, 1950-
  [DNLM: 1. Child Abuse, Sexual--diagnosis. 2. Child Abuse, Sexual--therapy. 3. Adolescent. 4. Child.
5. Forensic Medicine--methods. 6. Physical Examination--methods. WA 325]
  RJ507.S49M44 2011
  618.92'85836--dc22

                        2010045973

CONTRIBUTORS

Michelle I. Amaya, MD, MPH
ABP Board Certified, Child Abuse Pediatrics
Associate Professor
Department of Pediatrics
Medical University of South Carolina
Charleston, South Carolina

Craig L. Barlow, JD
Assistant Attorney General
Division Chief
Children's Justice Division
Utah Attorney General's Office
Salt Lake City, Utah

Kathy Bell, MS, RN, SANE-A, SANE-P
Forensic Nursing Administrator
Tulsa Police Department
Tulsa, Oklahoma

Robert W. Block, MD, FAAP
Professor and Daniel C. Plunket Chair
Department of Pediatrics
School of Community Medicine
The University of Oklahoma-Tulsa

Daniel D. Broughton, MD
Professor of Pediatric and Adolescent Medicine
Mayo Clinic
Rochester, Minnesota

Michelle Clayton, MD, MPH, FAAP
Assistant Professor of Pediatrics
Eastern Virginia Medical School
Children's Hospital of The King's Daughters
Norfolk, Virginia

Judith A. Cohen, MD
Medical Director
Center for Traumatic Stress in Children & Adolescents
Allegheny General Hospital
Professor of Psychiatry
Drexel University College of Medicine
Pittsburgh, PA

Sharon W. Cooper, MD, FAAP
Adjunct Professor of Pediatrics
University of North Carolina School of Medicine
Chapel Hill, North Carolina

Allan R. De Jong, MD
Medical Director
Children at Risk Evaluation (CARE) Program
Nemours - Alfred I. duPont Hospital for Children
Wilmington, Delaware

Karen J. Farst, MD, MPH
Assistant Professor
Department of Pediatrics
College of Medicine
University of Arkansas for Medical Sciences
Little Rock, Arkansas

Martin A. Finkel, DO, FACOP, FAAP
Professor of Pediatrics
Medical Director
Child Abuse Research Education & Service (CARES)
Institute
School of Osteopathic Medicine
University of Medicine and Dentistry of New Jersey
Stratford, New Jersey

Lori Frasier, MD
Professor of Pediatrics
Medical Director
Medical Assessment Team
Primary Children's Center for Safe and Healthy Families
Salt Lake City, Utah

Roberta A. Hibbard, MD
Professor of Pediatrics
Director
Section of Child Protection Programs
Indiana University School of Medicine
Indianapolis, Indiana

Jerry G. Jones, MD
Professor of Pediatrics
University of Arkansas for Medical Sciences
Director
Center for Children at Risk
University of Arkansas for Medical Sciences
Arkansas Children's Hospital
Little Rock, Arkansas

Nancy D. Kellogg, MD
Division Chief and Professor of Pediatrics
Division of Child Abuse Pediatrics
UT Health Science Center, San Antonio
San Antonio, Texas

Anthony C. Leonard, PhD
Assistant Professor
Biostatistician
Department of Public Health Sciences
University of Cincinnati College of Medicine
Cincinnati, Ohio

Kathi L. Makoroff, MD
Assistant Professor of Pediatrics
University of Cincinnati College of Medicine
Mayerson Center for Safe and Healthy Children
Cincinnati Children's Hospital and Medical Center
Cincinnati, Ohio

Anthony P. Mannarino, PhD

Marcellina Mian, MDCM, FRCPC, FAAP
Adjunct Professor of Pediatrics
Weill Cornell Medical College in Qatar
Doha, Qatar
Lecturer in Pediatrics
Harvard Medical School
Boston, Massachusetts

Laura K. Murray, PhD
Assistant Professor of International Health
Boston University School of Public Health
Boston, Massachusetts

Vincent Palusci, MD, MS, FAAP
Professor of Pediatrics
New York University School of Medicine
New York, New York

Carol A. Plummer, PhD
Associate Professor
Myron B. Thompson School of Social Work
University of Hawaii
Honolulu, Hawaii

Robert A. Shapiro, MD
Professor of Clinical Pediatrics
University of Cincinnati College of Medicine
Medical Director
Mayerson Center for Safe and Healthy Children
Cincinnati Children's Hospital Medical Center
Cincinnati, Ohio

John Stirling, Jr., MD
Director
Center for Child Protection
Santa Clara Valley Medical Center
Medical Director
Santa Clara County's Children Shelter
San Jose, California
Clinical Professor
Stanford University
Lucile Packard Children's Hospital
Palo Alto, California

Supplemental Photo Contributions

Michelle Ditton, RN, FNE, SANE-A, SANE-P
Diana Faugno, MSN, RN, CPN, SANE-A, SANE-P, FAAFS, DF-IAFN
Margie Jessen, RN, FNP
Marilyn Kaufhold, MD
Carolyn Levitt, MD
Arne Myhre, MD
Lynn Sheets, MD
Mary Spencer, MD

FOREWORD

Substantiation of reports of sexual abuse of children has been declining since 1990, reduced by 51%, according to Jones (*Childhood Victimization: Violence, Crime, and Abuse in the Lives of Young People*). Researchers in this field expressed doubt that this steep decline could be real, and this prompted further investigation (*Child Abuse Negl.* 2001;25:1139-1158). The findings of this research suggested the decline was real and did not reflect changed standards by agencies or other artifactual explanations (*Explanations for the Decline in Child Sexual Abuse Cases*). They found that this decline paralleled other social improvements: the fall in teen suicides, teenage births, numbers of children living in poverty, youth runaways, juvenile drug use, and improvements in child behavior problems and competence scores on the Child Behavior Checklist.[1] While considering numerous factors to explain these trends, Finkelhor and Jones suggest that agents of social intervention "could well have curbed child victimization through a number of mechanisms" (*Childhood Victimization: Violence, Crime, and Abuse in the Lives of Young People*). These agents include police, victim advocates, legal advocates, teachers who educate about maltreatment and domestic violence as well as the media, who have raised awareness of victimization by reporting on maltreatment and portraying it in film and on television.

I believe another factor involved: more highly developed professional skills at all levels of the diagnostic process. Over the last 25 years, the evidence base in child sexual abuse has grown exponentially. Since 1994, over 300 peer-reviewed articles have been published in medical journals alone, and this figure doesn't include research published in the social sciences, mental health, legal and law enforcement publications. In addition, the education and training of professionals for this field of practice has improved substantially. This ensures more accurate diagnosis in these cases and avoids confusing normal variants or other mimics of sexual abuse for true cases.

This is where this up-to-date, well-written book is so helpful. The authors of the various chapters in *Medical Response to Child Sexual Abuse* are truly experts in the field, with clinical experience and research to bolster their writing. There are chapters in this volume that are not available in other books on sexual abuse: the background and history of the field, special problems of adolescent patients, qualifications of medical examiners, child sexual abuse as a global issue, child sexual abuse as a symptom, an approach to the disabled child who may have been abused, and sexual abuse prevention strategies, to name just a few. These, in addition to the basics about anatomy and the medical approach to diagnosis, will equip the child abuse professional to be more proficient and precise in the performance and interpretation of a child sexual abuse evaluation.

Robert M. Reece, MD
Clinical Professor of Pediatrics
Tufts University School of Medicine
Director
Child Protection Program
The Floating Hospital for Children
Tufts New England Medical Center
Boston, Massachusetts
Editor
The Quarterly Update
North Falmouth, Massachusetts

FOREWORD

We may never truly know exactly how many children are sexually abused during their childhood years, but we do know that the numbers are enormous. Child sexual abuse is more common than childhood cancer, juvenile diabetes, and congenital heart disease combined. Despite this, public discussion or even acknowledgement of this issue was not commonplace throughout most of history. This is no longer the case today. In fact, public awareness of the problem has never been higher. Internet predators, clergy abuse scandals, and cases involving child pornography regularly make local and national headlines alongside countless other stories of children being sexually abused by family members or other close contacts. Many of the television crime dramas watched by children and parents alike now routinely include stories about the sexual abuse of children. As our collective awareness of the problem of child sexual abuse has grown, so has the recognition that the response of the professional community must involve a collaborative, multidisciplinary approach in order to be successful. Law enforcement, social services, mental health, and medical providers now routinely work closely together to respond to cases of child sexual abuse, each providing their own specific services and expertise to respond to this problem. Of particular importance in this multidisciplinary approach to the care of sexually abused children is the medical component. There have been many changes over the past several decades with regard to what "having a medical evaluation" means for sexually abused children. Much has been learned about anatomy, interpretation of findings, evidence collection, medical management, therapy, and prevention. Consequently, the current standards of care for the medical management of sexually abused children are quite different today than in decades past. It is critical that all professionals who work with sexually abused children are familiar with what the medical response should involve.

It is in this context that Dr. Rich Kaplan has brought together many of the world's leading authorities regarding child sexual abuse to create *Medical Response to Child Sexual Abuse*. Dr. Kaplan brings his vast experience and his unique perspective to this text, having worked with abused children for over 30 years—first as a social worker and then as a pediatrician. His thoughtful, thorough, objective, meticulous, and hopeful approach to providing care to children is reflected throughout the book. Dr. Kaplan and his co-authors cover a vast amount of material in a clear and easily accessible manner. Although written from a medical perspective, *Medical Response to Child Sexual Abuse* is intended as a comprehensive resource for both medical as well as non-medical professionals. To know what the current, state-of-the-art standard of care approach to the medical evaluation of sexually abused children is, this text will serve as a primary resource.

The chapters that address basic anatomy of the genitalia and anus as well as the medical evaluation when sexual abuse is suspected should be mandatory reading not only for every clinician who provides medical care to children, but also to any other professional who works with sexually abused children. This book clarifies and demystifies the examination process, and most importantly, addresses what exams can and cannot "tell" us. We recognize that when children disclose sexual abuse, they do so in various timeframes, having experienced a wide variety of abuse. How does the care of a child who discloses an event that occurred yesterday differ from that of one who discloses an event from last summer? How does the care of an adolescent differ from that of a young child? What kind of medical management is required? We have learned that there is no "one exam fits all" response to child sexual abuse. This text addresses all these issues at length and allows the clinician to provide the best possible care to their patients. One of the most important issues in the medical evaluation of child sexual abuse is to ensure that physical findings are identified correctly for what they are. Dr. Kaplan's text addresses these issues at great length as well. *Medical Response to Child Sexual Abuse* also assists providers in working with children and families with the long term consequences of sexual abuse.

Quite simply, this text provides everything that professionals who work with sexually abused children and adolescents need to understand the medical response to child sexual abuse. Medical providers who are familiar with this information will provide even better care to the children they serve and will be more effective members of their community's multidisciplinary team. The non-medical professionals who use this book will better understand exactly what it is that medical providers can do for children and for them. We owe Dr. Kaplan and his co-authors a debt of gratitude for creating such a singularly useful text for all professionals who work with these children and their families.

James E. Crawford-Jakubiak, MD, FAAP
Medical Director
Center for Child Protection
Children's Hospital & Research Center Oakland
Oakland, California

FOREWORD

Medical Response to Child Sexual Abuse is a carefully crafted compendium of chapters taking the reader from an initial review of history to a glimpse of hope for the future. Along the way, we learn a great deal about what is known about child sexual abuse from basic anatomy to 5 chapters focused on medical evaluation issues, and other chapters presenting information on evidence-based literature review, the description and value of multidisciplinary teams, collaborative practice models, the importance of prevention and expanding perspectives for the way we think about and react to the sexual maltreatment of children.

As the field of child abuse pediatrics has recently evolved into a pediatric subspecialty, we plan to increase the education of all health professionals in the many facets of violence and abuse involving children. The goal is to have informed health care providers at many levels, from those delivering primary care and those with increased knowledge and clinical competencies in child abuse to the pediatricians who are board certified in the subspecialty.

We have learned a great deal over the last several years about the lifelong consequences of maltreatment. If we can properly discover, treat, and remedy the effects of sexual abuse, we cannot only foster healthy lives, but we can also dramatically affect the huge economic costs of morbidity and mortality created by unrecognized abuse followed by health behaviors and physiologic responses to the stress created by the abuse.

An important outcome of having a uniformly informed cadre of clinicians evaluating children who may have been sexually abused will be consistency with the process of initial evaluation and treatment, follow-up care, documentation of important findings, and collaboration between physicians and other professionals. This text, complete with up-to-date information on interpretations of physical findings including conditions that may mimic sexual abuse, sexually transmitted infections, and forensic interpretation, is a template for the consistency we desire. The reader will find well-referenced chapters, allowing easy access to the literature supporting authors' opinions and advice. Case scenarios and clear examples of clinical situations as well as reports of successful approaches to child abuse prevention and intervention will assist readers in evaluating their own programs and/or developing new programs.

The contributors chosen by the authors are well known in the field and collectively have a great amount of experience, paving the way for the next generations of dedicated professionals that have a desire to work with children to both prevent their abuse and to intervene with an appropriate evaluation and diagnosis of sexual abuse when necessary.

We know now that most physical examinations of children alleging sexual abuse will be normal. Descriptions of these examinations are not only important medically, but legally as well. This is also true for descriptions of injuries when they are found. Appropriate treatment, whether for the emotional stability of the child, or for injuries or infections is an important facet of our work. *Medical Response to Child Sexual Abuse* clearly defines practical, evidence-informed advice for documenting and managing a variety of cases. When we are confronted with substantiating our findings and opinions in court, it is helpful to know that this text will be an accepted authority to support our work. For those future pediatricians who will bravely enter into fellowships in child abuse pediatrics, this book will pave the way to successful passage of certification examinations. For other health care providers, incorporating the information provided in the text will enable them to practice in an equivalent, evidence-based style consistent with the best practices all our children deserve. After all, it is our children for whom we seek the knowledge and skills necessary for their care.

Robert W. Block, MD, FAAP
Professor of Pediatrics
School of Community Medicine
The University of Oklahoma College of Medicine
Tulsa, Oklahoma

PREFACE

The concept of medical care for children who are possible victims of child sexual abuse is relatively new. In the last decade, we have seen the medical care for these children undergo a significant evolution in which we now see these children as patients who require medical attention and care. The focus of this book is to address the medical care for these children from a variety of perspectives.

Our central goal has been to demystify the medical care of these children, and it is emphasized that while there are special competencies involved, this is much more similar to medical care for other conditions than it is different. When caring for a child who is a possible victim of child sexual abuse, the same principles and standards of medical care exist, such as obtaining a complete and well-documented history and physical examination, performing an appropriate and scientifically driven laboratory evaluation, and forming a medical diagnosis to guide the ongoing care needs of the child. This is the definition of good pediatric medical care. It should be clear that the medical component is simply one part of the response to possible maltreatment, but we hope that this text will help crystallize the elements that make this component such an important part of the community response.

While the legal issues certainly are important for the safety and well-being of children, the focus of this text primarily will be on the medical and therapeutic care these children need to heal and, hopefully, to have a happy and productive life.

In *Medical Response to Child Sexual Abuse*, we have brought together national experts and scholars with a variety of expertise in the scientific fields that relate to the care of young victims. This group of contributors has created an impressive and helpful text that covers the entire range of the medical response to child sexual abuse. While the focus of this book is medical care, it is our hope that other members of the multidisciplinary team will find this a useful reference.

We would like to thank all the wonderful contributors for their hard work and their patience in the development of this text. Collaboration with them has been both gratifying and educational, and hopefully it will be the same for those who use this text as a reference.

Rich Kaplan, MSW, MD, FAAP
Joyce A. Adams, MD
Suzanne P. Starling, MD, FAAP
Angelo P. Giardino, MD, PhD, MPH, FAAP

REVIEWS

This text is destined to be an excellent resource for novices as well as experienced providers of medical care to victims of sexual abuse. In addition, investigators and social workers without medical backgrounds will benefit from increased understanding of the nature, importance, and value of these medical assessments. Clinicians faced with the seemingly never-ending stream of victims will find the last chapter on prevention particularly helpful, providing hope that we can effect change.

Deborah Lowen, MD
Associate Professor of Pediatrics
Director
Child Abuse Pediatrics
Vanderbilt University School
of Medicine
Nashville, Tennessee

This textbook offers a comprehensive and detailed accounting of the medical assessment of the alleged childhood sexual abuse victim. It serves as an excellent resource for the multidisciplinary team responsible for the evaluation of these complex cases. Both Martin Finkel and Allan De Jong have provided the clinician with a well-referenced guide for how to accurately and effectively medically assess, interpret, and document sexual abuse or assault in children and adolescents. Anyone working in the field of child maltreatment should add this publication to their annals.

Barbara L. Knox, MD, FAAP
Medical Director
Child Protection Program
University of Wisconsin American
Family Children's Hospital
Assistant Professor
Department of Pediatrics
University of Wisconsin School of
Medicine and Public Health
Madison, Wisconsin

This is a valuable, exhaustive resource combining anatomic, epidemiologic, therapeutic, and preventative strategies for children and young adults. Beginning with historical context and moving through basic anatomy, physiology, and pathology, the reader quickly learns best practices in health services for sexual abuse, assault, and exploitation. Team approaches, collaboration, telemedicine, training, treatment, and mental health services are reviewed in great detail, and there is a superlative discussion of research methods and the state of knowledge in the field topped off with legal and international issues and prevention. This book should be read by any professional who wants to responsibly provide services for children and families facing these difficult problems.

Vincent J. Palusci, MD, MS, FAAP
Professor of Pediatrics
New York University School
of Medicine
New York, New York

This comprehensive text will be an invaluable resource to any medical provider who has contact with children. With topics ranging from basic genital anatomy to court testimony and future directions for prevention, it is an excellent resource not only for those whose careers are primarily focused on child sexual abuse but also to those who simply desire a basic understanding. In recent decades, there have been tremendous advances in medicine related to child sexual abuse, and this book synthesizes all of this information.

Mark Hudson, MD
Midwest Children's Resource
Center
Children's Hospitals and Clinics
of Minnesota
St. Paul, Minnesota

This comprehensive text ought to be available to each multidisciplinary team member tasked with treating and/or investigating child and adolescent sexual abuse and assault. Diverse topics are carefully addressed including interviewing children with impairments, commercial sexual exploitation, and efficacious mental health therapies. Dr. Allan De Jong's chapter on acute sexual abuse should be required reading for physicians and sexual assault nurse examiners tasked with forensic evidence collection and acute medical treatment. Dr. Martin Finkel details the highest standards to which clinicians should adhere as they elicit histories, conduct physical exams, and complete medicolegal documentation. This text is an excellent resource for both novice and established clinicians who serve child sexual abuse survivors and their families.

Tanya Hinds, MD, FAAP
Child Abuse Pediatrician
Children's National Medical
Center
Washington DC

Dr. Kaplan's new text is much more than a "how to do a sexual abuse exam" or a "how to interpret the exam" handbook. The book includes chapters on how to talk with families after the examination, the history and future of child sexual abuse prevention, and child and youth prostitution and pornography. This is both a reference book and a thoughtful stimulus to broaden our thinking about the causes and effects of child sexual abuse and the role of the medical professional in caring for our patients and for the community.

Naomi F. Sugar MD
Clinical Professor of Pediatrics
University of Washington
Medical Director
Center for Sexual Assault and
Traumatic Stress
Harborview Medical Center
Seattle, Washington

CONTENTS IN BRIEF

CONTENTS IN DETAIL

Medical Response to

Child Sexual

Abuse

A Resource for Professionals
Working with Children and Families

STM Learning, Inc.

Leading Publisher of Scientific, Technical, and Medical Educational Resources
Saint Louis
www.stmlearning.com

Chapter 1

THE MEDICAL RESPONSE TO CHILD SEXUAL ABUSE: AN HISTORICAL OVERVIEW

Rich Kaplan, MSW, MD, FAAP

It is fitting for a textbook on medical care for victims of child sexual abuse to begin with a view toward the past. The social, scientific, and clinical factors that have evolved are briefly reviewed in this chapter in order to provide an historical context in which to view current practice and perhaps a vantage point from which to view the future.

FROM THE DAWN OF CIVILIZATION

The sexual maltreatment of children appears to be as old as civilization. Claude Levi-Strauss[1] described the incest taboo as being present from the "dawn of culture." There are many descriptions of child sexual abuse from a variety of ancient cultures. The description of Lot being seduced by his daughters in Genesis suggests that both sexual contact with children and incest were social issues in ancient times. In a fascinating depiction of the sexual mistreatment of young children in the Byzantine Empire from 324-1453 CE, the abuse of children from both peasant and royal classes is described.[2] The authors conclude that "child sexual abuse is an ancient social phenomenon" and despite political and religious prohibitions, "the problem seems to have remained endemic in all social classes." Likewise, references to child sexual abuse among ancient Greeks, Romans, Egyptians, Hebrews, and others have been reported.[3]

Through the Renaissance, Enlightenment, and Modern Era, maltreatment—including sexual abuse—showed no evidence of abating. Accounts of sexual abuse from early 20th-century Scotland[4] and Canada[5] give disturbing insights into the response to child sexual abuse in the relatively recent past. Even as society articulates its abomination of child sexual abuse, there is no doubt that it persists and, with the advent of modern technology, has added new forms.

THE EARLY MEDICAL RESPONSE

As pervasive as the sexual maltreatment of children has been throughout recorded time and as widespread the religious, political, and cultural sanctions against such abuse have been, people may conclude that the medical community has, with equivalent consistency and vigor, responded to this abuse as it has to other major health concerns. However, the medical response to child sexual abuse has been, for the better part of modern history, absent or—at best—sputtering and sporadic.

There was an attempt at a response early in the second half of the 19th century when a visionary French pathologist named Ambroise Tardieu wrote the remarkably accurate and essentially first modern medical descriptions of both child physical and sexual abuse.[6,7] Tardieu described and analyzed over 900 cases of sexual abuse of both boys and girls. His drawings of genital findings (**Figures 1-1** through **1-5**) are extremely accurate and hold up well even in the colposcopic age. Like so many scientific visionaries, Tardieu's work was remarkably underappreciated by his contemporaries. Rather than becoming the observational cornerstone for a burgeoning line of scientific inquiry and clinical practice, it faded into obscurity for well over a century.

It is not entirely fair to say that Tardieu was completely alone. Several other French physicians addressed the issue of child sexual abuse during this brief enlightenment. Masson[8] describes works by Lacassagne, Garraud, and Bernard that support Tardieu's work and elaborate on the incidence and nature of the sexual abuse of children.[9] In fact, in *Des Attentatts a la puduer sur les petites filles (The Sexual Assault on Young Girls)*, Bernard noted 36 176 reported cases of "rape and assault on the morality of young children" between 1827 and 1870. These works notwithstanding, considering the prevalent social and medical response to child sexual abuse, Tardieu was essentially a voice in the wilderness that was quickly forgotten.

Figure 1-1.
Tardieu's drawings of genital findings. Reproduced from Tardieu A. E'tude me'dico-le'gale sur les attentats aux moeurs. 7th ed. Paris: Librairie JB Baille`re et Fils;1878.

What stands as perhaps the best example of the 19th century's social and medical ambivalence toward the sexual abuse of children comes from a man who was certainly no stranger to ambivalence—Sigmund Freud. Long a source of great speculation and debate, it is clear that in less than 3 years, Freud—at least publicly—abandoned his revolutionary seduction theory, which essentially identified sexual abuse as a cause of hysteria, in favor of the now-famous Oedipal complex. Whether Freud's reversal was the result of social and professional pressure[8,10] or because of a natural evolution of psycho-analytic theory[11] is well beyond the scope of this chapter. Suffice it to say that at least on one level, the child victim became a seductress.[12] Postulating that children have sexual feelings toward a parent essentially made them coconspirators in any incestuous abuse.

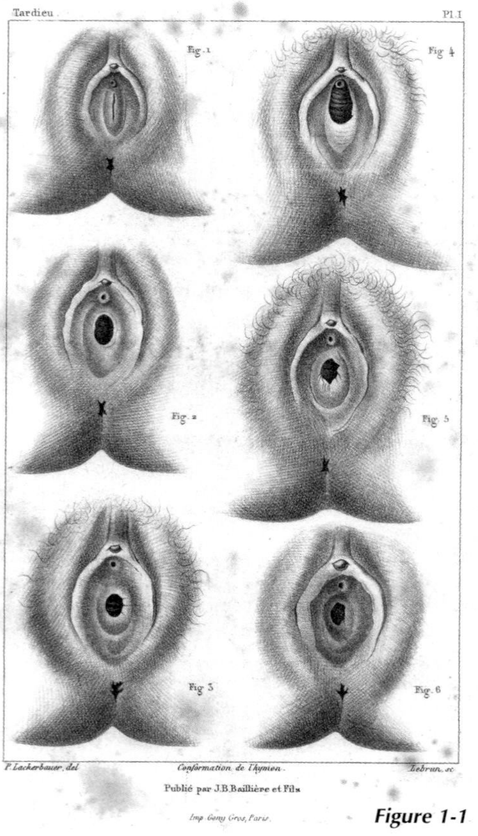

Figure 1-1

If Tardieu's unappreciated pioneering and Freud's about-face serve as metaphors for 19th century medicine's inability to respond scientifically to child sexual abuse, then we need to look no further than the issue of childhood gonorrhea for a metaphor for the same inability for the early part of the 20th century. By the early 20th century, the science of medicine had clearly established a causal link between sexual contact and venereal diseases, including gonorrhea. However, it was not until the 1970s that there was general acceptance of the role of sexual abuse in the etiology of childhood gonococcal infections. Evans pointed out that, with respect to children, for the better part of the century, "physicians consistently downplayed and often denied the possibility of sexual transmission, providing other, less plausible explanations."[13] Arguments about differences in prepubertal anatomy and physiology that supported nonsexual transmission were proposed from multiple credible sources. Even when sexual transmission was acknowledged, it was not thought to occur in good families. As late as

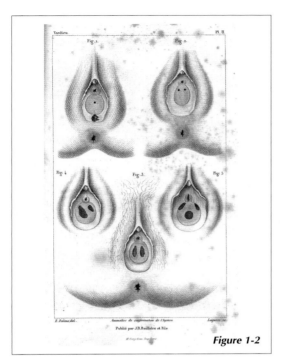

Figure 1-2

Figures 1-2 through **1-5.** *Tardieu's drawings of genital findings. Reproduced from Tardieu A. E'tude me'dico-le'gale sur les attentats aux moeurs. 7th ed. Paris: Librairie JB Baille`re et Fils;1878.*

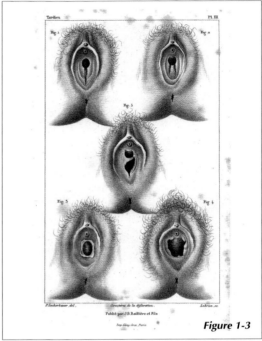

Figure 1-3

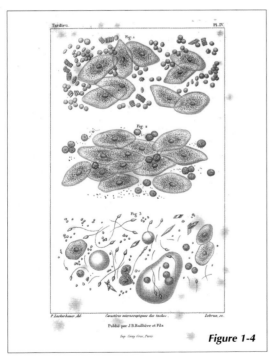

Figure 1-4

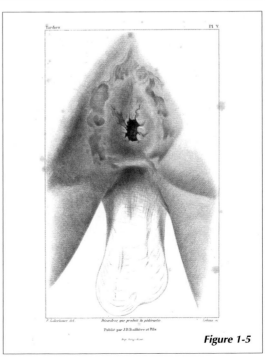

Figure 1-5

1973, physicians were not urged to consider child abuse in cases of gonococcal pharyngitis in prepubertal children.[14] In 1975, the sexual transmission of gonorrhea to children was described as a result of voluntary sex.[15]

In the 20th century, there was an awakening to the notion of child abuse in general. While it is true that the sentinel American child abuse case, that of Mary Ellen Wilson, occurred in 1874, the medical community truly awoke with a start on the occasion of the publication of Kempe's *The Battered-Child Syndrome*.[16] Child physical abuse was acknowledged as a legitimate diagnosis, and additional medical research and other scholarly work began to appear in the medical literature. Sixteen years later, Kempe described another hidden form of abuse.[17] In delivering the 1977 C. Anderson Aldrich lecture, Kempe "hoped to stimulate broader awareness among pediatricians about the problem of sexual abuse."

THE MODERN RESPONSE

A groundswell of interest in child sexual abuse had developed by the time Kempe gave his lecture. Sgroi was publishing a landmark article on childhood venereal disease[18] and would soon publish a second article on the same subject that would rebuke the medical community for burying its head in the sand.[19] She was compiling the first US clinical handbook on child sexual abuse.[20] Shortly thereafter, Fontana, who had already made his mark as a medical pioneer in the area of physical abuse, entered into the discussion and added energy to the effort.[21] As a result, around 1980, the medical community was alerted to the age-old horror of child sexual abuse.

Nonmedical pioneers were at work as well, providing key psychological and epidemiologic underpinnings to the scientific understanding of this complex and troublesome "new" medical problem. In *Child Sexual Abuse Accommodation Syndrome*,[22] Roland Summit provided an insightful view into the sometimes counterintuitive behavior of young victims. At about the same time, David Finkelhor was beginning his remarkable and ongoing work in the epidemiology of sexual abuse and exploitation.[23]

As authorities were receiving reports of suspected child sexual abuse, there was an increase in requests to physicians to evaluate these children for medical signs of this abuse. An early article[24] reported on the utility of the colposcope to provide magnified views of the genital and anal tissues of children. The colposcope, equipped with a camera to document the examination findings, was purported to detect minute injuries not visible to the naked eye. The hymen in the prepubertal girl, a previously obscure and nearly mystic tissue, was now being seen, literally, in an entirely new light. With magnification, never before seen findings and an entire new lexicon of mounds, bumps, notches (both *u* and *v* shaped), folds, ridges, clefts, and innumerable other terms appeared. The concept of *intact* was considered too vague, given these new observations.

Physicians who evaluated children and used a colposcope for magnification and documentation of their findings began to publish in the pediatric and gynecologic literature. The first papers were descriptive studies, usually of children who were referred for suspected sexual abuse to specialty centers. McCann and associates published the results of the first study of perianal[25] and genital[26] findings in children who had been selected for nonabuse.

These new clinical data led to the question of whether any of these physical findings could be useful in an evidentiary way. In other words, could this newfound understanding of hymenal morphology provide clear evidence to prove or disprove sexual abuse? With the asking of this question, the nature of the medical role in sexual abuse cases veered in an entirely new direction. The primary role of the medical evaluator of a sexually abused child became the discovery and documentation of physical—genital or perianal—evidence to confirm or disprove abuse. In many cases the medical caregiver's role had much less to do with the provision of care and much more to do with legal proceedings. In many ways, this trend has persisted, at times compromising children's access to much-needed medical care.

THE ROLE OF LAW ENFORCEMENT

As the role of the physician was gearing up, the legal, law enforcement, and child protection communities were gearing up as well. These cases were difficult legally from the beginning. It was difficult for the community at large and for the juror in particular to accept that these horrendous things actually happened. At about the same time, famous and scandalous sexual abuse cases such as the McMartin daycare center case in California and the debacle in Jordan, Minnesota, contributed to the public's skepticism. These early attempts at interviewing possible child victims were so leading that it was not possible to garner the truth. Prosecutors and detectives looked to the medical examination as probative help in breaking through the denial. This was found to be rarely helpful. Community professionals were forced to look in another direction—and the medical role was often limited to performing forensic examinations. In some communities, this is still the case.

At the same time that the medical caregiver role was being redefined, another force came into play. A Huntsville, Alabama, prosecutor and later Alabama Congressman, Robert E. "Bud" Kramer, noting the difficulties of prosecuting child sexual abuse cases, founded the nation's first child advocacy center in Madison County, Alabama. Not long afterward, with collaboration from national child abuse experts including medical child abuse pioneer Dr. Carolyn Levitt, the National Network of Child Advocacy Centers was born. This organization has evolved into the National Children's Alliance (NCA). The NCA has become the accrediting body for more than 500 child advocacy centers across the country. These centers utilize medical services in a variety of ways. Some centers are hospital based and thus focus on medical care for young victims. Others are associated with prosecutors' offices, and decisions regarding medical care are often made by individuals with no medical training. There are a host of models in between.

SCIENTIFIC ADVANCES

There is good news on the scientific side. Building on the pioneering work of Heger and McCann and associates, researchers such as Berenson[27-31], Adams[32], and Kellogg[33,34] have provided strong evidence-based support for the notion that the vast majority of child sexual abuse victims will have no diagnostic genital findings even on magnified exam. This finding begs a new and more difficult question: why examine these children at all? The answer, which must be given in the context of appropriate medical care, follows.

MEDICAL CARE OF THE CHILD ABUSE VICTIM: NOW AND BEYOND

Even at the beginning of the 21st century, the role of the child sexual abuse medical provider is still being defined. This special practice swelled with potential in 19th-century France only to literally disappear in the face of denial, ambivalence, and downright deception for the next 100 years. A medical reawakening of sorts has occurred, but many questions still need to be answered. Confusion exists about the medical care of these young victims. Should they be seen as patients, or are they potential witnesses who simply need a hymen check? The medical community is struggling with these questions.

There is an ongoing and concerted effort to answer these questions. This process has taken several forms. In 2002, a group of pediatric child abuse consultants began meeting in an effort to develop consensus on the medical care of possible sexual abuse victims. Blending current evidence-based research on physical findings with consensus on best practice, the work of this group led to the development of an article entitled "Guidelines for Medical Care of Children Who May Have Been Sexually Abused."[32] The American Academy of Pediatrics' Committee on Child Abuse and Neglect (COCAN) has, with the help of Dr. Nancy Kellogg, reissued an updated edition of "The Evaluation of Sexual Abuse in Children."[34] The National Association of Children's Hospitals and Related Institutions (NACHRI) has issued guidelines for the response to child abuse among member institutions with language that reinforces the position taken by the preceding 2 documents. Finally, the American Board of Pediatrics and the American Board of Medical Specialties have both approved Child Abuse Pediatrics as a pediatric subspecialty.

What does all this mean for the future of the medical response to child sexual abuse? It means several steps forward and one critical step back. The new subspecialty is certainly a major step forward. It will allow for the further development of the child abuse research infrastructure and an increase in support of child abuse fellowships. It should also serve to enhance embryonic efforts at professional peer review and continuous quality improvement among child abuse centers and medical providers. NACHRI's action is also a step in the right direction. By strongly encouraging their constituent children's hospitals to develop medical child abuse services, they will be helping to ensure the regional and local availability of medical child abuse expertise. The work by the guidelines consensus group and COCAN also takes us a step forward as they summarize the current state of the science of child sexual abuse and provide structure to the conduct of the medical evaluation.

The step back may be the most critical step of all. It is the return to the concept that the evaluation of the possibly sexually abused child is, first and foremost, the provision of medical care. Comprehensive care of the sexually abused child is much more than looking at a magnified hymen for evidence or swabbing for a perpetrator's bodily fluids. It is more than forensic interviews and court testimony. It includes a good history, a thorough physical examination, appropriate tests, referrals to and collaboration with other health care professionals including psychotherapists, and appropriate follow-up. It also includes providing patient and family education, anticipatory guidance, and, when indicated, much-needed reassurance. Certainly, there are special competencies and a specific knowledge base, but it is more similar to other pediatric care than it is different.

CONCLUSION

There is great potential for the evolution of medical care for the young sexual abuse victim. Bolstered by a legal climate that grants increased credibility to the provider of medical diagnosis and treatment, there can be a return to the professional practice that launched this specialized care—the practice of medicine.

REFERENCES

1. Levi-Strauss C. *The Elementary Structure of Kinship.* London, United Kingdom: Eyne & Spotterswood; 1969.

2. Lascaratos J, Poulakou-Rebelakou E. Child sexual abuse: historical cases in the Byzantine Empire (324-1453 AD). *Child Abuse Negl.* 2000;24(8):1085-1090.

3. Kahr B. The sexual molestation of children: historical perspectives. *J Psychohistory.* 1991;19(2):191-224.

4. Davidson R. This pernicious delusion: law, medicine, and child sexual abuse in early-twentieth-century Scotland. *J Hist Sex.* 2001;10(1):62-77.

5. Sangster J. Masking and unmasking the sexual abuse of children: perceptions of violence against children in "the Badlands" of Ontario, 1916-1930. *J Fam Hist.* 2000;25(4):504-526.

6. Labbé J. Ambroise Tardieu: the man and his work on child maltreatment a century before Kempe. *Child Abuse Negl.* 2004;29(4):311-324.

7. Roche EA. The work of Ambroise Tardieu: the first definitive description of child abuse. *Child Abuse Negl.* 2005;29(4):325-334.

8. Masson J. *The Assault on Truth: Freud's Suppression of the Seduction Theory.* New York, NY: Penguin; 1984.

9. Olafson E, Corwin DL, Summit RC, et al. Modern history of child sexual abuse awareness: cycles of discovery and suppression. *Child Abuse Negl.* 1993;17(1):7-24.

10. Powell RA, Boer DP. Did Freud mislead patients to confabulate memories of abuse? A reply to Gleaves and Hernandez (1999). *Psychol Reports.* 2004;95(3 Pt 1):863-877.

11. Gleaves DH, Hernandez E. Wethinks the author doth protest too much: a reply to Esterson (2002). *Hist Psychol.* 2002;5(1):92-98.

12. Birken L. From seduction theory to Oedipus complex: a historical analysis. *New German Critique.* 1988;43:83-96.

13. Evans, H. Physician denial and child sexual abuse in America. In: Warsh CK, Strong-Boag V, eds. *Children's Health Issues in Historial Perspective.* Waterloo, Canada: Wilfrid Laurier University Press; 2005:327-352.

14. Abbott SL. Gonococcal tonsillitis-pharyngitis in a 5-year-old girl. *Pediatrics.* 1973;52(2):287-289.

15. Israel KS, Rissing KB, Brooks GF. Neonatal and childhood gonococcal infections. *Clin Obstet Gynecol.* 1975;18(1):143-151.

16. Kempe CH, Steele BF. The battered-child syndrome. *JAMA.* 1962;181:17-24.

17. Kempe CH. Sexual abuse, another hidden pediatric problem: the 1977 C. Anderson Aldrich lecture. *Pediatrics.* 1978;62(3):382-389.

18. Sgroi SM. Pediatric gonorrhea beyond infancy. *Pediatr Annals.* 1979;8(5): 326-336.

19. Sgroi SM. *Handbook of Clinical Intervention in Child Sexual Abuse.* Lexington, MA: Lexington Books; 1981.

20. Sgroi, SM. Pediatric gonorrhea and child sexual abuse: the venereal disease connection. *Sex Transm Dis.* 1982;9(3):154-156.

21. Fontana VJ. When systems fail: protecting the victim of child sexual abuse. *Child Today.* 1984;13(4):14-18.

22. Summit RC. The child sexual abuse accommodation syndrome. *Child Abuse & Negl.* 1983;7(2):177-193.

23. Finkelhor, D. How widespread is child sexual abuse? *Child Today.* 1984;13(4): 18-20.

24. Woodling BA, Heger A. The use of the colposcope in the diagnosis of sexual abuse in the pediatric age group. *Child Abuse Negl.* 1986;10(1):111-114.

25. McCann J, Voris JS, Wells R. Perianal findings in prepubertal children selected for nonabuse: a descriptive study. *Child Abuse Negl.* 1989;13:179-193.

26. McCann J, Wells R, Voris JS. Genital findings in prepubertal children selected for nonabuse: a descriptive study. *Pediatr.* 1990;86:428-439.

27. Berenson AB. Appearance of the hymen at birth and one year of age: a longitudinal study. *Pediatrics.* 1993;91(4):820-825.

28. Berenson AB. The prepubertal genital exam: what is normal and abnormal. *Curr Opinion Obstet Gynecol.* 1994;6(6):526-530.

29. Berenson AB. A longitudinal study of hymenal morphology in the first 3 years of life. *Pediatrics.* 1995;95(4):490-496.

30. Berenson AB, Chacko MR, Wiemann CM, et al. Use of hymenal measurements in the diagnosis of previous penetration. *Pediatrics.* 2002;109(2):228-235.

31. Berenson AB, Grady JJ. A longitudinal study of hymenal development from 3 to 9 years of age. *Pediatrics.* 2002;140(5):600-607.

32. Adams JA, Kaplan RA, Starling SP, et al. Guidelines for medical care of children who may have been sexually abused. *J Pediatr Adol Gynecol.* 2007;20(3):163-172.

33. Kellogg ND, Menard SW, Santos A. Genital anatomy in pregnant adolescents: "normal" does not mean "nothing happened." *Pediatrics.* 2004;113(1 Pt 1): e67-69.

34. Kellogg ND, Committee on Child Abuse and Neglect. The evaluation of sexual abuse in children. *Pediatrics.* 2005;116(2):506-512.

Chapter 2

Basic Anatomy of the Genitalia and Anus

Joyce A. Adams, MD

In order to recognize signs of child sexual abuse, it is necessary to first be familiar with normal genital anatomy, its variations, and its development. While this may seem obvious, the lack of understanding of the many variations in normal appearance of the genital and anal tissues in children has led to misunderstandings among medical and non-medical professionals alike. Even after the publication of the first detailed descriptions of anal and genital anatomy in non-abused prepubertal children,[1-3] some physicians and nurses who perform child sexual abuse medical evaluations are not familiar with the findings from those and subsequent studies.[4-9]

When a child's examination is thought to show signs of injury or abuse but actually represents normal findings or evidence of another medical condition, the medical provider may contact child protection and/or law enforcement officials to report the suspicions. The child and family would then be unnecessarily traumatized by a referral and investigation of those suspicions.

It is also important for medical and nursing professionals, as well as non-medical professionals, to be able to speak the same language when describing features of genital and anal anatomy in children and adolescents. Anatomy courses in medical and nursing school rarely provide the necessary detail about the features of genital anatomy in children, usually focusing on adults and on pathology common to adult patients rather than children.

In the early 1990s, a group of physicians met at conferences to agree on proper terminology for describing features of genital and anal anatomy, and the results of a 4-year consensus development process was published by the American Professional Society on the Abuse of Children in 1995. Some of the definitions were taken from standard medical dictionaries and anatomy textbooks, but, out of necessity, other definitions were created by specialists working in the field of sexual abuse medical evaluation.

Table 2-1 is a list of terms and definitions from that publication.[10]

Table 2-1. Basic Genital Anatomy, Related Terminology, and Definition of Terms.[10]
ANATOMICAL STRUCTURES IN THE FEMALE:
— **Mons pubis:** The rounded, fleshy prominence, created by the underlying fat pad that lies over the symphysis pubis (pubic bone).
— **Vulva:** The external genitalia or pudendum of the female. Includes the anterior commisure, clitoris, labia majora, labia minora, vaginal vestibule, urethral orifice, vaginal orifice, hymen, and posterior commisure. *(continued)*

Table 2-1. Basic Genital Anatomy, Related Terminology, and Definition of Terms. *(continued)*

ANATOMICAL STRUCTURES IN THE FEMALE:

— *Anterior commisure:* The union of the two labia minora anteriorly/superiorly.

— *Clitoris:* A small, cylindrical, erectile body, situated at the anterior (superior) portion of the vulva, covered by a sheath of skin called the clitoral hood; homologous with the penis in the male.

— *Labia majora (singular: labium majus):* Rounded folds of skin forming the lateral boundaries of the vulva.

— *Labia minora (singular: labium minus):* Longitudinal thin folds of tissue enclosed within the labia majora. In the prepubertal child, these folds extend from the clitoral hood to approximately the midpoint on the lateral walls of the vestibule. In the adult, they enclose the structures of the vestibule.

— *Vaginal vestibule:* An anatomic cavity containing the opening of the vagina, the urethra, and the ducts of Bartholin's glands. Bordered by the clitoris superiorly, the labia minora laterally, and the posterior commisure inferiorly.

— *Urethral orifice:* External opening of the canal (urethra) from the bladder.

— *Vestibular bands:* Small bands of tissue lateral to the urethral orifice that connect the periurethral tissues to the anterior lateral walls of the vestibule (urethral support ligaments), or bands of tissue lateral to the hymen connecting to the vestibular wall.

— *Vaginal orifice:* The opening to the uterovaginal canal.

— *Vagina:* The internal structure extending from the uterine cervix to the inner edge of the hymen.

— *Hymen:* A membrane that partially, or rarely completely, covers the vaginal orifice.

— *Fossa navicularis/posterior fossa:* Concavity on the lower part of the vestibule situated inferiorly to the vaginal orifice and extending to the posterior commisure or posterior fourchette.

— *Posterior commisure:* The union of the two labia majora inferiorly (toward the anus).

ANATOMICAL STRUCTURES IN THE MALE:

— *Penis:* Male sex organ composed of erectile tissue through which the urethra passes; homologous with the clitoris in the female.

— *Glans penis/balanus:* The cap-shape expansion of the corpus spongiousum at the end of the penis. It is covered by mucous membrane and sheathed by the prepuce (foreskin) in uncircumcised males.

— *Scrotum:* The pouch that contains the testicles and their accessory organs.

— *Median raphe:* A ridge or furrow that marks the line of union of the two halves of the perineum.

(continued)

Table 2-1. *(continued)*

DESCRIPTIVE TERMS RELATED TO THE PERINEUM AND ANUS:

— ***Perineum:*** The external surface or base of the perineal body, lying between the vulva and the anus in the female, and the scrotum and the anus in the male. Underlying the external surface of the perineum is the pelvic floor and its associated structures occupying the pelvic outlet, which is bounded anteriorly by the pubic symphysis (pubic bone), laterally by the ischial tuberosity (pelvic bone), and posteriorly by the coccyx (tail bone).

— ***Perineal body:*** The central tendon of the perineum located between the vulva and the anus in the female and between the scrotum and anus in the male.

— ***Anus:*** The anal orifice, which is the lower opening of the digestive tract, lying in the fold between the buttocks through which feces is extruded.

— ***Anal skin tag:*** A protrusion of anal verge tissue that interrupts the symmetry of the perianal skin folds.

— ***Anal verge:*** The tissue overlying the subcutaneous division of the external anal sphincter at the most distal portion of the anal canal (anoderm) and extending exteriorly to the margin of the anal skin.

— ***Pectinate/dentate line:*** The sawtoothed line of demarcation between the distal (lower) portion of the anal valves and the pectin; the smooth zone of stratified epithelium that extends to the anal verge. This line may be apparent when the external and internal anal sphincters relax and the anus dilates.

Definitions taken from "Practice Guidelines: Descriptive Terminology in Child Sexual Abuse Medical Evaluations" published by the American Professional Society on the Abuse of Children, 1995. Adapted and reprinted with permission from the American Professional Society on the Abuse of Children.

EMBRYOLOGY

An appreciation of the wide variation in the appearance of the genital and anal tissues in children requires an understanding of embryology and how the external genital tissues develop. For the first 6 weeks of development, the genital structures of the human embryo are in an undifferentiated state. In males, a transcription factor encoded on the sex-determining region of the Y chromosome (SRY) is produced during the seventh week, which triggers male development. In the absence of a Y chromosome and SRY production, female development progresses.

Figures 2-1 and **2-2** show the development of the male and female external genital structures from the indifferent stage (4 to 7 weeks) through the 12th week. The genital tubercle differentiates into the glans and shaft of the penis in the male, and into the glans and shaft of the clitoris in the female. The definitive urogenital sinus develops into the penile urethra in the male and the vestibule of the vagina in the female. The urethral fold becomes the penis surrounding the penile urethra in the male or the labia minora in the female. The labioscrotal fold develops into either the scrotum in the male or the labia majora in the female.[11]

A detailed study of the development of the perineum was published in 2005, which provided a new understanding of the formation of the vagina and hymen.[12] In the undifferentiated state, the distal ends of the fused paramesonephric ducts are separated from the urogenital sinus by the dense stroma of the Mullerian tubercle. In females, the mesonephric ducts regress and the fused paramesonephric ducts form the uterus and vagina. The mesonephric orifices are incorporated into the orifice of the developing vagina, and the epithelium is replaced by the epithelium from the Mullerian tubercle.

The vagina expands and extends downward to bulge into the vestibulum, and the paramesonephric epithelium is transformed into vaginal epithelium. The glycogen-filled cells begin to disintegrate, which forms the lumen of the vagina.

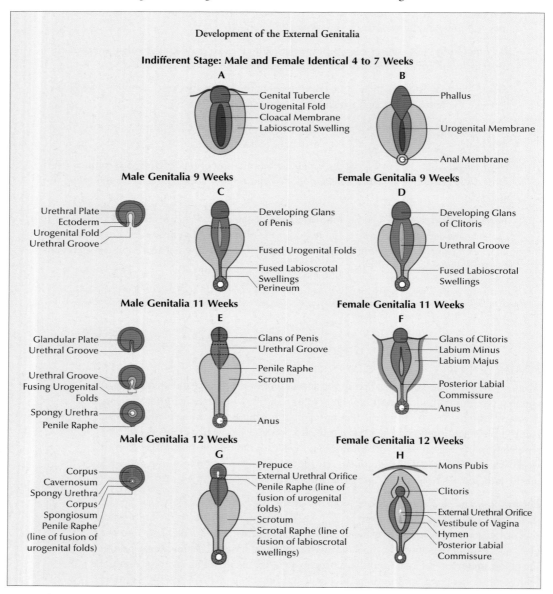

Figure 2-1. *Development of the external genitalia. Diagrams A and B illustrate the appearance of the genitalia during the indifferent stage (fourth to seventh weeks). Diagrams C, E, and G illustrate stages in the development of the male external genitalia at 9, 11, and 12 weeks, respectively. To the left are schematic transverse sections of the developing penis, illustrating the formation of the spongy urethra. Diagrams D, F, and H illustrage stages in the development of the female external genitalia at 9, 11, and 12 weeks, respectively. Figures and legend reprinted with permission from Moore KL, Persaud TVN, The Developing Human, Clinically Oriented Embryology, Sixth Edition. Philadelphia: WB Saunders;1998, p332.*

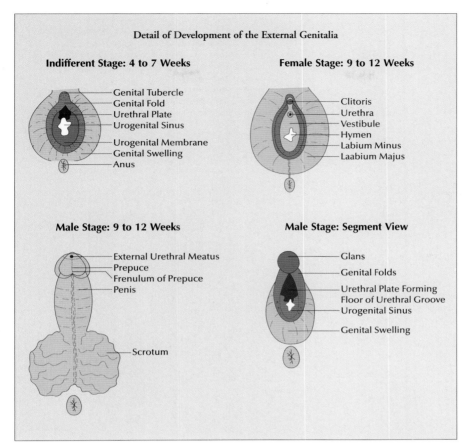

Detail of Development of the External Genitalia

Indifferent Stage: 4 to 7 Weeks
- Genital Tubercle
- Genital Fold
- Urethral Plate
- Urogenital Sinus
- Urogenital Membrane
- Genital Swelling
- Anus

Female Stage: 9 to 12 Weeks
- Clitoris
- Urethra
- Vestibule
- Hymen
- Labium Minus
- Laabium Majus

Male Stage: 9 to 12 Weeks
- External Urethral Meatus
- Prepuce
- Frenulum of Prepuce
- Penis
- Scrotum

Male Stage: Segment View
- Glans
- Genital Folds
- Urethral Plate Forming Floor of Urethral Groove
- Urogenital Sinus
- Genital Swelling

Figure 2-2.
Detail of development of the external genitalia in the female and the male. Reprinted with permission of Lippincott Williams & Wilkins, from: Snell RS, Clinical Anatomy for Medical Students. Baltimore, Philadelphia: Lippincott Williams & Wilkins; 2004

Figures 2-3-a, b, c, d, and **e** are diagrams of the microscopic appearance of tissues taken from female fetuses at varying stages of development. The data from the study by van der Putte provide support for the theory that the vagina is formed mainly from paramesonephric epithelium, not from the urogenital sinus.[12] Alternate theories postulated prior to this study held that the inferior portion of the vagina was formed from a portion of the urogenital sinus called the sinuvaginal bulb.[11]

The lengthening of the vagina into the vestibulum, where it meets the dense stromal tissue of the Mullerian tubercle, forms the hymen.[12] Folds in the urogenital sinus contribute to the lateral folds of the hymen. The deepening of the dorsal vestibular groove (shown in **Figure 2-4**) accentuates the dorsal segment of the hymen, which in clinical terms is referred to as the posterior or inferior rim. Both the inner side and the outer side of the hymen are made up of sinus epithelium. Van der Putte reports that primordial urethral glands were occasionally found on the inner side of the hymen, which he believes could be the origin of the hymenal cysts described by Merlob et al.[13] Another finding from this study is that the hymen itself is "… built of finely fibrillar connective tissue without the smooth muscle element predominant in all of its surrounding tissues."[12]

The opening in the hymen develops as the stromal tissue between the descending vagina and the urogenital sinus regresses. It is postulated that the denser the column of stromal tissue, the more likely it is that the tissue will not completely regress, which leads to a microperforate or imperforate hymen. See **Figure 2-5** for details of female external genital anatomy. If the tissue is denser in some areas than others, the uneven regression could also produce a septate or cribriform hymen.

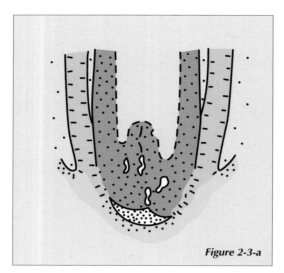

Figure 2-3-a

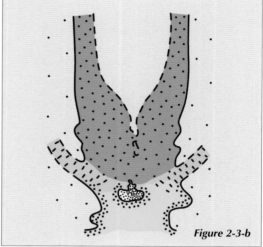

Figure 2-3-b

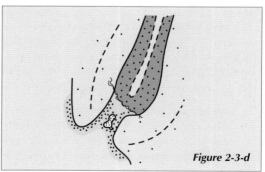

Figure 2-3-d

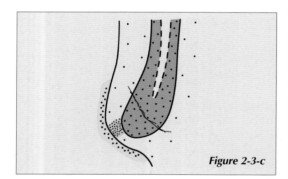

Figure 2-3-c

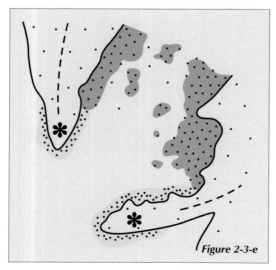

Figure 2-3-e

Figures 2-3-a to e. *Development of the vagina. Schematic drawings of transverse and median sections through female fetuses, showing the relationships between the epithelia of the paramesonephric structures (red), the mesonephric structures (pink), the Mullerian tubercle (blue) and the urogenital sinus (yellow). Figures adapted (by van de Putte) and reprinted by permission of Springer Verlag, from van der Putte SCJ. "The Development of the Perineum in the Human," Advances in Anatomy, Embryology and Cell Biology, 2005; 177:46.*

Figure 2-3-a. *The sexually indifferent complex demonstrates the fused paramesonephric ducts with their solid distal ends in direct contact with the mesonephric epithelium, but still separated from the epithelium of the urogenital sinus.*

Figure 2-3-b. *The distal paramesonephric epithelium has thickened into lateral "wings" of solid stratified epithelium, while sinus epithelium extends over a short distance into the orifices of the regressing mesonephric ducts.*

Figure 2-3-c. *Structures shown as median section.*

Figure 2-3-d. *The lateral wings of the paramesonephric epithelium have greatly broadened, the central lumen narrowed, and the epithelium transformed into stratified squamous epithelium; the stromal column has further regressed.*

Figure 2-3-e. *The volume of the vagina has greatly increased while its glycogen-rich epithelium disintegrates centrally to form the definitive lumen of the vagina, leaving remnants of tissue that will become the hymen (marked with an *).*

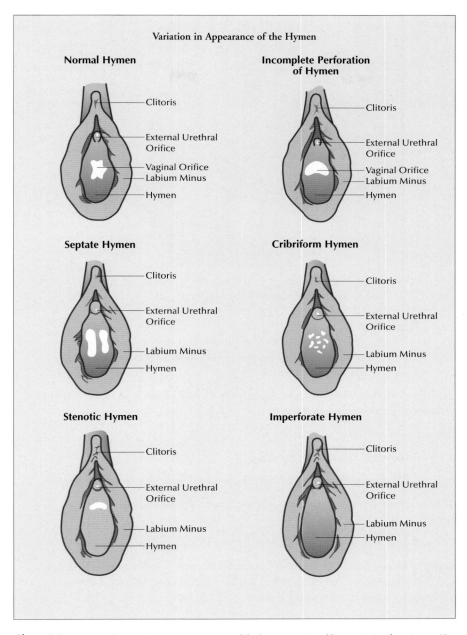

Figure 2-4. Drawings show variations in appearance of the hymen, reprinted by permission from Moore KL and Persaud TVN. The Developing Human: Clinically Oriented Embryology, Sixth Edition. Philadelphia: WB Saunders; 1998.

NORMAL VARIATIONS

The increasing societal awareness of the problem of child sexual abuse, beginning in the 1980s, and the involvement of physicians in the evaluation of children with suspected child sexual abuse, stimulated interest in the appearance of the hymen in neonates. A study by Jenny et al[14] identified the presence of a hymen in all 1131 neonates examined, and Berenson et al[15] described the morphology of the hymen and anatomical variations in 449 neonates who were examined and photographed in the first week of life. **Table 2-2** summarizes terminology related to the hymen.[10]

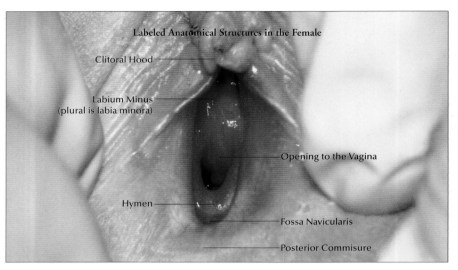

Figure 2-5.
Labeled anatomical structures in the female. Photograph of a 5-year-old girl, examined in the supine position using labial separation. See Table 2-1 for definitions.

Labeled Anatomical Structures in the Female

Clitoral Hood

Labium Minus
(plural is labia minora)

Opening to the Vagina

Hymen

Fossa Navicularis

Posterior Commisure

Table 2-2. Descriptive Terms and Definitions Related to the Hymen.[10]

ANATOMICAL STRUCTURES IN THE FEMALE:

— *Annular:* Variation in morphology where the hymenal membrane tissue extends completely around the circumference of the vaginal orifice.

— *Crescentic:* Hymen with attachments at approximately the 11 and 1 o'clock positions with no tissue present between the two attachments.

— *Cribiform:* Hymen with multiple small openings.

— *Imperforate:* Hymenal membrane with no opening.

— *Septate:* Hymen with two or more openings, caused by bands of tissue that bisect the opening.

— *Fimbriated:* Hymen with multiple projections and indentations along the edge, creating a ruffled appearance.

— *Redundant:* Abundant hymenal tissue that tends to fold back upon itself or protrude.

— *Hymenal mound or bump:* A solid elevation of hymenal tissue that is wider or as wide as it is long, located on the edge of the hymenal membrane. This structure may be seen at the site where an intravaginal column attaches to the hymen.

— *Hymenal tag:* An elongated projection of tissue arising from any location on the hymenal rim.

— *Hymenal cyst:* A fluid-filled elevation of tissue, confined within the hymenal tissue.

— *Hymenal cleft:* An angular or v-shaped indentation on the edge of the hymenal membrane.

— *External hymenal ridge:* A midline longitudinal ridge of tissue on the external surface of the hymen. May be either anterior or posterior and usually extends to the edge of the hymen.

Definitions taken from "Practice Guidelines: Descriptive Terminology in Child Sexual Abuse Medical Evaluations" published by the American Professional Society on the Abuse of Children, 1995. Adapted and reprinted with permission from the American Professional Society on the Abuse of Children.

The neonates were found to have primarily annular hymens; that is, the hymenal tissue extended 360 degrees around the opening to the vagina. Hymenal clefts, cysts, tags, mounds, external ridges, and intravaginal ridges were noted. See **Appendix Figures 2-1** through **2-21** for examples of anatomical variations of the hymen. The location of various features was described using a clock face, with the 12 o'clock position defined as directly below the urethra and the 6 o'clock position in the midline above the posterior commisure. In a follow-up study of 62 infants examined at 1 year, Berenson et al[4] noted that 10 of 13 infants who had an annular hymen with a notch in the 12 o'clock position as neonates had a crescentic hymen at 1 year. A crescentic hymen is defined as a configuration in which the attachments of the hymen are at the 1 to 2 o'clock and 10 to 11 o'clock positions, with an absence of hymenal tissue in between. At 1 year, 28% of infants had crescentic hymens compared to none in the neonate period; the frequency of external hymenal ridges decreased from 82% to 14% at 1 year.

Table 2-3 summarizes the changes in the frequency of various features of hymenal morphology among the children who were followed by Berenson et al from birth to 3 years[5] and those followed from 3 to 9 years.[6]

Table 2-3. Changes in Hymenal Features by Age.[4-6,10,14,15]

	PERCENTAGE OF SUBJECTS HAVING SPECIFIC HYMENAL FEATURES LISTED BY AGE					
FEATURE	NEWBORN N=486	1 YEAR N=57	3 YEARS N=134	5 YEARS N=93	7 YEARS N=80	9 YEARS N=61
Annular hymen	100	52	41	23	18	10
Crescentic hymen	0	28	50	77	82	90
Redundant hymen	100	42	25	N/A	N/A	N/A
Hymen tags	13	10	7	13	10	10
Hymen bump/mound	0	5	44	53	78	69
Intravaginal ridges	54	66	83	86	90	92
External hymenal ridge	82	17	7	3	1	0
Notch/cleft	38	19	14	7	9	11
Mean horizontal diameter of opening (mm)	N/A	3.8 +/- 1.1	4.7 +/- 1.2	4.6 +/- 1.6	5.5 +/- 1.9	6.1 +/- 2.3
Range of horizontal diameter of opening	N/A	2.5 - 6.0 mm	2.8 - 8.0 mm	1.0 - 8.0 mm	1.75 - 10.5 mm	1.75 - 12.25 mm
Width of posterior hymenal rim, range	N/A	2 - 4 mm	2.5 - 4.0 mm	1.0 - 6.5 mm	0.75 - 5.5 mm	1.25 - 4.75 mm

The longitudinal study supported the clinical observation that hymenal opening width increases with the age of the child. The mean horizontal diameter of the opening increased from 3.8 mm at 1 year to 6.1 mm at 9 years, with the width of the hymenal opening ranging from 2.5 to 6.0 mm at 1 year to 1.75 to 12.25 mm at 9 years. The other trend noted in the follow-up study was the decrease in the mean width of the posterior/inferior rim of hymen. The range of measurements of the posterior rim was 2 to 4 mm at 1 year, but changed to 0.75 to 5.5 mm at 7 years.

Cross-sectional studies of children selected for non-abuse, examined using colposcopy and photographs, reported a similar range of measurements of the diameter of the hymenal opening and the width of the posterior rim of hymen. McCann et al[1] reported measurements of the horizontal diameter of the hymenal opening, using labial traction, of 2 to 8 mm in girls 2 to 5 years, 1 to 9 mm in girls 5 to 7 years, and 2.5 to 10.5 mm in girls 8 years through Tanner Stage 2 development. While there were not enough girls in each age group to compare width of the posterior hymenal rim by age, researchers reported that among girls who were examined in the prone knee-chest position, the range of posterior rim width was 1 to 8 mm, with a mean of 2.8 mm.

A cross-sectional study of 211 girls from 1 month to 7 years by Berenson et al[2] also found that the mean horizontal diameter of the hymenal opening varied significantly by age (2.5 +/- 0.8 mm to 3.6 +/- 1.2 mm) and that the measurement of the posterior rim of hymen was as small as 0.9 to 1.0 mm in girls between 1 and 7 years who were considered to be non-abused. A study of 195 non-abused girls between 5 and 7 years by Myhre et al[7] also found that the range of measurement of the posterior hymenal rim, using labial traction, was 1.1 to 7.9 mm wide.

Appendix Figures 2-22 and **2-23** are examples of cases where the opening in the hymen may seem wide and the posterior rim relatively narrow, but in both cases the measurements from the photographs showed that they were within the normal range for a child of that age.

EFFECTS OF PUBERTY

THE HYMEN

With the onset of puberty, the hymen and other genital tissues show the effects of hormonal influence, especially estrogen. The hymen becomes thicker, paler, less sensitive to touch, and more likely to fold upon itself. These changes are illustrated in the following 3 cases. In a follow-up study of girls examined at 5 to 7 years,[7] Myhre et al re-examined a subset of subjects at 10 to 13 years. The hymen, vagina, and labia show the effects of development, as seen in **Appendix Figures 2-24** through **2-27**.[16]

Adolescent girls, from 13 to 19 years, with and without a history of penile-vaginal intercourse, were examined in a study to compare the appearance of the hymen.[17] **Appendix Figures 2-28** through **2-31** show some of these variations, from a very thick, tulip-shape hymen with an anterior opening (**Appendix Figures 2-28-a** and **b**) to a relatively narrow rim of hymen in a girl who denies intercourse (**Appendix Figure 2-31**).

Because estrogen causes the tissues of both the hymen and vagina to thicken and become pale, it is sometimes difficult to identify the edge of the hymen. The use of a large swab covered by a balloon for color contrast (**Appendix Figure 2-29**), or a regular cotton-tipped applicator to stretch out the edge of the hymen (**Appendix Figures 2-30** and **2-31**) can assist the examiner in determining the integrity of the hymenal rim.

THE VAGINA

As pubertal development progresses, all the tissues and structures of the vaginal vestibule show the effects of estrogen. **Appendix Figure 2-32** is an example of the fossa groove that develops in some patients during early puberty due to the effect of estrogen on the inner aspect of the labia minora. The external surface of the labia affected by androgenic hormones in the same way the scrotal skin changes in males. The skin becomes darker, thicker, and develops folds or rugae. For reasons not fully understood, the labia minora can be affected on one side more than another, which causes an asymmetry that can be quite pronounced (see **Appendix Figures 2-33** and **2-34**).

THE CERVIX

The cervix may also take on a different appearance as puberty progresses (**Appendix Figure 2-35**). In the younger adolescent, the columnar epithelium of the endocervix is visible on the outer surface, which gives it a darker red, sometimes pebbled appearance (**Appendix Figure 2-36**). This pattern changes as the neck of the cervix lengthens and the endocervical tissues regress inward.

THE ANUS

The skin around the anus, when the external anal sphincter is contracted and the anus is closed, takes on a wrinkled appearance. The tighter the contraction of the sphincter, the more wrinkles or folds are seen. In some children, there is a gap in the subcutaneous division of the external sphincter muscle, which causes an area in the midline, usually at the 6 o'clock position, to be smooth and free of folds. This condition was named *diastasis ani* (**Appendix Figure 2-37**) by Dr. John McCann[3] who observed this finding in 26% of the children in his study of perianal findings in non-abused children. Berenson et al,[8] in a study of 89 female infants under 18 months, also noted this *smooth area* in 26% of subjects. Myhre et al[9] studied children 5 to 7 years with no history or suspicion of sexual abuse and noted that more boys than girls were found to have *diastasis ani*, and that it was more commonly observed in the prone knee-chest position than in the left lateral position. In the knee-chest position, 12% of subjects had the finding.

Anal tags and thickened midline skin folds are common findings in children who have not been abused. Tags were seen in 11% of the subjects in the study by McCann et al[3] and in 6% of subjects in the study by Myhre et al.[9] **Appendix Figure 2-38** is an example of a midline tag.

The skin in the perianal area may have darker pigmentation than elsewhere on the body. This was first described in the study by McCann et al,[3] where the prevalence varied by ethnicity. Among white children, 22% had hyperpigmentation of the perianal skin, compared to 53% of the African American children and 58% of the Hispanic children (**Appendix Figures 2-39** and **2-40-a**).

When the external anal sphincter relaxes but the internal sphincter remains closed, the anal opening may have an irregular appearance. This is shown in **Appendix Figure 2-40-b**. When both the internal and external anal sphincters relax, the anal canal is visualized, and in some views, the pectinate line can be seen. The pectinate line is the line of demarcation between the skin of the anal canal (pectin) and the anal mucosa, and can have a jagged appearance due to the anal columns and crypts. These structures are shown in **Appendix Figures 2-41** and **2-42**.

Anal dilation, with both internal and external sphincters relaxed, was found in 49% of 267 children selected for non-abuse in the study by McCann et al[3] in which all children were examined in the prone knee-chest position, some for as long as 4 minutes (**Appendix Figure 2-43**). A smaller number of children showed complete anal dilation within 30 seconds (14.6%). Myhre et al[9] reported the frequency of complete anal dilation seen in 100 boys and 167 girls between the ages of 4 and 6 years who were examined in the prone knee-chest position for 30 seconds as part of a study of findings in non-abused children. Complete anal dilation was seen in 3% of the boys and 5.6% of the girls, for a rate of 4.7% overall. In the Myhre study, complete anal dilation was very rare (0.7%) when the child was examined in the left lateral position.

Another feature described in the studies by McCann et al[3] and Myhre et al[9] is that of venous pooling or venous congestion of the blood vessels in the perianal area. McCann et al reported that at the midpoint of the examination in the knee-chest position, 52% of the subjects had venous pooling. In the Myhre et al study, children were not kept in the knee-chest position as long as in the McCann et al study (average time 30 seconds compared to up to 4 minutes), and venous congestion was documented in 20% of subjects. The perianal area has a rich blood supply, and the veins become engorged when the child is positioned so that venous return from the plexus is impaired. This can lead to a rather alarming purple/blue coloration of the surrounding skin, which should not be mistaken for trauma. See **Appendix Figures 2-44** through **2-45** for examples of venous pooling.

The congenital defect known as failure of midline fusion, or perineal groove, is another finding on anogenital examination that may cause concern if it is not recognized. In 1984, Dr. Anthony Shaw published photos of 6 children with this defect in the "Picture of the Month" section of the *American Journal of Diseases of Childhood*.[18] His report stated that the condition required no treatment, and that the defect would eventually fill in. The defect was also described in a textbook of surgery[19] as having the following features: "normal formation of the vestibule, urethra and vagina, hypertrophic minoral tails which skirt the perineum and course posteriorly to join at the anus or surround it, and a wet groove in the perineum between the fourchette and the anus." **Appendix Figures 2-46-a, b,** and **c** are from a case report published in 1989 describing a child who was referred for suspected sexual abuse because of the unusual genital finding.[20]

A 2006 report described the results of a surgical correction of a perineal groove in a 6-month-old girl.[21] Histological analysis of the excised tissue revealed squamous epithelial tissue at both ends, with rectal mucosa in between. There was also edema, patchy hemorrhage, and scattered inflammatory cell infiltrate in lamina propria surrounding normal rectal crypts. The authors postulate that the anomaly represents an embryologic remnant of the urorectal septum rather than a failure of midline fusion.

CONCLUSION

It should not be surprising that there is considerable variation in the appearance of the structures of the external genitalia and anal tissues in non-abused children. Every child is a unique individual, and while there may be common patterns in how tissues develop, there is much not understood about anatomic variations. For example, it is not clear exactly why the hymen changes from primarily annular to primarily crescentic as a child grows and estrogen effect regresses, or what factors are involved in the development of the septate, microperforate, or imperforate hymen.

Additional studies of children with no history or concern for abuse are needed, especially studies of the appearance of the genital tissues in girls between 9 and 13 years. Further studies are also needed of the appearance of the anal tissues in children of different ages and of the prevalence of dilation in children with and without a history of constipation. Further research will help to answer some of the remaining questions regarding what is normal when it comes to the appearance of the genital and anal tissues in children.

APPENDIX 2-1: FEATURES OF GENITAL AND ANAL ANATOMY

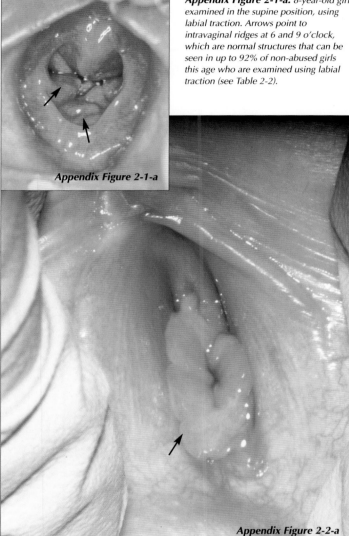

Appendix Figure 2-1-a. *8-year-old girl examined in the supine position, using labial traction. Arrows point to intravaginal ridges at 6 and 9 o'clock, which are normal structures that can be seen in up to 92% of non-abused girls this age who are examined using labial traction (see Table 2-2).*

Appendix Figure 2-1-a

Appendix Figure 2-1-b

Appendix Figure 2-1-b. *Same patient examined in the prone, knee-chest position. Arrow points to an intravaginal ridge. The hymen is smooth and without interruption. This type of normal examination is common in children who describe being molested and are examined some time distant from the last episode of abuse. Touching or rubbing of the genital area, contact between a perpetrator's hand or penis and the external genital structures, and oral-genital contact would not be expected to cause any injury.*

Appendix Figure 2-2-a

Appendix Figure 2-2-a. *2-year-old girl examined using labial separation. The hymen at 7 o'clock location is thick and shows the effects of estrogen. The hymen is redundant and folded, and in this view neither the hymenal edge nor the hymenal opening can be seen.*

Appendix Figure 2-2-b. *Using labial traction, with the examiner grasping the labia majora and gently pulling forward, the hymen at 7 o'clock opens as does the urethral orifice shown at 12 o'clock, and an intravaginal ridge at 5 o'clock can be visualized extending into the vagina at the 8 o'clock location.*

Appendix Figure 2-2-b

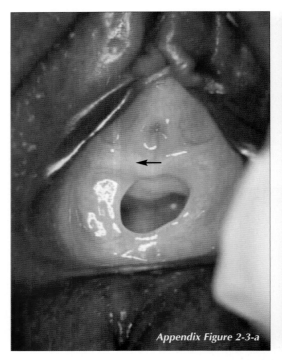

Appendix Figure 2-3-a

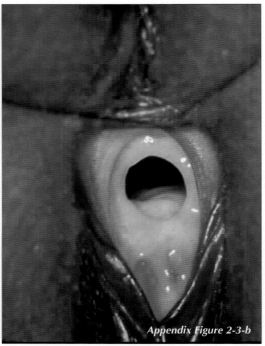

Appendix Figure 2-3-b

Appendix Figure 2-3-a. *6-year-old girl with no suspicion of sexual abuse. The photograph shows an annular hymen with tissue all the way around the hymenal opening, including at the 12 o'clock position. This is the most common hymen configuration in newborns and girls up to age 3 years, from the longitudinal studies by Berenson, et al (see Table 2-2).*

Appendix Figure 2-3-b. *In the prone knee-chest position, the smooth, non-interrupted edge of the hymen is clearly demonstrated.*

Appendix Figure 2-4. *11-year-old girl with no history of sexual abuse. This photo shows a normal, crescentic hymen, with attachments at the 2 o'clock and 10 o'clock position. The arrow points to periurethral support bands, which are normal structures.*

Appendix Figure 2-5. *2-year-old Hispanic girl brought for suspicion of sexual abuse. The hymen is sleeve-like, with a ventral opening and an external hymenal ridge in the midline at 6 o'clock. The redness in the fossa is not specific for sexual abuse.*

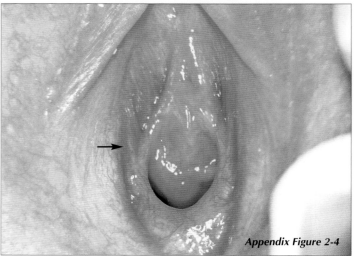

Appendix Figure 2-4

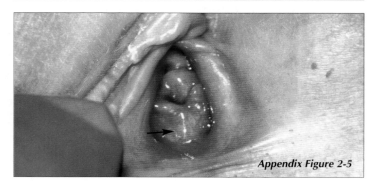

Appendix Figure 2-5

Appendix Figure 2-6. *Annular hymen in a 6-month-old Caucasian female, showing the thick appearance typical of estrogen effect.*

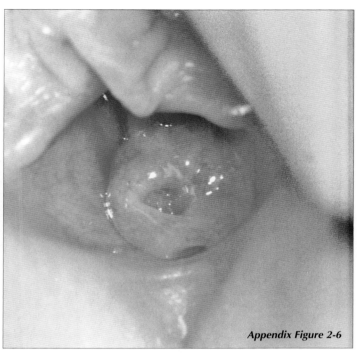

Appendix Figure 2-6

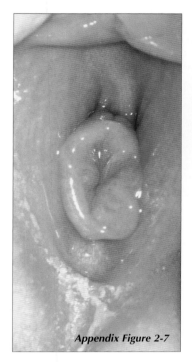

Appendix Figure 2-7

Appendix Figure 2-7. *Annular hymen in a 16-month-old girl, shown using labial separation.*

Appendix Figure 2-8-a. *3-year-old girl, examined using labial traction. The hymen is thick, suggesting estrogen effect, and the inner edge of the hymen is smooth.*

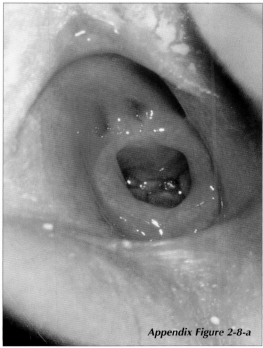

Appendix Figure 2-8-a

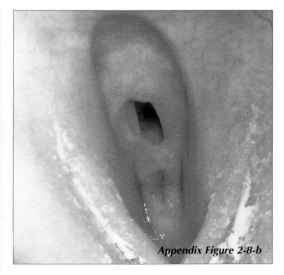

Appendix Figure 2-8-b

Appendix Figure 2-8-b. *In the knee-chest position, the hymen edge looks sharper, but the rim is smooth and without interruption.*

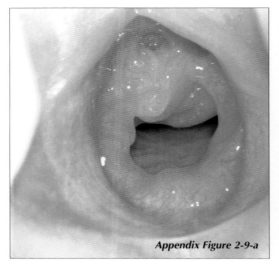

Appendix Figure 2-9-a. *2-year-old Caucasian girl, examined using labial traction. The crescentic hymen has attachments at 11 o'clock and 2 o'clock. There is a small mound or bump on the hymen at 6 o'clock and at 9 o'clock.*

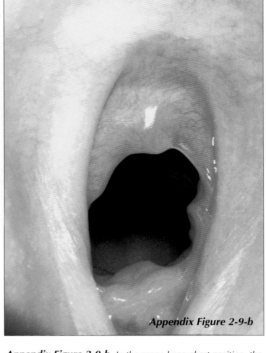

Appendix Figure 2-9-b

Appendix Figure 2-9-b. *In the prone knee-chest position, the mound at 6 o'clock is now seen at 12 o'clock, and the mound at 9 o'clock is seen at 3 o'clock.*

Appendix Figure 2-10-a. *This 4-year-old girl, examined using labial traction, has a thick, redundant hymen. The edge is not well defined. She has no history or suspicion of sexual abuse.*

Appendix Figure 2-10-b. *Using labial traction, the hymenal opening is easily seen, and the inner edge of hymen is smooth except for a mound or tag at 6 o'clock. While the opening may appear "large" to a caregiver or inexperienced medical provider, it is normal for the labial traction technique to produce the largest measurements of the horizontal diameter of the hymenal opening. The measurement on this child was within the normal range, according to studies of non-abused children.*

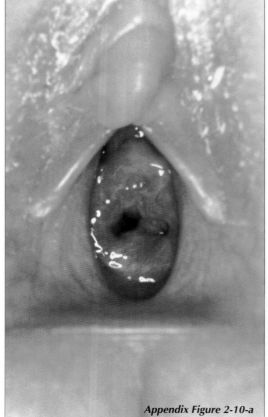

Appendix Figure 2-10-a

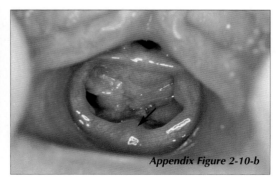

Appendix Figure 2-10-b

Appendix Figure 2-10-c. *In the prone knee-chest view, the mound on the hymen appears as a thickening, possibly a resolving hymenal tag from birth. This is a normal variation in the hymen.*

Appendix Figure 2-11-a. *This 8-year-old African American girl gave a history of penile-vaginal contact by an uncle. Using supine labial traction, the hymen appears to have a superficial cleft at the 3 o'clock location.*

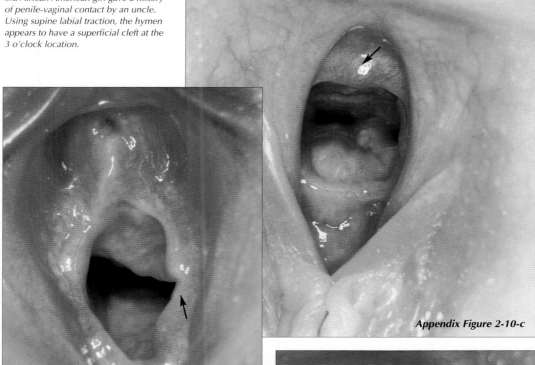

Appendix Figure 2-10-c

Appendix Figure 2-11-a

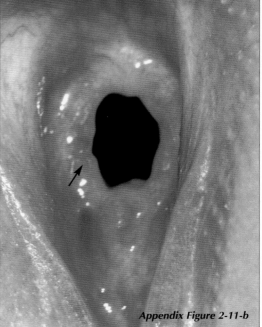

Appendix Figure 2-11-b. *In this prone knee-chest view, there is not a notch in the hymen at the 9 o'clock location, which would correlate with the 3 o'clock location when she was examined supine. A mound caused by an intravaginal ridge can give the impression of a notch adjacent to the mound, so additional techniques are needed to stretch out the edge of the hymen for a better view.*

Appendix Figure 2-11-b

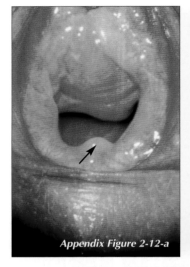
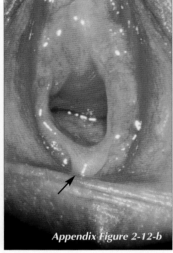
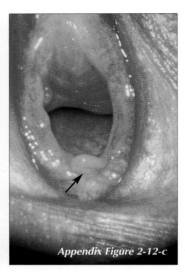

Appendix Figure 2-12-a. *Appendix Figure 2-12-b.* *Appendix Figure 2-12-c.*

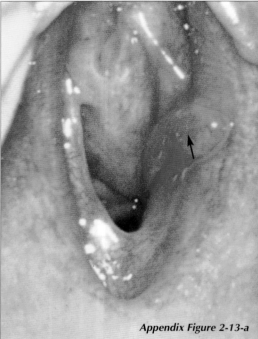

Appendix Figure 2-13-a

Appendix Figure 2-12-a. *3-year-old girl with no complaint of abuse, examined using labial traction. There is a small mound on the hymen at the 6 o'clock location, but otherwise the hymen is smooth and normal in appearance.*

Appendix Figure 2-12-b. *In this view, the mound appears to be a tag on the hymen, which is now folded outward.*

Appendix Figure 2-12-c. *The midline tag has again folded inward, causing the appearance of a mound.*

Appendix Figure 2-13-a. *This 3-year-old girl also has a tag on the hymen, at the 3 o'clock location, which is folded outward against the vestibular wall on the patient's left side.*

Appendix Figure 2-13-b. *By using labial traction to separate and then oppose the labia majora, the tag has been released and is now folded across the hymenal opening, touching the vestibular wall at the 9 o'clock location.*

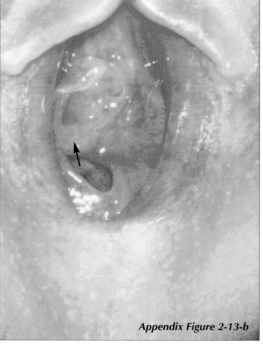

Appendix Figure 2-13-b

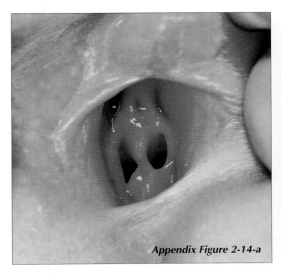

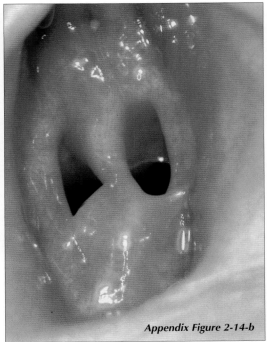

Appendix Figure 2-14-a. *3-year-old girl with a septate hymen.*

Appendix Figure 2-14-b. *Showing the septum extending from 12 to 6 o'clock across the vaginal opening. In order to be sure this is only a hymenal septum and not a vaginal septum, a small swab or probe should be passed behind the septum.*

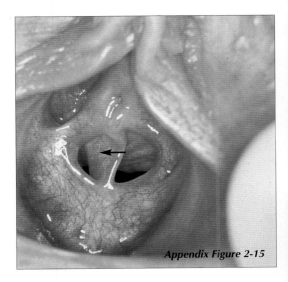

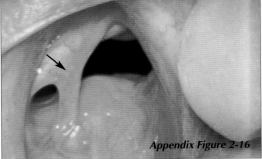

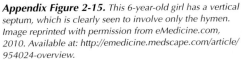

Appendix Figure 2-15. *This 6-year-old girl has a vertical septum, which is clearly seen to involve only the hymen. Image reprinted with permission from eMedicine.com, 2010. Available at: http://emedicine.medscape.com/article/ 954024-overview.*

Appendix Figure 2-16. *This 3-year-old girl had an unusual appearance to the hymen. In the prone knee-chest position, a vertical septum is seen extending across the introitus, resulting in two asymmetric hymenal openings.*

Appendix Figure 2-17. *Normal periurethral support bands in a 16-year-old girl with a redundant, closed hymen.*

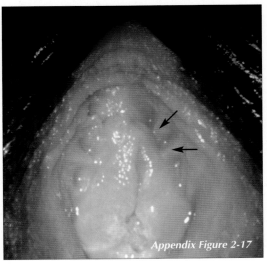

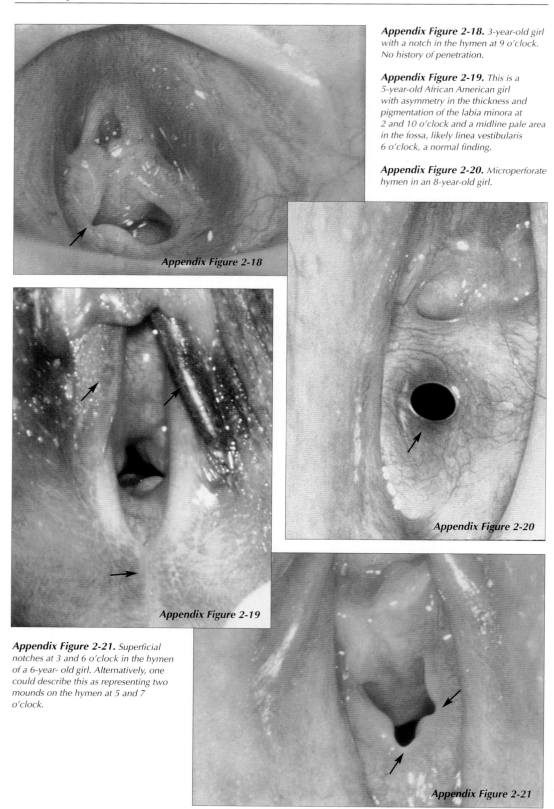

Appendix Figure 2-18. *3-year-old girl with a notch in the hymen at 9 o'clock. No history of penetration.*

Appendix Figure 2-19. *This is a 5-year-old African American girl with asymmetry in the thickness and pigmentation of the labia minora at 2 and 10 o'clock and a midline pale area in the fossa, likely linea vestibularis 6 o'clock, a normal finding.*

Appendix Figure 2-20. *Microperforate hymen in an 8-year-old girl.*

Appendix Figure 2-18

Appendix Figure 2-20

Appendix Figure 2-19

Appendix Figure 2-21. *Superficial notches at 3 and 6 o'clock in the hymen of a 6-year- old girl. Alternatively, one could describe this as representing two mounds on the hymen at 5 and 7 o'clock.*

Appendix Figure 2-21

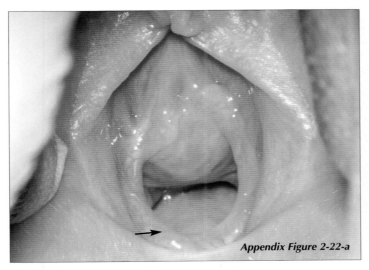

Appendix Figure 2-22-a

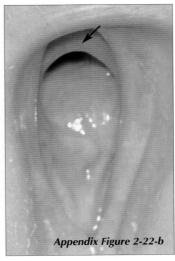

Appendix Figure 2-22-b

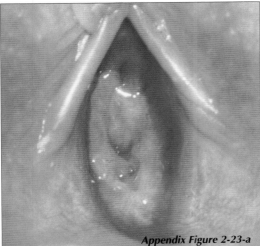

Appendix Figure 2-23-a

Appendix Figure 2-22-a. *8-year-old girl who describes "sex" with an 11-year-old boy. In the supine position, using labial traction, the hymen is crescentic, with a smooth edge.*

Appendix Figure 2-22-b. *In the prone knee-chest position, the posterior rim of the hymen is smooth and without interruption.*

Appendix Figure 2-23-a. *This 2-year-old girl was referred because of sexual acting out behaviors. Using labial separation, the hymen is closed.*

Appendix Figure 2-23-b. *Using labial traction, both the urethral opening at 12 o'clock and the hymenal opening at 7 o'clock are revealed. It is difficult to assess the integrity of the posterior hymenal rim.*

Appendix Figure 2-23-c. *In the prone knee-chest position, the posterior rim, while relatively narrow for a child of this age, is smooth and without signs of injury.*

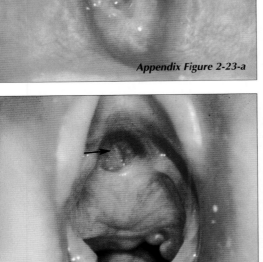

Appendix Figure 2-23-b

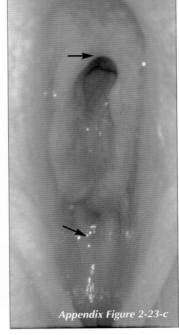

Appendix Figure 2-23-c

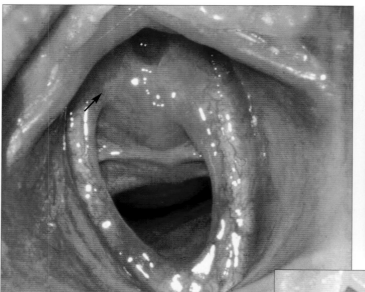

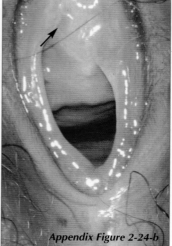

Appendix Figure 2-24-b

Appendix Figure 2-24-a

Appendix Figure 2-24-a. *7-year-old girl examined as part of a study of normal anatomy in nonabused children, done in Trondheim, Norway. This is a crescentic hymen with the attachment at 11 and 2 o'clock. Contributed by Arne K. Myhre, MD; Trondheim, Norway.*

Appendix Figure 2-24-b. *Reexamined child as part of a follow-up study, now age 12 years, 9 months. The hymen has a very similar appearance, but now is thicker and paler in color. Contributed by Arne K. Myhre, MD; Trondheim, Norway.*

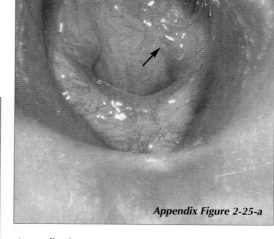

Appendix Figure 2-25-a

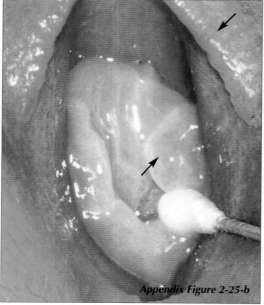

Appendix Figure 2-25-b

Appendix Figure 2-25-a. *6 year, 9 month old girl examined as part of the study by Myhre et al. Note the appearance of the labia minora at 1 o'clock. There is a flap of hymen noted at 2 to 3 o'clock. Contributed by Arne K. Myhre, MD; Trondheim, Norway.*

Appendix Figure 2-25-b. *Same child, seen at follow-up at age 12 years, 7 months. The labia minora at 1 o'clock are thicker, longer, and more pigmented. The flap of hymen is more prominent with the effect of endogenous estrogen shown at 3 o'clock. Contributed by Arne K. Myhre, MD; Trondheim, Norway.*

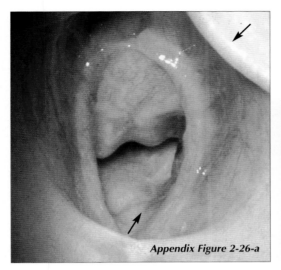

Appendix Figure 2-26-a

Appendix Figure 2-26-a. *This child is 5 years, 11 months old at the time of her first examination. The labium minus, seen here, is thin and smooth at the 1 o'clock position. The hymenal edge at 7 o'clock is not seen clearly, but there is an intravaginal ridge at that location.*

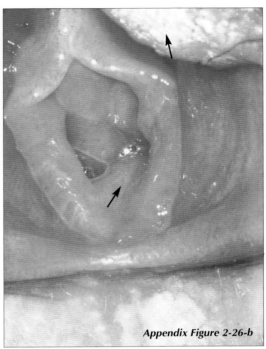

Appendix Figure 2-26-b

Appendix Figure 2-26-b. *At her follow-up examination, the child is now 11 years, 8 months old. The labium minus is thicker and darker at 3 o'clock. The intravaginal ridge is seen at the same location as in the first examination at 1 o'clock, and the hymen is thicker, paler, and folds outward.*

Appendix Figure 2-27-a. *8-year-old Mexican American girl, examined in the supine position, using labial traction. Periurethral support bands are seen bilaterally at 2 and 10 o'clock. The hymen is thick and pale at 6 o'clock, reflecting the effect of estrogen. The child has begun breast development, but does not yet have pubic hair. Image reprinted with permission from eMedicine.com, 2010. Available at: http://emedicine.medscape.com/article/ 954024-overview.*

Appendix Figure 2-27-b. *In the prone knee-chest position, the hymen retains its thick, pale appearance.*

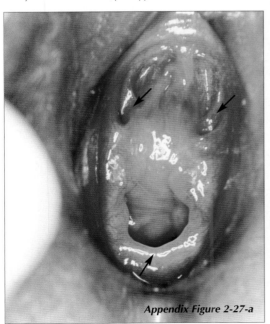

Appendix Figure 2-27-a

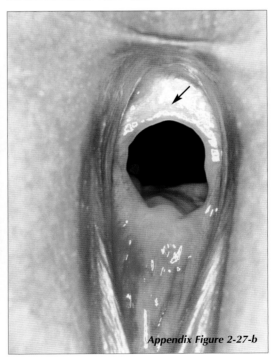

Appendix Figure 2-27-b

Appendix Figure 2-28-a. *Tulip-shaped, estrogenized hymen in a 14-year-old girl examined as part of a study of the appearance of the hymen in adolescent girls with no history of sexual activity. This girl described difficulty inserting a tampon, likely due to the shape of her hymen.*

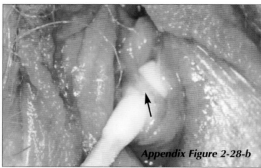

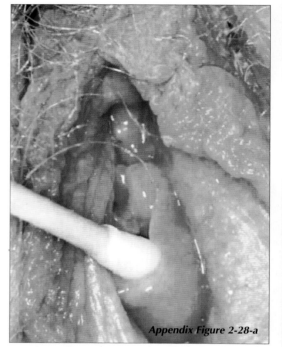

Appendix Figure 2-28-a

Appendix Figure 2-28-b. *Same 14-year-old girl with a swab showing the presence of a hymenal septum.*

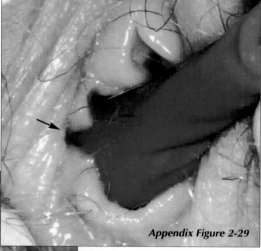

Appendix Figure 2-29

Appendix Figure 2-29. *18-year-old girl, consensually sexually active, with a complete cleft in the hymen at the 9 o'clock position. A large swab, covered by a latex balloon, provides contrast and stretches out the hymen to identify the cleft.*

Appendix Figure 2-30. *16-year-old girl, part of the study of the hymen in adolescents, with the hymen stretched out with a regular cotton swab. The width of the wooden handle of the swab is 2 mm, which is the same apparent width of the posterior hymen rim in this patient.*

Appendix Figure 2-30

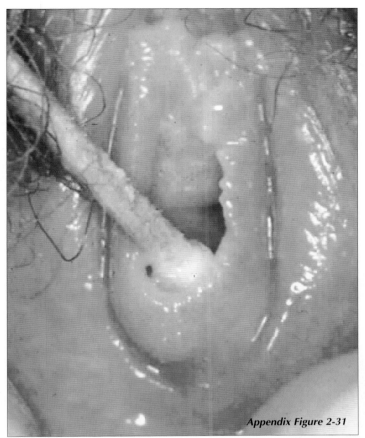

Appendix Figure 2-31. *This 14-year-old girl has a wider rim of hymen at the 6 o'clock location. She denies intercourse and does not use tampons.*

Appendix Figure 2-32. *This 13-year-old girl's hymen shows the thick, pale color typical of estrogen effect at 9 o'clock. A groove in the fossa is also noted at 6 o'clock. This is a common finding in girls during the first stages of pubertal development, as the tissues of the vulva thicken in response to hormone levels. Image reprinted with permission from eMedicine.com, 2010. Available at: http://emedicine.medscape.com/article/954024-overview.*

Appendix Figure 2-31

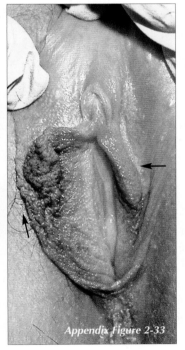

Appendix Figure 2-33

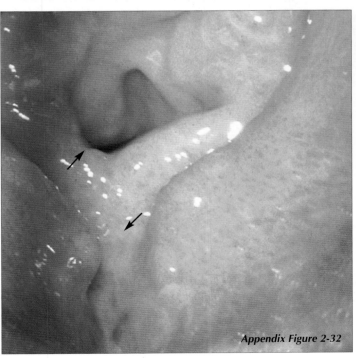

Appendix Figure 2-32

Appendix Figure 2-33. *This 14-year-old Mexican American girl shaves her vulva (a very common practice in adolescents, whether or not they are sexually active). She also has asymmetric development of her labia minora, with the right labium minus longer, thicker, and more pigmented than the left. Patients may request cosmetic surgery to reduce the size of the larger labium minus.*

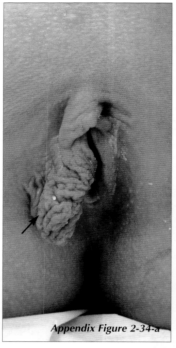

Appendix Figure 2-34-a. *The mother of this 11-year-old girl with Down syndrome was worried about molestation because of the unusual appearance of her genital tissues. The mother had not seen the child for 2 years, and in the interval the girl had begun menstruation and needed help with hygiene. This is a dramatic example of asymmetric development of the labia minora, with the right labium minus showing thickening, wrinkling and hyperpigmentation caused by the androgenic hormones of puberty. On the right, the labium minus has the appearance typical of a prepubertal girl. It is not known why the tissues of the genitalia respond in this asymmetric manner.*

Appendix Figure 2-34-b. *Using further labial traction, the estrogenized hymen is seen. Although this child had no pubic or axillary hair, she did have breast development and was having regular monthly menstrual cycles.*

Appendix Figure 2-34-a

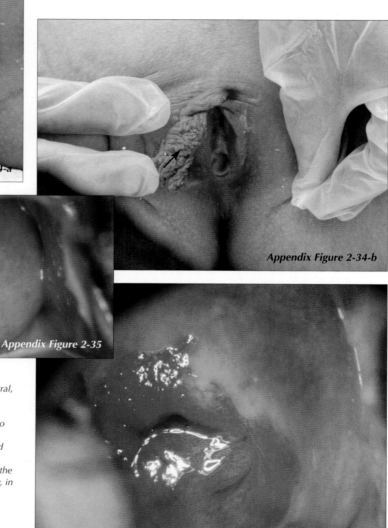

Appendix Figure 2-34-b

Appendix Figure 2-35

Appendix Figure 2-35. *This is a normal-appearing cervix with a central, round os in a 17-year-old girl.*

Appendix Figure 2-36. *This is also a normal cervix, showing cervical ectropion. This appearance is caused by the columnar epithelium of the endocervix extending outward onto the surface of the cervix in early puberty, in this case in a girl age 14.*

Appendix Figure 2-36

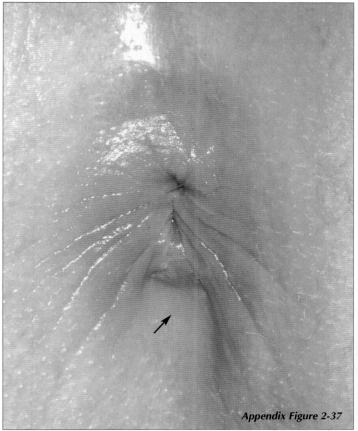

Appendix Figure 2-37. *Normal pattern of anal folds in a 5-year-old girl, showing a smooth area at 6 o'clock, called diastasis ani. This appearance is thought to be caused by a break in the fibers of the subcutaneous division of the external anal sphincter muscle. It is the contraction of the external sphincter that caused the circular pattern of folds in the perianal skin.*

Appendix Figure 2-37

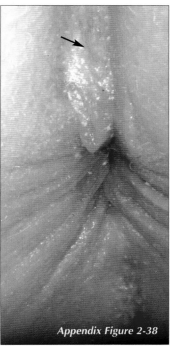

Appendix Figure 2-38. *This 3-year-old boy has a thickened perianal fold in the midline, which can appear as a tag.*

Appendix Figure 2-39. *This 3-year-old African American girl has normal anal folds and normal increased pigmentation of the perianal skin. Hyperpigmented skin in the perianal area and vulva is common in children of color.*

Appendix Figure 2-38

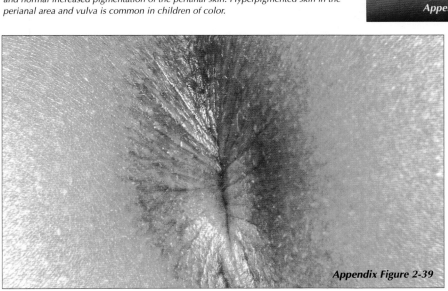

Appendix Figure 2-39

Appendix Figure 2-40-a. *This 5-year-old Mexican American girl had given a history of being fondled. The perianal folds are normal.*

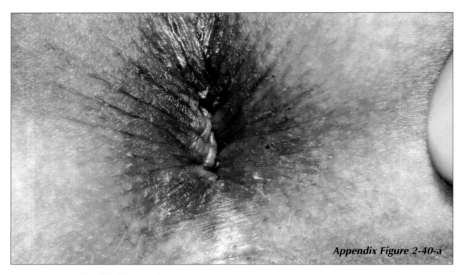

Appendix Figure 2-40-a

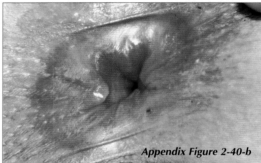

Appendix Figure 2-40-b

Appendix Figure 2-40-b. *With separation of the buttocks, the external anal sphincter relaxes, while the internal sphincter remains closed. This causes an irregular appearance that should not be mistaken for trauma.*

Appendix Figure 2-41. *This drawing shows the relationship of the branches of the internal and external anal sphincter muscles and the structures of the anus and rectum. Reprinted by permission from: Snell RS. Clinical Anatomy for Medical Students. Baltimore, MD: Lippincott Williams & Wilkins; 2004.*

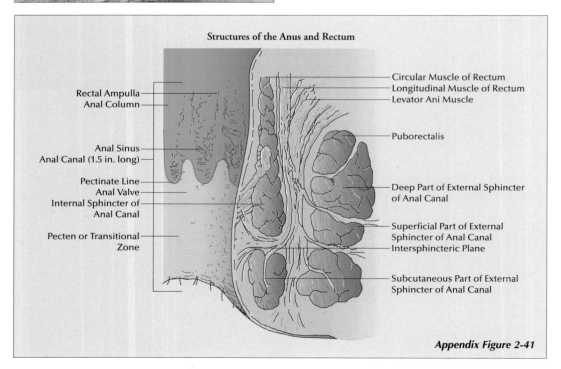

Structures of the Anus and Rectum

Rectal Ampulla
Anal Column

Anal Sinus
Anal Canal (1.5 in. long)

Pectinate Line
Anal Valve
Internal Sphincter of Anal Canal

Pecten or Transitional Zone

Circular Muscle of Rectum
Longitudinal Muscle of Rectum
Levator Ani Muscle

Puborectalis

Deep Part of External Sphincter of Anal Canal

Superficial Part of External Sphincter of Anal Canal
Intersphincteric Plane

Subcutaneous Part of External Sphincter of Anal Canal

Appendix Figure 2-41

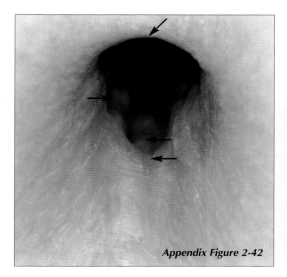

Appendix Figure 2-42.

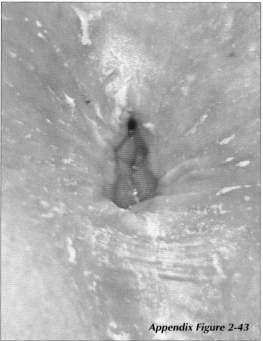

Appendix Figure 2-42. *Photograph of the anus of a 4-year-old child in the prone knee-chest position who is relaxed enough for the anus to dilate; both external and internal anal sphincters are relaxed. The arrows show the anal verge at 12 o'clock, the pectin at 6 o'clock upper, the pectinate line at 6 o'clock lower, and an anal column at 9 o'clock.*

Appendix Figure 2-43. *9-year-old female who reported fondling. The anus shows the appearance when the external sphincter is relaxed, but the internal sphincter is closed. This is normal.*

Appendix Figure 2-44. *2-year-old female with no complaints of anal discomfort or constipation. The dark ring around the anus is pooling of blood in the plexus of veins and is a normal finding.*

Appendix Figure 2-43

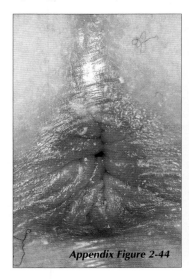

Appendix Figure 2-44

Appendix Figure 2-45. *11-year-old male with venous pooling and flattening of the anal folds due to partial relaxation of the external anal sphincter.*

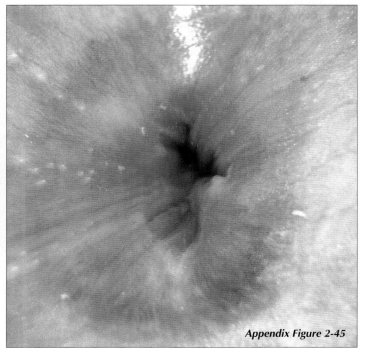

Appendix Figure 2-45

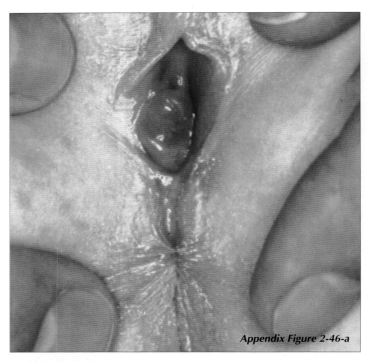

Appendix Figure 2-46-a

Appendix Figure 2-46-a, b, and **c.** Reprinted with permission from Adams JA, Horton M. Is it sexual abuse? Confusion caused by a congenital anomaly of genitalia. Clin Pediatr. 1989;28(3):146-148. 1989 Copyright by Sage Publications, Inc.

Appendix Figure 2-46-a. Photograph taken with a 35mm camera of the genital area of a 15-month-old girl who was referred for possible sexual abuse due to the finding of a defect in the perineum.

Appendix Figure 2-46-b. At 16 months of age, the patient was examined using a colposcope for magnification. Part of the hymen is seen superiorly, with the perineal groove descending from the fossa to the anus. The skin at the border of the defect has a rolled appearance.

Appendix Figure 2-46-c. View of the perianal tissues, with the groove seen extending to the anal verge.

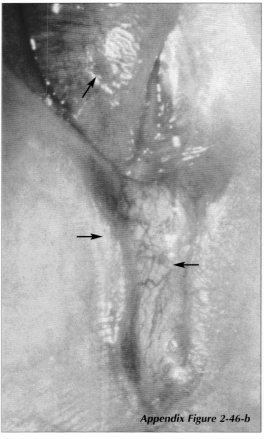

Appendix Figure 2-46-b

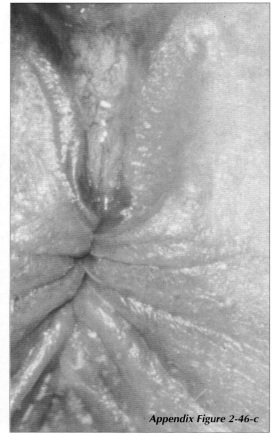

Appendix Figure 2-46-c

REFERENCES

1. McCann J, Wells R, Simon M, Voris J. Genital findings in prepubertal girls selected for non-abuse: a descriptive study. *Pediatrics*. 1990;86(3):428-439.

2. Berenson AB, Heger AH, Hayes JM, Bailey RK, Emans SJ. Appearance of the hymen in prepubertal girls. *Pediatrics*. 1992;89(3):387-394.

3. McCann J, Voris J, Simon M, Wells R. Perianal findings in prepubertal children selected for nonabuse: a descriptive study. *Child Abuse Negl*. 1989;13(2):179-193.

4. Berenson AB. Appearance of the hymen at birth and one year of age: a longitudinal study. *Pediatrics*. 1993;91(4):820-825.

5. Berenson AB. A longitudinal study of hymenal morphology in the first 3 years of life. *Pediatrics*. 1995;95(4):490-496.

6. Berenson AB, Grady JJ. A longitudinal study of hymenal development from 3 to 9 years of age. *J Pediatr*. 2002;140(5):600-607.

7. Myhre AK, Berntzen K, Bratlid D. Genital anatomy in non-abused preschool girls. *Acta Paediatr*. 2003;92(12):1453-1462.

8. Berenson AB, Somma-Garcia A, Barnett S. Perianal findings in infants 18 months of age or younger. *Pediatrics*. 1993;91(4):838-840.

9. Myhre AK, Berntzen K, Bratlid D. Perianal anatomy in non-abused preschool children. *Acta Paediatr*. 2001;90(11):1321-1328.

10. Adams JA, et al. *Practice Guidelines: Descriptive Terminology in Child Sexual Abuse Medical Evaluations*. Chicago, IL: American Professional Society on the Abuse of Children; 1995:1-8.

11. Moore KL, Persaud TVN. *The Developing Human, Clinically Oriented Embryology*, 6th ed. Philadelphia, PA: WB Saunders; 1998.

12. van der Putte SCJ. The development of the perineum in the human. *Adv Anat Embryol Cell Biol*. 2005;177:46.

13. Merlob P, Bahari C, Liban E, Reisner SH. Cysts of the female external genitalia in the newborn infant. *Am J Obstet Gynecol*. 1978;132(6):607-610.

14. Jenny C, Kuhns MLD, Arakawa F. Hymens in newborn female infants. *Pediatrics*. 1987;80(3):399-400.

15. Berenson AB, Heger A, Andrews S. Appearance of the hymen in newborns. *Pediatrics*. 1991;87(4):458-465.

16. Myhre AK, Myklestad K, Adams JA. Changes in genital anatomy and microbiology in girls between age 6 and age 12 years: a longitudinal study. *J Pediatr Adolesc Gynecol*. 2010;23:77-85.

17. Adams JA, Botash AS, Kellogg N. Differences in hymenal morphology between adolescent girls with and without a history of consensual sexual intercourse. *Arch Pediatr Adolesc Med*. 2004;158(3):280-285.

18. Gellis SG, Feingold M, Shaw A, Dewitt GW. Picture of the month: perineal groove. *Am J Dis Child*. 1977;131:921-922.

19. Stephens FD, Smith ED. *Ano-Rectal Malformations in Children*. Chicago, IL, Year Book Medical Publishers; 1971:114-116.

20. Adams JA, Horton M. Is it sexual abuse? Confusion caused by a congenital anomaly of the genitalia. *Clin Pediatr.*1989;28(3):146-148.

21. Mullassery D, Turnock R, Kokai G. Perineal groove. *J Pediatr Surg.* 2006;41:e41-e43. doi:10.20/j.jpedsurg.2005.12.068

Chapter 3

THE MEDICAL EVALUATION OF AN ALLEGED CHILDHOOD SEXUAL ABUSE VICTIM

Martin A. Finkel, DO, FACOP, FAAP

Sexual abuse is a common childhood experience with the potential for serious long-term consequences. Those who participate in the assessment of a child suspected of experiencing sexual abuse must do so with knowledge, skill, and sensitivity that comes from understanding the "disease of sexual victimization."[1-4] The medical evaluation of a child suspected to have experienced inappropriate sexual contact is not all that dissimilar from the evaluation of a child with an illness. The process of coming to a diagnostic assessment incorporates all of the traditional components of the evaluation of any complex medical condition. The subject matter, however, requires an understanding of the clinical expression of sexual victimization, just as the diagnosis of any disease is not possible without understanding its clinical presentation. Many of the dynamics of sexual abuse are not intuitive, and they may be counterintuitive to those who are misinformed.[5-8] The tools to create a medical evaluation begin with building on the knowledge of the dynamics of sexual victimization and developing the necessary skills to obtain a history in a manner that is nonjudgmental, facilitating, and empathizing. The medical record must precisely reflect the details of the questions asked and the child's verbatim response.[9-10]

The medical record articulates the clinical encounter of the health care providers, child or adolescent patient, and caregiver. The medical record of children who may have experienced abusive sexual contact shares most of the core elements of the standard medical record/consultation format found in either an office-based or a hospital-based practice. Acceptable medical practice dictates that clinicians assessing a child in this circumstance follow a standard set of assessment parameters, similar to what would be anticipated in the evaluation of any medical condition. When a patient sees a doctor, a current medical history is obtained, including a detailed review of systems (ROS) and appropriate developmental and social history. Verifying the medical history affords an opportunity to understand the chronology of events from the possibly abusive contact to the circumstances that resulted in disclosure.

In suspected sexual abuse examinations, the examiner should presume that there is a significant probability that state child protective services (CPS), law enforcement, prosecutors, and defense counsel will review the record. In contrast, most office records are reviewed only in a peer review situation or a malpractice action. In anticipation of external scrutiny, one must construct the medical record with exacting attention to detail. The medical record must be legible, well constructed, and educational, with defensible conclusions.[10] The medical record should carefully chronicle the medical history, anatomic findings (even when normal), and laboratory test results. The medical record is the instrument the clinician will use to make the diagnosis and treatment recommendations.[11] The credibility of the diagnostic assessment will be questioned if the record is incomplete or poorly formulated.[12-13]

This chapter will describe core elements of conducting a comprehensive evaluation as well as the types of information that need to be obtained, the how-to's of obtaining information, and the documentation of the medical history and physical examination. Intertwined throughout the chapter will be a few inescapable legal concepts that have general applicability to a patient's medical record and that take on special significance in children suspected of having been sexually abused. The end of this chapter will provide some suggestions on how to tie all of the pieces together to formulate a clear and balanced diagnosis.

DOCUMENTING THE CLINICAL EVALUATION

Clinicians document their interactions with their patients in a variety of ways. Documentation can take the form of precise language reflecting details of the medical history or of a synthesis of the information gathered. For example, in most busy practices, the clinician may ask a series of questions, listen to the patient's responses, and, either after the history or the examination, summarize the interaction and record salient points. Although a style that synthesizes and organizes information and deletes irrelevant information may be acceptable for general medical practice, this method is not the standard procedure for documentation of the medical history in cases of suspected child sexual abuse.

When a medical history is obtained, a clinician must take care to record verbatim the questions asked and the responses provided by the child or caregiver (or both). It is precisely the idiosyncratic statements of children that provide the greatest insight into what they may have experienced. Their responses to questions highlight an age-inappropriate understanding of sexual activities or knowledge of symptom-specific complaints temporally related to events; therefore, it is critically important that the medical record reflect the exact details of the history obtained. This can be accomplished by contemporaneously recording in writing the questions asked and the responses provided. It is helpful for children to understand that everything they have to say is important and therefore everything will be written down. Clinicians should indicate that the child may be asked to wait until everything said is written down before telling more of what happened.

Children respond best to and are most likely to provide the richest contextual details when asked questions that are developmentally appropriate and that follow a style that is not leading or suggestive. Clinicians should attempt to avoid questions that allow the child to respond with a short answer in preference to questions that encourage the child to provide a narrative response. A simple self-test is to review the history obtained by reading only the responses to the questions. If the narrative that emerges is understandable and cohesive, then a limited number of leading and suggestive questions were used. There is a clear continuum regarding leading, suggestive, and coercive questioning.[10] Open-ended questions that lack suggestibility tend to provide the clearest understanding of what a child may have experienced.

CHILDREN'S ADVOCACY CENTERS AND THE MULTIDISCIPLINARY APPROACH

Child advocacy centers throughout the United States were developed to coalesce limited resources into the co-location of investigative, child protection, medical, and mental health services, as well as to reduce the number of times a child may have to repeat the account of an experience. Reducing the number of "interviews" reduces the potential for inconsistency in historical details. In some communities and medical centers, the health care provider relies on the videotaped investigative interview conducted either by CPS or law enforcement agents (and sometimes both). The medical professional then has the opportunity to view the videotaped interview. With this approach, the health care provider who obtained background information from the videotaped interview asks limited questions of the child that address medically pertinent concerns. There are advantages to understanding a child's experience through the process of a physician-obtained, detailed medical history from the child. This may result in additional insights into the case. The physician's role is to diagnose any adverse effects of potential abusive sexual contact and to treat patients believed to have experienced such abuse. The physician is not an investigator, yet a thorough and skilled medical history and examination may have great investigatory value when viewed through the lenses of CPS and law enforcement.

THE MEDICAL RECORD

The medical record crystallizes the information-gathering process that leads to the formulation of a diagnosis. In allegations of child sexual abuse, it is best to envision a puzzle in which several disciplines can and will provide valuable information not readily accessible to the health care provider. In some cases, the medical piece of this puzzle may stand on its own; whereas in other cases, the collective observations and information-gathering provide an understanding of what a child may have experienced. The medical record not only serves as the vehicle for a diagnostic assessment for the clinician, but also as a tool to inform caseworkers, law enforcement, and the courts that will statutorily have access to the medical record. The medical record will most likely be reviewed in the context of case management discussions in a multidisciplinary team review.

ESTABLISHING THE DIAGNOSING AND TREATING PHYSICIAN RELATIONSHIP

When a child or adolescent is brought to a medical provider, it is because the child has independently recognized a need for health care, a guardian has recognized a need for medical attention, or either a CPS agent or law enforcement professional who understands the potential medical consequences of inappropriate sexual contact has referred the child to obtain medical care. It is therefore important to explain to the patient in a developmentally appropriate way that he or she is being seen for the purpose of diagnosis and treatment. Explanation of the purpose of the examination and documentation that the child understood that he or she is being seen for diagnosis and treatment will enhance the potential admissibility of the child's medical history under the exception to hearsay for purposes of medical diagnosis and treatment.[10] The admissibility of out-of-court statements is important because it will allow the clinician to fully explain the basis on which the diagnostic assessment was formulated. Many medical conditions are diagnosed without confirmatory laboratory tests or specific examination findings but rather a constellation of presenting history, symptoms, and signs.

The purpose of the examination can be explained in variety of ways depending on the child's age. The following serves as an example of how this issue can be explained to most children. The clinician might begin with an introductory comment such as:

You know that when you have gone to the doctor in the past and not felt well, the doctor asks you all kinds of questions, like 'Does your tummy hurt? Do you have a headache or have you had a fever?' The reason the doctor asks questions is simply to understand what may have been bothering you. Then the doctor can decide what parts of your body to take a look at. The doctor can also decide whether you will need any special tests or medicines to get you better. I will be asking you some questions about what happened. The questions I am going to ask are not to embarrass you or make you uncomfortable but simply to help me understand what happened. If I understand what happened, I can do a better job of taking care of you and deciding whether you need any special tests or medicines to get you better.

The clinician should allow the child to express any special concerns. Once it is clear that the child understands the purpose of taking the medical history, the clinician should ask the child, "Is it important to tell the doctor the truth?" The child will usually answer "yes." The response should be followed by asking the child to explain why it is important to tell the truth. The child might respond by saying, "That way the doctor can help me get better." A natural transitional question will be to inquire whether the child has any worries or concerns that he or she would like to share.

Children may appreciate the need to see a doctor if they have been injured but would not be expected to fully understand the potential consequences of sexual interactions. In addition, parents may not fully appreciate the potential consequences of the sexual interactions and should receive guidance that encourages seeking diagnostic and treatment services. It is incumbent on medical professionals to educate parents, colleagues in child protection, and mental health and law enforcement regarding the potential medical consequences of sexual abuse and the benefits of diagnostic and treatment services.

MEDICAL HISTORY DOCUMENTATION

The old maxim that "if it is not in the record, it wasn't done or considered" is as appropriately applied to the medical record as it is to any other type of documentation. In the assessment of children for possible maltreatment, the clinician cannot rely on an independent recollection of an interaction with a patient supported only by limited notations. The medical record must be an accurate reflection of the evaluation and stand on its own. A well-structured and comprehensive record is a testament to the thoroughness with which the clinician obtained the medical history, conducted the examination, and formulated a diagnosis.

Information regarding the presenting symptoms will be obtained from a variety of sources, each of which must be weighed for their relevance. When individuals other than the child provide information, it will generally be considered hearsay and therefore should not be used in the formulation of the clinical diagnosis. The clinician making the diagnosis will rely on the interpretation and integration of the following: the medical history, physical examination findings, and laboratory test results. When obtaining a medical history from the child and caregiver, all information is recorded verbatim. It is inadequate to simply provide a summary note because it fails to capture the nuances of the history. Documentation should reflect all introductory comments, along with the exact questions asked and the child's verbatim response. In part, the basis for the hearsay treatment exception is their presumption that when a patient goes to the doctor, he or she will tell the truth as it is in his best interest to do so. Logically, the patient tells the truth to the doctor so the doctor can make the diagnosis and get the patient better more quickly. Therefore, the treatment exception allows for admissibility of the child's description of symptoms, sensations, or pain associated with the presenting concern. The child's description of the cause of the injury or "illness" may also provide idiosyncratic details that would otherwise be difficult to explain in terms of the child's developmentally appropriate knowledge: for example, a symptom related to a specific event without experience of the event. If the child states that the injury or contact was at the hands of a particular individual, the clinician must explain why the identity of that individual would be important to the diagnosis at hand.[10]

Information provided by child protection, law enforcement, or a non-offending parent regarding the presenting concerns is important but should not be relied upon as the sole source of data when formulating a diagnosis. Background information from sources other than the child does not negate the need to speak to the child independently. Background information is often helpful in understanding the context in which a suspected event occurred.

In some communities, clinicians have been discouraged from obtaining a medical history from children about their suspected experiences. The basis for this practice is the presumption that the retelling will be traumatic to the child, and there is concern that there may be new information that might be discrepant with the initial disclosure. In regard to the first issue, children can find it therapeutic to retell the details to a medical professional who understands and can help them express their worries or concerns. As one child said to me, "I can tell you because you're a doctor."[14] In regard to the issue of potential discrepancies in details from subsequent histories, the clinician should not compromise his or her ability to conduct a complete and thorough assessment and thus should obtain a medical history from the child. If discrepancies arise, then there will be a need to address these. Many of the questions asked by the clinician for medical diagnostic purposes are not expected to have been addressed by nonmedical professionals, and the history obtained by the clinician has the potential to enhance the understanding of what a child might have experienced.

COMPONENTS OF THE MEDICAL HISTORY AND RECORD

The medical record in sexual abuse cases is not dissimilar to the traditional medical record. In most pediatric assessment settings, basic information regarding the child's medical history is appropriately obtained from a parent, usually the mother. The same is the case in suspected sexual abuse cases. The clinician may begin with a review of the child's medical history, including a detailed ROS. If the child is present in the room when the medical history is being reviewed, it is best not to discuss any of the details of the child's suspected experiences but to reassure the child that he or she will be spoken to independently and will have an opportunity to share any potential worries or concerns prior to the examination. Children can be asked to think about any worries or concerns they might have while Mom is being asked all these boring questions. After the medical history is obtained, the child should be asked to leave the room and the non-offending parent/caregiver should then share an understanding of the concerns as heard or observed, either first-hand or through a third party. The information obtained from the caregiver is important to frame the issue but generally should not be used in formulating a diagnosis because it will be considered hearsay. When hearsay is used in the formulation of a diagnosis, the use of such information should be qualified and appropriately noted. Whenever possible, information about the chief complaint or history of the possible contact should be obtained from the child alone, not from the caregiver.

The medical history should consist of the following components:

— Birth history

— Family history

— Social history

— Developmental history

— Hospitalizations/emergency department visits

— Past surgery

— Medications/allergies

— Review of body systems with particular attention to genitourinary (GU) and gastrointestinal (GI) symptoms

— History obtained from the caregiver regarding presenting concerns

— History obtained from the child

When the child's caregiver is unavailable to provide the medical history, the clinician should ask the referring agency to try to obtain medical records for review. The history obtained from the caregiver should be structured in a way to obtain the best possible chronology of events and observations. The clinician should ask questions that encourage the caregiver to provide contextual detail regarding observations and statements. For example, if the child made a statement to a caregiver in a manner that was spontaneous and idiosyncratic, it would be important to understand the circumstances under which the statement was made. The caregiver should be asked to provide as exact a recollection of the child's disclosure or observed behavior as possible and the reaction to the disclosure. Few caregivers anticipate that their child will disclose inappropriate sexual interactions, and thus few have developed a thoughtful response. Too frequently a caregiver may respond by being upset, showing disbelief, or questioning the child in a manner that might suggest to the child that he or she was responsible for what occurred. Depending upon the manner in which the caregiver responds, the child may be more or less likely to repeat the initial disclosure. The disclosure process is just that—a process over time in which children share increasingly greater details depending on their level of comfort and perceived consequence to them and the suspected perpetrator.

Review of Systems (ROS)

All body systems should be included in the medical history; however, the GU and GI review of systems will take on special importance. The GU and GI systems can provide information that may have special relevance to the issue of sexual contact. The importance of the ROS in part stems from the need to identify any current or preexisting medical conditions that should be considered when assessing GU or GI symptoms that may have an association with sexual contact. Routine medical practice requires consideration of a differential diagnosis whenever signs and symptoms that may have a variety of causes are present. If the child has had either GI or GU symptoms for reasons unrelated to the suspected sexual contact, preexisting knowledge of such symptoms will be used to determine the presence of the same symptoms when they result from sexual contact.

When children experience genital fondling, vulvar coitus, or coitus, they may be able to provide important historical details of postfondling dysuria or postvulvar coital dysuria that can confirm with medical certainty that they have experienced genital trauma.[15] Dysuria results from rubbing and resultant superficial trauma to the periurethral or vestibular structures (or both). The injuries incurred from fondling or vulvar coitus are generally superficial and heal very quickly without demonstrative residual.[16]

When the child's ROS reveals a history of urinary tract infections and the child has experienced dysuria associated with such, it should be anticipated that it may be suggested that knowledge of this symptom is the result of a prior infection and not abusive contact. The clinician can address these challenges by conducting a thorough ROS. When considering preexisting conditions, the clinician carefully evaluates the temporal relationship between a set of symptoms and the child's symptom(s) referable to the contact. Questions about the GU system should include a discussion of the following: history of urinary tract infections, vaginal discharges, vaginal odor, vaginal bleeding, diaper dermatitis, urinary incontinence, use of bubble baths, treatment for any sexually transmitted diseases, menstrual history, use of tampons, abortions, accidental genital injuries, vaginal foreign bodies, prior examinations of the genitalia for any reason other than routine health care, and self-exploratory activities/masturbation.

The GI ROS should include the following: the age of toilet training and whether there were any difficulties with such; use of rectal suppositories, enemas, or medications for stooling; history of constipation or painful bowel movements; frequency and character of stools; and history of recurrent vomiting, diarrhea, hematochezia, hemorrhoids, fecal incontinence, rectal itching, pinworms, and surgical procedures involving the GI tract.

Myers[10] has identified a number of issues that if addressed will result in a more thorough and defensible medical record. Key components of the medical record from a legal perspective are as follows:

— Document of the child's age at the time of the statement.

— Note the duration of elapsed time between the suspected abuse and the child's statement.

— Specify who was present when the child made the statement, where the statement was made, and to whom it was made.

— Document whether specific statements are made in response to questions or are spontaneous.

— Note whether the child's responses are made to leading or nonleading questions.

— Note whether the child's statement was made at the first opportunity that the child felt safe to talk.

— Document the emotional state of the child. Note if the child was excited or distressed at the time of the statement and, if so, what signs or symptoms of excitement or distress were observed.

— Document whether the child was calm, placid, or sleeping prior to making the statement or soon thereafter.

— Use the exact words that the child uses to describe the characteristics of the event.

— Document the child's physical condition at the time of the statement.

— Note any suspected incentives for the child to fabricate lies or to distort the truth.

Conducting the Physical Examination

The physical examination will differ slightly depending on the length of time between the last episode of suspected abuse and the time the child is brought in for evaluation. In cases in which the police or another agency requests the collection of forensic evidence, a standard protocol should be followed to collect samples for analysis, sometimes called the "rape kit." The acute sexual assault evaluation is described in detail in Chapter 11. For children who are examined outside the time frame of an acute evaluation, often defined as 72 hours since the episode of abuse, a complete physical examination is still needed, and the findings will be documented in much the same manner.[17] Chapter 5 reviews the approach to conducting the non-emergent medical evaluation.

The accurate interpretation of medical and laboratory findings in cases of suspected child sexual abuse requires that the medical provider be familiar with normal anatomy, congenital variations, findings caused by conditions other than abuse, and findings due to trauma.[18] Some infections, for example, can be transmitted by sexual contact but can also be transmitted by nonsexual contact. It is essential that the medical provider have access to the latest recommendations from organizations such as the American Academy of Pediatrics and the Centers for Disease Control and Prevention (CDC) when there is a suspicion or confirmed case of infection caused by a sexually transmissible organism.[19-23] Guidelines for the interpretation of medical and laboratory findings are discussed in detail in Chapter 8.

Purpose and Timing of the Medical Examination

Children who are suspected of having experienced age-inappropriate sexual activities are at risk for incurring both anogenital and extragenital trauma and sexually transmitted diseases. In addition, children and adolescents may express significant concerns about their sense of body intactness that can be addressed only in the context of a complete medical history and head-to-toe examination. The medical history and examination are essential components of the complete assessment of any child suspected of being sexually abused and are critical in addressing the health concerns of both the child and the caregiver. All children can benefit from a comprehensive medical evaluation, even when the last suspected contact may have been years earlier. For the physician, the question should not be if the child should have an examination but rather when. An appropriately conducted medical evaluation should have great therapeutic value to the child and non-offending parent and is one of the first steps in the process of healing following sexual abuse.

When children disclose abusive sexual contact, one of the very first questions by the physician should be, "When was the last time something happened?" The disclosure or suspicion of sexual abuse almost always precipitates a crisis and, for the parent, an emergent need to know, which frequently result in a call to the primary care doctor and possibly a trip to the emergency department. In many communities, the emergency department is the least optimal place to conduct a sexual abuse examination. Once a child arrives in an emergency department, the prudent action is first to determine when the last time something of a sexually inappropriate nature occurred; if more than 5 days subsequent, the examination should be deferred to colleagues in the community who are skilled in evaluating children who are suspected to have experienced sexual abuse. This would be no different than seeking a cardiologist for the assessment of a patient with arrhythmia or unknown origin, because that cardiologist is best equipped owing to special training and experience.

The evaluation of a child suspected of having been abused dictates the need for clinicians to work in a collaborative fashion with professionals from child protection, mental health, and law enforcement. In great part, this is the case because of statutorily mandated reporting of child abuse and the investigation that is required. Although the examination and the medical report may prove to have investigative value, the clinician must make it clear to child protection and law enforcement agents that the purpose of examining a child suspected of being abused is to diagnose and treat any residual to the suspected sexual contact, should there be such. The medical professional's primary concern is the patient's health and well-being, and thus all aspects of the examination are conducted in a manner that is therapeutic to the child. This includes anticipating and addressing anxieties and fears, providing reassurance, and treating acute injuries or sexually transmitted diseases.

The clinician's diagnosis and recommendations not only serve the needs of the child directly, but they also help nonmedical colleagues understand the child's specific treatment needs and facilitate the child receiving attention for such needs.

The examination is conceptualized as serving the purposes of diagnosing and treating both abnormality (residual to concerns) and confirming normality (wellness). Under this rubric, all children suspected of being abused deserve the benefit of an examination. For many children and parents, the issue of normality will be equal in importance to concerns about abnormality. Physicians treat patients either through the direct provision of medicine or the time-honored benefit of reassuring patients and addressing their rational and at times unrealistic concerns. After a thorough history is taken, the child's and the caregiver's concerns are heard, and an examination is conducted, the health benefit of reassurance by a clinician that a child's body is okay demonstrates both to the child and caregiver that their concerns were heard and addressed. When children and caregivers can be assured that there will be no long-term adverse health consequences of the abuse, the child and caregivers can focus on addressing the mental health issues that ultimately are the key to overcoming any abuse experience.

Preparing Caregiver and Child for the Physical Examination
In preparation for the examination, it is important to anticipate both the fears and anxieties of the child or adolescent and of the caregiver. In introductory comments to the caregiver, it is important to take the time to explain what the caregiver should anticipate during the evaluation. For example, the physician may say the following to the caregiver:

I am a kids' doctor, and one of the things I do that is different than most kids' doctors is every day I have the opportunity to examine children when there has been a concern that they may have experienced something inappropriate or seen something inappropriate or both. I understand those concerns have been raised with your child. Let me tell you what we hope to accomplish today. I will review with you your child's medical history and ask you to tell me the concerns that bring you here in a chronological manner and any of your worries, concerns, or observations. I will then speak to your child alone, and when I am done speaking with your child, you will come back into the room and have your child change into a gown for a head-to-toe examination with you present throughout.

For a prepubertal female child, the physician may add:

I don't anticipate doing anything that is physically uncomfortable to your daughter. Because of your daughter's age, she won't experience an adult gynecologic examination as you think of it. There won't be the use of an instrument or speculum.

For male patients, the physician may explain that the use of an anoscope will only occur if necessary. The physician may sum up by saying:

If appropriate, cultures from the rectum and mouth using a small cotton swab to test for sexually transmitted infections will be obtained. Following the examination, I will meet with you again and provide my opinion, answer any questions, and discuss the next steps necessary to assess the mental health impact of what your child experienced and how to obtain appropriate mental health services.

In a developmentally appropriate way, it is equally important to anticipate and address the fears and anxieties that the child or adolescent might have prior to proceeding with the examination. Young children may be concerned that they are going to get a vaccination and are relieved when they find out that is not the case. Whenever possible, explain to the child what will be happening next in the examination. If the child desires, encourage the child to touch instruments; this tangible step helps to demystify the examination and provides an opportunity for the child to have a sense of participation and control throughout the examination. Video colposcopy is an excellent tool that allows the child to watch the anogenital examination if desired. With young children, ask if they would like to see their belly button or finger on the television first. This serves as a way of demonstrating that there is nothing invasive about the scope. Maintain an active dialogue with the child throughout the examination, and proceed at a pace that is comfortable for the child.

The physical examination begins with a general assessment of the child's health, including vital signs and appropriate measurements. The examination will generally proceed in a head-to-toe fashion, and the record should note findings relevant to the concerns at hand as well as any medical conditions that need attention. Children should not have just an anogenital examination without attention to their general well-being. Children who have experienced sexual abuse may also have suffered physical abuse and neglect and have findings on examination that may need to be addressed in concert with the disclosure of sexual abuse. See Chapter 5 (non-emergent assault) and Chapter 11 (acute assault) on how to conduct the physical examination.

Recording the Physical Examination and Findings

In a review of the documentation of an examination conducted on a child believed to have been sexually abused, the manner in which the record is structured and the details provided should reflect that a complete and thorough assessment was conducted. Introductory statements show the purpose of the examination and present background information regarding how the child appeared at the time of the examination. The record should include the overall medical condition of the child, the general physical examination findings, and a detailed description of the appearance of all genital and anal structures and any relevant extragenital findings. A detailed report demonstrates that the examiner understands the importance of being thorough and has reflected such in recording the examination findings in a precise manner. Any physical findings interpreted to be either diagnostic or supportive of the diagnosis should have visual documentation to augment the written record. Photographic and video documentation will help eliminate the opportunity for an adversary to request that a child undergo a repeat examination if a second opinion is sought. I believe that all examinations should include objective documentation of the genital and anal structures whether diagnostic findings are present or not. The justification for such a rigorous examination is that children remain at risk for something of an inappropriate nature to occur in the future. Thus, the baseline documentation of an initial examination may prove to be a useful reference should there be a concern in the future. Baseline documentation can be of particular value in those circumstances in which a child is seen in the context of a custody dispute or the allegations are unsubstantiated but are of concern. Photographic, colposcopic, and videocolposcopic methods of documentation have become routine, and they are the standard of care in the evaluation of suspected sexual abuse.[11]

Because the physical examination will infrequently demonstrate diagnostic residual, it is important to formulate an opinion that explains the absence of findings.[24] Although it is "normal to be normal" as evidenced by the absence of physical findings, in most cases, there are ways that this finding can be explained in a manner that informs the reader.[25,26] Rather than using truncated summary words or phrases such as "normal" examination, "no physical evidence of sexual abuse," "the examination neither confirms nor denies the history provided," or "consistent with the history of sexual abuse," the clinician should provide a clear description of the examination findings and explain the reasons for the absence of acute or chronic residual when historical details support the concern that the child experienced something of a sexually inappropriate nature. The diagnostic assessment should integrate the physical examination findings, laboratory results, and medical history in a manner that is clear and descriptive.

Reliance on a preformed check-off list that designates findings as either normal or abnormal without an opportunity to write a narrative should be avoided. The following example, which is only an excerpt of a report, illustrates an alternative way of describing the genital and anal examination findings.

Description of the Anogenital Examination Component of a Consultative Report When Diagnostic Findings Are Not Present

The child was examined in both the supine frog-leg and knee-chest position by using labial separation and traction. The examination was enhanced with the use of videocolposcopy at 4, 6, 10, and 16 magnifications with white and red-free light, and it was also recorded. The child is Tanner stage 1 for both breast and pubic hair development and Huffman stage 1 for estrogen effect of the external genitalia. The clitoral hood, labia majora, and labia minora are well formed without acute or chronic signs of trauma. Through use of labial separation and traction, the structures of the vaginal vestibule were visualized. There was no abnormal degree of redness, vaginal discharge, or malodor. There was some redundancy to the tissue surrounding the urethral meatus. The hymenal membrane orifice had a crescentic configuration with an uninterrupted velamentous border along its edge from 2 to 10 o'clock with the child supine.

The external surface of the hymenal membrane, inner aspects of the labia minora, fossa navicularis, and posterior fourchette did not demonstrate any acute or chronic signs of injury. There was a fine, lacy vascular pattern to the vestibular mucosa. The appearance of the hymenal membrane orifice was unchanged in the knee-chest position. There were no signs of sexually transmitted infections. The external anal verge tissues and perineum were examined in the supine knee-chest position with the legs flexed onto the abdomen. There was a symmetric rugal pattern, normal sphincter tone, and a constrictive response to separation of the buttocks. Slight venous pooling was evident during the later part of the examination and disappeared with anal constriction. There were no acute or chronic signs of trauma to the external anal verge tissues, the distal portion of the anal rectal canal, or the perineum.

INTEGRATION OF PHYSICAL EXAMINATION FINDINGS AND MEDICAL HISTORY: FORMULATING A DIAGNOSIS

The medical record is the sum and substance of the medical evaluation. The diagnosis must be formulated in a manner that is clear and defensible. The clinician must consider and incorporate salient aspects of each of the following when formulating a diagnosis:

— Historical details and behavioral indicators reflective of the contact

— Symptoms that can be directly associated with the contact

— Acute and healed genital/anal injuries

— Extragenital trauma

— Forensic evidence

— Sexually transmitted diseases

An important purpose of the medical record is to educate all who review issues with respect to the following: (1) why there may be discrepancies between a child's perception of their experience and what actually happened, (2) why children who provide clear histories of pain and/or bleeding as a result of the contact may not have diagnostic physical findings, and (3) which types of symptoms secondary to trauma might be anticipated when a child experiences genital fondling, genital-to-genital contact, or anal trauma. Throughout the diagnostic and treatment process and report writing, the clinician must be objective, know the limitations of clinical observations, incorporate differential considerations, and formulate a diagnosis in a manner that is unbiased.

The following examples reflect common clinical scenarios, each of which will require the formulation of very different diagnostic assessments:

— Inappropriate sexual contact by history and/or behaviors is described; however, there are no diagnostic physical findings on examination.

— Diagnostic findings are present that are reflective of inappropriate contact (ie, trauma, sexually transmitted diseases, and/or seminal products) and are supported by descriptive history/behavior.

— Diagnostic findings are present that are reflective of inappropriate contact (ie, trauma, sexually transmitted diseases, and/or seminal products) without descriptive history/behavior.

— Inappropriate sexual contact that can be confirmed with medical certainty without healed residual symptoms.

— Insufficient historical or behavioral details to support a concern of inappropriate sexual contact, and the physical examination is nondiagnostic.

Although the constellation of historical, behavioral, and examination findings will vary from patient to patient, the following serve as examples of how one component of the diagnostic assessment could be formulated in each of the following common scenarios:

1. Inappropriate sexual contact by history/behavior is described; however, there are no diagnostic physical findings on examination.

Case Scenario

The medical history presented by an 8-year-old girl reflects progression of a variety of inappropriate sexual activities over time initially represented to her in a caring and loving context. Although the initial interactions were described as playful, the activities progressed with correspondingly escalating threats to maintain secrecy. The young girl did not report experiencing any physical discomfort following the genital fondling or the stroking of her uncle's genitalia. During the medical history, she asked what that icky stuff was that came out of his "pee pee" and explained that she had to wipe it from her "peach" by using a tissue. In addition, she said that she was worried that people could tell just by the way that they looked at her that she had to do those disgusting things. In light of the history regarding contact with genital secretions, she is at risk for contracting a sexually transmitted disease. I have evaluated this girl for sexually transmitted diseases. Treatment and follow-up will be initiated should any of the test results be positive. Her physical examination does not demonstrate any acute or chronic symptoms residual to the sexual contact, nor would they be anticipated in light of her denial of discomfort associated with the contact. Her body image concern is common among children who experience sexual abuse. I do not believe there is any alternative explanation for this child's history of progressive engagement in sexual activities, threats to maintain secrecy, detailed description of a variety of sexually explicit interactions, and concerns about body image other than from experiencing sexual abuse. The most significant impact of her inappropriate sexual experiences is psychological. She needs to be evaluated by a clinical child psychologist to assess the impact of her inappropriate experiences, develop a therapeutic plan, and provide anticipatory guidance regarding body safety.

2. Diagnostic findings are present that are reflective of inappropriate contact (ie, trauma, sexually transmitted diseases, and/or seminal products) and supported by descriptive history/behavior.

Case Scenario

A 7-year-old girl provided a clear and detailed medical history reflecting her genital-to-genital contact with her father and coercion into placing her mouth onto her father's genitalia. She perceived the genital-to-genital contact to involve penetration into her vagina. She reported a history of bleeding and pain following the genital-to-genital contact. Although her disclosure occurred 1 month following the last stated contact, her physical examination demonstrated diagnostic residual to this contact. On physical examination, a well-defined healed transection of the posterior portion of her hymen is found that extends to the base of its attachment on the posterior vaginal wall. This finding is diagnostic of blunt-force penetrating trauma and reflects the introduction of a foreign body through the structures of the vaginal vestibule, the hymenal orifice, and into the vagina. She did not report physical discomfort associated with the history of oral-genital contact, although she stated that white stuff from her father's penis got into her mouth. Her contact with ejaculate places her at risk for a sexually transmitted disease. She has been evaluated for sexually transmitted diseases. Should any of the tests be positive, treatment and follow-up will be initiated.

3. Diagnostic findings are present that are reflective of inappropriate contact (ie, trauma, sexually transmitted diseases, and/or seminal products) without descriptive history/behavior.

Case Scenario

A 10-year-old girl was unable to provide adequate details through a history to fully understand the scope of sexually inappropriate activities for which there has been a concern. Although seminal products were found on her underwear, none were found on examination nor would be anticipated because the last suspected contact was 2 weeks earlier. This child's disclosure to her best friend regarding sexual interactions with a family "uncle" resulted in an investigation and the request for an examination to diagnose and treat any symptoms residual to the suspected sexual abuse. During attempts to obtain the medical history, this girl appeared very withdrawn and would not make eye contact or engage in meaningful conversation. Throughout the examination she appeared as if she were dissociating herself from the examination process.

Her genital examination did not demonstrate any acute or chronic signs of trauma or signs of sexually transmitted diseases. The anal-rectal examination demonstrated a well-defined linear scar at 5 o'clock in the knee-chest position. With anoscopy, the scar was observed to extend from the external anal verge tissues across the anoderm and to the pectinate line. The appearance of the scar was enhanced with the use of a red-free filter and recorded on 35 mm film and through video colposcopy.

Although this young girl appeared emotionally unavailable to provide historical details regarding inappropriate sexual activities, the recovery of seminal products in her underwear and the presence of a healed laceration of the anal tissues confirms with medical certainty that she experienced blunt-force penetrating trauma. This girl would benefit from being seen by a child psychiatrist who could assess the emotional impact of her experience, provide appropriate medication, and develop a treatment plan.

4. Inappropriate sexual contact that can be confirmed with medical certainty without healed residual symptoms.

Case Scenario

A 9-year-old girl provided a detailed history of a variety of sexually inappropriate interactions with her stepfather spanning a 6-month time frame. The initial activities were represented to her as a special game in a loving context. The most recent event 10 days prior to the disclosure involved her stepfather placing his "stuff" into her "coochie." Using an anatomically detailed model, the child clarified to me that "stuff" referred to a penis and "coochie" referred to the vagina. When asked to explain what she meant by inside with the use of an anatomic model of the female genitalia, she demonstrated that she thought his "stuff" was placed inside in the adult sense of penetration. On physical examination, no acute or chronic signs of trauma or sexually transmitted diseases were found. The edge of the hymenal membrane was without interruption. The orifice diameter was 5 mm with traction and insufficient to have allowed introduction of a foreign body such as a penis into the vagina. Although this young girl perceived the genital-to-genital contact to involve penetration into the vagina, penetration was limited to the structures of the vaginal vestibule.

When asked how the genital-to-genital touching felt, she said that it hurt when he rubbed his "stuff" on her "coochie." When asked in what way it hurt, she stated that it hurt her after her stepfather stopped touching her when she went to the bathroom afterwards to "go pee." When asked to describe the discomfort she had when she went to pee, she stated that it stung. When asked if she had ever felt anything like that before, she said "no." When asked if she ever saw anything to make her know she was hurt, she responded "no." When asked how long the discomfort with peeing lasted, she said "just that day." A review of systems was negative for any alternative medical history explanation for knowledge of the symptom of dysuria. The symptom of dysuria temporally related to the genital-to-genital contact reflects trauma to the periurethral area as a result of rubbing. The only way this young girl could know about the symptom of dysuria temporally related to the genital-to-genital contact is by experiencing this condition. The trauma she incurred to the periurethral area and/or vestibular mucosa was superficial and has since healed without residual symptoms, as anticipated. The extent of genital-to-genital contact was limited to penetration within the structures of the vaginal vestibule.

5. Insufficient historical or behavioral details to support a concern of inappropriate sexual contact, and the physical examination is nondiagnostic.

Case Scenario

A 2-year-old boy was examined to address the concern that he may have been touched in a sexually inappropriate manner. This concern arose because of a diaper rash, intermittent self-stimulatory behaviors, and some resistance to having his diaper changed. His mother raised the question whether her son may have been touched in a sexually inappropriate manner to account for the genital irritation, increased genital touching, and resistance to having his diaper changed. His mother stated that she had been sexually abused by her father as a child and wanted to protect her son from the same. The maternal grandparents occasionally babysit her son. His physical examination is positive for diaper dermatitis due to Candida albicans, and he has secondary impetiginous lesions. The historical and behavioral details that have been provided are insufficient to confirm with medical certainty that this boy has experienced anything of a sexually inappropriate manner. The constellation of behavioral changes can be attributed to his diaper dermatitis and are not the result of any sexually inappropriate contact. This child, and all children, should receive anticipatory guidance regarding body safety in a developmentally appropriate manner. I have obtained baseline documentation of the appearance of his anogenital anatomy that will serve as a reference should there be any concerns in the future. The present concerns afford an opportunity for this child's mother to address any unresolved issues concerning her own experience and exercise caution in leaving her child in the care of any individual with whom she has concern.

Less frequent clinical presentation scenarios may include the following:

— Identification of a healed injury on examination with no prior suspicion of abuse in the absence of historical or behavioral indicators.

— A child who is evaluated with a concern without clear historical or behavioral details to support the concern, which may be a reflection of hypervigilance due to a caregiver's personal experience.

— A sexually transmitted disease is diagnosed in a young child for whom no explanation for how the child contracted the disease is available following a complete investigation.

— Fabricated or misinterpreted behaviors and/or history alleging sexual abuse generally in young children. This form of presentation may be seen in adversarial caregiver relationships such as custody disputes.

— Fabrication of lies or distortion of historical details by adolescents.

The diagnostic assessments presented as case examples in this chapter represent a few ways in which the clinician can articulate findings and interpret them for those who will need to reference the consultative report. A clear and detailed medical record will reduce the likelihood that the clinician will need to appear in court to explain the record. The medical report should make appropriate recommendations for any follow-up medical care and mental health services.

CONCLUSION

When children are believed to have experienced sexually inappropriate activities, the health care provider plays a very important role in that child's care. The health care provider's primary focus is the diagnosis and treatment of symptoms residual to suspected sexual abuse. As discussed earlier, the examination is both for the detection and treatment of "abnormality" with regard to symptoms and the determination of "normality." It should be conducted for both purposes.[27]

The clinician has a responsibility to gather the information necessary to formulate a diagnosis in an objective manner. The responsibility also extends to the formulation of a clear, descriptive report that states the basis upon which the clinical diagnosis was made and can be supported. The manner in which the consultative report is constructed and supported by appropriate documentation speaks to the level of skill of the clinician. The clinician's assessment should be informative for colleagues in child protection and law enforcement who must interpret the medical evaluation and consider the information within the context of a multidisciplinary perspective.

A clearly written and defensible report will serve clinicians well in any legal proceedings for which they may be required to testify. Detailed consultative reports can reduce the chance of court appearances because the record can stand on its own.

Substantiation of sexual abuse is within the purview of child protection. The medical component remains an important and frequently ordinal piece when attempting to understand what a child might have experienced. A mental health clinician's assessment can provide additional insights into understanding a child's experience, particularly when interpreting the limited statements and behaviors of young children or when custody matters appear to be prominent components of the presenting concern.[28-31]

The final decision regarding the outcome of a case ultimately rests on the integration of medicine, mental health, child protection, law enforcement, and the courts. From a clinician's perspective, the gold standard for the best outcome for the patient focuses on meeting the medical, mental health, and protection needs of the child and family.

REFERENCES

1. Finkelhor D. Sex among siblings: a survey on prevalence, variety, and effects. *Arch Sex Behav*. 1980;9:171-194.

2. Finkelhor D. Boys as victims: review of the evidence. In: Finkelhor D. *Child sexual abuse: new theory and research*. New York: Free Press; 1984:150-170.

3. Finkelhor D, Hotaling G, Lewis IA, Smith C. Sexual abuse in a national survey of adult men and women: prevalence, characteristics, and risk factors. *Child Abuse Negl*. 1990;14:19-28.

4. Finkelhor D, Dziuba-Leatherman J. Children as victims of violence: a national survey. *Pediatrics*. 1994;94(4 pt 1):413-420.

5. Finkelhor D, Browne A. The traumatic impact of child sexual abuse: a conceptualization. *Am J Orthopsychiatry*. 1985;55:530-541.

6. Finkelhor D. The victimization of children: a developmental perspective. *Am J Orthopsychiatry*. 1995;65:177-193.

7. Sgroi SM. *Handbook of Clinical Intervention in Child Sexual Abuse*. Lexington, MA: D.C. Heath and Co; 1982.

8. Summit RC. The child sexual abuse accommodation syndrome. *Child Abuse Negl.* 1983;7:177-193.

9. Myers JE. Role of physician in preserving verbal evidence of child abuse. *J Pediatr.* 1986;109:409-411.

10. Myers JEB. Investigative interviewing regarding child maltreatment. In: Myers JEB. *Legal issues in child abuse and neglect practice.* 2nd ed. Thousands Oaks, CA: Sage; 1998:102-152.

11. Finkel MA, Ricci LR. Documentation and preservation of visual evidence in child abuse. *Child Maltreat.* 1997;2:322-330.

12. Boyce MC, Melhorn KJ, Vargo G. Pediatric trauma documentation. Adequacy for assessment of child abuse. *Arch Pediatr Adolesc Med.* 1996;150:730-732.

13. Parra JM, Huston RL, Foulds DM. Resident documentation of diagnostic impression in child sexual abuse evaluations. *Clin Pediatr (Phila).* 1997;36:691-694.

14. Finkel, MA. "I can tell you because you're a doctor"; Commentary on girls who disclose sexual abuse: signs and symptoms following genital contact. The importance of the pediatricians detailed medical history when evaluating suspected child sexual abuse. *Pediatrics.* 2008;122(8):422.

15. DeLago C, Deblinger ED, Schroeder, et al. Girls who disclose sexual abuse: urogenital symptoms and signs following sexual contact. *Pediatrics.* 2008;122(8): e221-226

16. Finkel MA. Anogenital trauma in sexually abused children. *Pediatrics.* 1989; 84:317-322.

17. Christian CW, Lavelle JM, De Jong AR, Loiselle J, Brenner L, Joffe M. Forensic evidence findings in prepubertal victims of sexual assault. *Pediatrics.* 2000;106(1 Pt 1):100-104.

18. Adams JA, Kaplan RA, Starling SP, et al. Guidelines for medical care of children who may have been sexually abused. *J Pediatr Adolesc Gynecol.* 2007;20(3): 163-172.

19. Centers for Disease Control. *Sexually transmitted diseases: treatment guidelines 2006. Sexual assault or abuse of children.* Centers for Disease Control and Prevention Web site. http://www.cdc.gov/std/treatment/2006/sexual-assault.htm#children. Updated April 13, 2007. Accessed October 28, 2008.

20. Kellogg N; American Academy of Pediatrics Committee on Child Abuse and Neglect. The evaluation of sexual abuse in children. *Pediatrics.* 2005;116:506-512.

21. Siegel RM, Schubert CJ, Myers PA, Shapiro RA. The prevalence of sexually transmitted diseases in children and adolescents evaluated for sexual abuse in Cincinnati: rationale for limited STD testing in prepubertal girls. *Pediatrics.* 1995;96:1090-1094.

22. US Department of Justice. *A National Protocol for Sexual Assault Medical Forensic Examination: Adults/Adolescents: President's DNA Initiative.* Washington, DC: Office on Violence Against Women; 2004. Report NCJ 206554.

23. Giardet RG, Lahoti S, Howard LA et al. Epidemiology of sexually transmitted infections in suspected child victims of sexual assault. *Pediatrics.* 2009;124(1):79-86.

24. Heger A, Ticson L, Velasquez O, Bernier R. Children referred for possible sexual abuse: medical findings in 2384 children. *Child Abuse Negl.* 2002;26:645-659.

25. Adams JA, Harper K, Knudson S, Revilla J. Examination findings in legally confirmed child sexual abuse: it's normal to be normal. *Pediatrics.* 1994;94:310-317.

26. Kellogg ND, Menard SW, Santos A. Genital anatomy in pregnant adolescents: "normal" does not mean "nothing happened." *Pediatrics.* 2004;113(1 Pt 1):e67-e69.

27. Finkel MA, Giardino AP. *Medical evaluation of child sexual abuse: a practical guide.* 3rd ed. American Academy of Pediatrics; Chicago, IL: 2009.

28. Friedrich WN, Beilke RL, Urquiza AJ. Behavior problems in young sexually abused boys: a comparison study. *J Interpers Violence.* 1988;3:21-28.

29. Friedrich WN, Grambsch P, Broughton D, Kuiper J, Beilke RL. Normative sexual behavior in children. *Pediatrics.* 1991;88:456-464.

30. Friedrich WN. Sexual victimization and sexual behavior in children: a review of recent literature. *Child Abuse Neglect.* 1993;17:59-66.

31. Friedrich WN, Jaworski TM, Huxsahl JE, Bengston BS. Assessment of dissociative and sexual behaviors in children and adolescents with sexual abuse. *J Interpers Violence.* 1997;12:155-171.

Chapter 4

THE SEXUAL ABUSE POSTEXAMINATION CONFERENCE WITH FAMILIES

Jerry G. Jones, MD
Karen J. Farst, MD, MPH

The medical presentation and examination of child victims of sexual abuse and assault are described in Chapters 3 and 5. In the traditional model of management of medical disorders, the examination is followed by a discussion of findings, the significance of the findings, and any necessary subsequent care. However, that model is no longer adequate for the medical care of sexually abused children and their families. It does not meet their complex needs. As more becomes known about those needs, the role of the examiner is expanding into an extended postexamination conference.[1]

The characteristics of these conferences that take place after the medical evaluation for suspected sexual abuse vary and are driven by the age of the children, the perpetrators' relationships and means of engagement of the children, and the duration of contact. Throughout this chapter, *parent(s)* refers to the nonoffending custodial conference participants. The conference procedures are not different for other guardians as long as they have a legal right to the information.

CONFERENCE GOALS

The goals of the sexual abuse postexamination conference are medical, social, and mental health for the entire family. They are seldom evidentiary. Because most examination findings are normal, parents usually can be reassured their children have no injuries or physical evidence of infection; they can focus on safety and psychological needs. Parents should also understand the importance of meeting their own emotional needs, as each person in the family is a victim. They should understand the community system for investigation and management, how to access it, and what to expect from it. If possible, they should be empowered to become aggressive case managers for their children. The ultimate goal is to help children and their families become problem-solving, coping entities rather than patients.[2]

CONFERENCE PARTICIPANTS

The child sexual abuse examiner is always a participant in these conferences. Beyond the explanation of the medical findings, the examiner should be prepared to address some of the surrounding psychosocial issues of the child and parents. Differing levels of support personnel may be available to participate with the medical provider, depending on the size and resources of the medical facility. Social workers, nurses, family advocates, child protective services workers, law enforcement investigators, and mental health and other professionals may contribute in their areas of expertise. The examiner may not need to be present during the entire postexamination conference if other participants are available. If others are not available, however, the examiner should be prepared to attend the conference, still functioning within a team structure that includes other professionals readily available for assistance when needed.[3]

Ideally, both parents are present, although fathers are commonly absent despite staff encouragement to attend. Child victims old enough to receive information may also participate. Younger children may be involved only for reassurance of overall good health, because the sexual abuse examination is conducted in the context of a general examination. Parents should have time without their children present so they can discuss adult concerns or issues that may cause distress to the child if present. Older children deserve a conference without their parents to allow for a more open exchange of information.

CONFERENCE PROCEDURES

The postexamination conference should be held in an attractive room large enough to accommodate the participants comfortably without being intimidating in size. It should never be held in an examination or waiting room. Appropriate informational booklets for child and adult victims, printed material regarding referral resources, and paper for providing written instructions should be available. All participants should be present and introduced at the beginning of the conference.

The components of the postexamination conference are summarized in **Table 4-1**. The conference can be divided into 2 fields of health care: medical and psychosocial. The order of their discussion is dictated by the parents' perceived reason for presentation and the professional with whom they have had the most contact. If the parents brought their child for a medical evaluation, the examiner should generally proceed first to meet their medical expectations. The transition from one component of the conference to the next should be stated clearly. The parents should be told the reasons for discussion of concerns that the parents did not vocalize, such as a wish to be certain a child will grow up to be emotionally healthy.

Table 4-1. Outline of the Postsexual Abuse Examination Conference	
STEP	DESCRIPTION
Introduction	— Provide an appropriate room — Have all participants present and introduced at onset
Medical Component	— Describe and explain all findings — Provide the forensic and/or health significance of the absence or presence of findings of sexual abuse — Validate the child's feelings regarding the examination — Provide information that will enhance the child's body image and alleviate medical fears — Make follow-up recommendations
Psychosocial Assessment and Referrals	— Identify and alleviate sources of confusion, stress, fear, guilt, and shame — Identify children who need referral for counseling, possibly utilizing a child's symptom report tool

(continued)

Table 4-1. *(continued)*	
STEP	DESCRIPTION
Psychosocial Assessment and Referrals *(continued)*	— Identify parents' needs for counseling for stress, unresolved personal abuse issues, intimate partner violence, and substance abuse, possibly utilizing a parent's symptom report tool — Make reassessment and referral recommendations
Closure	— Summarize findings and reinforce recommendations — Provide written recommendations and resource material

MEDICAL ASPECTS

The examiner should explain the physical findings and their significance in lay terms. It is generally appropriate to assume the parents have little knowledge of genital anatomy. Parental understanding of the medical information is essential, whether or not findings of sexual abuse are present. Many patients and parents enter the medical evaluation with the belief that the examiner will be able to determine the presence, type, and severity of abuse that has (or has not) occurred. The examiner must be able to communicate the results and limitations of the examination findings with rationale clearly to lay people.

The reasons and research supporting an absence of physical findings indicative of abuse are covered in other chapters of this text. Some parents may use a lack of physical findings to decide the validity of their child's allegation of abuse. A parent's negative reaction to a child's disclosure may be heightened with the information that physical proof of the abuse is absent. The child who has made a credible disclosure that is not believed by the parent is at risk for reexposure to the abuser, lack of support in working through the victimization, and failure to receive counseling. Emotional support from a significant figure in a child's life is an important factor in development of resilience in the aftermath of sexual abuse.[4] A careful explanation of the implications of normal examination findings may prevent some of these safety and psychological risks.

The significance of abnormal findings should be explained. Parents need to understand that examinations are performed for both health and forensic purposes. Healed genital and anal injuries with forensic significance seldom have health significance. An explanation of the genital anatomy may help parents understand the location of an injury and the reasons for normal findings upon examination of a young child said to have been penetrated genitally. The analogy of a teacup can be useful. The rim and bowl of the cup are analogous to the separated labia and vestibule, while the hymen is at the bottom of the vestibule/cup. Just as penetration of the bowl may not reach the bottom of the cup, penetration of the vestibule may not include penetration of the hymen.

Parents should be encouraged to ask questions about the medical evaluation. Verification of the history of sexual abuse may occur at this time or before the examination, depending on the clarity and accuracy of the information initially available to the examiner. The child should not be reinterviewed unless that is part of an established community protocol. Because the examiner is providing a medical evaluation rather than a focused forensic examination, a complete past and family history and system review should be performed.[5] The examiner may uncover unmet health needs, past placement in foster care, physical or sexual abuse, or neglect.

Children's roles in accomplishment of their examinations should be praised vigorously and perhaps reinforced by asking them to provide a rating of the experience. A *terrible, bad, not so bad* scale can be used. Several standard measures have been suggested.[6] This expression of a child's feelings about the examination validates the child and gives some sense of control. Children's responses to appropriately performed examinations are usually positive, providing relief to parents. Children should be firmly reassured their examination findings are normal when that is true; no one, not even a physician, can tell that the sexual abuse occurred. Shame and poor body self-esteem can be harmful sequelae in the child who has been sexually abused.[7-9] For many children reassurance by a doctor or nurse that their body is normal and not damaged is the first step toward healing from the emotional trauma of the abuse.

When developmentally appropriate, postexamination explanations to children alone regarding the health of their bodies may answer questions that are too difficult for them to ask the examiner in the presence of their parents. Many children have fears about their bodies that may or may not be rational, such as irreparable damage, pregnancy, future inability to have children, and sexually transmitted infections. These fears may be elicited during the conference alone with the child and should be addressed. Information provided to children should be provided to the parents as well, so they can reinforce the information in the recovery process.

PSYCHOSOCIAL ASPECTS AND CRISIS INTERVENTION

The children and family victims of sexual abuse are almost always in crisis. The onset of the crisis for the child may be when the sexual event occurred or began, and it may be intensified or diminished after disclosure. For the family, the crisis begins when the sexual abuse is disclosed. Although the crisis event and disclosure are commonly of a circumscribed duration, the responses of the child, family members, and community agencies are not. When the coping mechanisms of the family members are overwhelmed, the effects of the crisis can last for weeks or years.[2]

Child sexual abuse examiners must have knowledge of common psychosocial factors and be prepared to offer guidance and referral; however, the psychosocial component does not involve psychotherapy. Crisis intervention in a single visit cannot substitute for the multiple visits commonly required for such treatment. It can be considered "psychological first aid."[3] Although medical professionals may perceive this aspect of the conference to be the responsibility of mental health or social work professionals, families in crisis look to medical providers for leadership. Sometimes the examiner may be the only child abuse professional available for the conference.

Crisis intervention historically has been designed to accomplish a single goal—the facilitation of recovery of relatively normal people following a single traumatic event. Similarly, a one-time postsexual abuse examination conference must have very limited psychosocial goals to be effective. The family in crisis should not be overwhelmed with information. Generally, 2 goals are sufficient. A goal for the parents and older children is to *identify and alleviate sources of confusion, concerns, and stress.* A goal for all is to identify those children and parents who require referral to mental health services.

Some family concerns are commonly expressed and the examiner must be prepared to address them. Usual questions and potential responses, to be adapted to the context and psychological status of the parents, are as follows.

The Disclosure and Its Reliability

Four frequently asked questions relate to the disclosure and its reliability:

1. Why did I not realize the sexual abuse was occurring?

2. Why did it take so long for my child to tell anyone?

3. Why did my child tell someone else and not me?

4. My daughter loves and misses her father and he loves her; doesn't that indicate that he could not have sexually abused her?

The answers to these questions are based on the dynamics of child sexual abuse. Parents may not realize that sexual abuse is occurring because it is secretly performed by people the parents and children trust. Children commonly do not disclose early because they fear retribution or anger directed at them or harm to someone else.[10] According to one report, fewer than half of sexual abuse victims told anyone at the time of the abuse.[11] The same fears may cause children to tell someone other than their parents. Children who provide a reliable disclosure of sexual abuse may still love and miss the perpetrator; they simply want the sexual abuse to stop.

The answers to these questions may provide clues that a parent does not believe a child's credible disclosure, and they warrant exploration with the parent. A parent's denial of the validity of a credible disclosure may be based on general distrust of the child's truthfulness, allegiance to the alleged perpetrator, or fear of consequences. The provider should attempt to ascertain whether the caregiver will protect the child from the alleged perpetrator during the investigation. If it appears likely the child will not be protected, the appropriate child protection agency should be contacted for a safety disposition. Beyond the immediate safety of the child, parental denial of the sexual abuse and anger at the child for having disclosed the abuse can have significant negative effects on the child's well-being, including an increased risk of suicide.[12,13] Mothers who are unsupportive of a child's disclosure of abuse have been found to have more problems with substance abuse, criminal behaviors, and problematic relationships with their male partners when compared to supportive parents.[14]

Conflict with Relatives

Questions regarding conflict with relatives are common:

— My parents say I should not have reported the sexual abuse by my brother, and they are attempting to get my daughter to change her disclosure. What should I do?

— Does this mean my child cannot visit her grandparents?

Parents should be praised for supporting their child in the face of pressure from family members. Children should never be subjected to adults who try to change their disclosure, and any exposure to them should be with strict supervision. Parents frequently become estranged from relatives who choose to believe the denial of an offender over the disclosure of a child, resulting in loss of family support for one of the parents. The parent who loses family support often requires counseling to deal with this loss as well as the sexual abuse of the child.

Safety of the Child

The following 3 questions relate to the safety of the child or family:

1. What can I do about court-ordered visitation with the alleged perpetrator this weekend?

2. He has a history of violence. How can I protect myself and my child?

3. The offender is my teenaged son. He has nowhere to live but in our home. How can I protect my daughter?

Protection of the child and family must be a priority. Visitation with an alleged perpetrator should cease until an investigation has been completed. However, the parent could become in violation of a court order if a visitation is denied. In many states, an order of protection is easily obtained and will prevent a parent from being held in contempt. A parent should also consult the child protective services investigator, who may be able to obtain the alleged perpetrator's agreement to forgo court-ordered visitation until an investigation is completed. An attorney should also be consulted. The parent who fears violence from an alleged perpetrator should receive recommendations similar to those for battered spouses. If possible, the parent should seek a place of shelter. If that is not a realistic option, the parent's locks should be changed and the concern reported to law enforcement for additional advice. When the perpetrator is a sibling of the child, the children must be separated. The offender should be taken into state custody, admitted for a psychiatric evaluation, or live with a family member who has no children. When a sibling remains in the home, concerns should be expressed to child protective services and another arrangement should be encouraged.

The Child's Behavior

Parents commonly ask at least 2 questions regarding their child's behavior:

1. Should I let my child talk about the sexual abuse?

2. Why did my child touch another child's genital area at childcare?

Some parents hope their child will forget the abuse and other parents have personal fears about confronting the abuse; however, parents should listen to the child who wishes to talk and acknowledge that their child's ability to speak about the abuse is brave. The child who asks questions deserves age-appropriate answers. Parents should not ask the child in-depth questions while an investigation is in progress; an investigator may fear the forensic interview has been contaminated or the child has been coached to provide false information. The child's expressed feelings should be validated. Sexually abused children often feel guilt and they should be reassured the abuse is the fault of the offender, not them. Most importantly, parents should reassure their children that they believe the disclosure and will keep them safe. Some children find the sexual abuse to be a secret too emotion-laden to articulate to a parent, perhaps due to feelings of guilt, fear of punishment, or a wish to protect the offender or parent. A parent's persistent silence may reinforce the child's perception that the subject is off-limits. The appropriate management, based on child and parental factors, can be recommended by the child's therapist.

Parents need to know that young sexually abused children frequently reenact the sexual act with toys, other children and adults, and themselves. Even highly focused behavior may resolve relatively soon after the sexual abuse ceases. If not, parents will need counseling in its management, and the child will need treatment if age appropriate. A common concern of parents is that their children may begin acting out sexually although they did not display such behavior at the time of the medical evaluation. The parents may become confused in attempting to differentiate between healthy and problematic sexual behaviors. Parents in general have been found to be in need of education on the range of age-appropriate sexual behaviors,[15] and they have voiced a desire to discuss the subject with their child's pediatrician.[16] The examiner should be prepared to describe the normal range of child sexual behaviors in relation to the developmental level of the child at the time of the examination. While no scale clearly defines normal and abnormal behavior, tools such as the Child Sexual Behavior Inventory have been normalized between sexually abused and nonabused groups to provide reference ranges for clinicians and parents.[17,18]

The Investigation

Parents commonly ask the following questions about the investigation:

1. How can I learn the status of the investigation?

2. My child would not talk to the investigator. Will that result in unsubstantiation of the abuse?

The multijurisdictional nature of a child abuse investigation can be confusing and stressful to a family that is already in crisis. A brief account of the local child protection and law enforcement/judicial structure can be helpful to the caregivers as they attempt to navigate an unfamiliar process. Studies of investigations performed with a coordinated, multidisciplinary approach versus segregated agencies show that both patient satisfaction[19] and legal outcomes are better with a coordinated response.[20,21] This may be partially attributable to the level of support the family unit receives in the coordinated process. Providing a summary of the investigation process and status, as well as resources such as investigator or victim advocate contact telephone numbers, may help bridge gaps between the family in crisis and the system.

If a child does not disclose abuse to an investigator, the likelihood that sexual abuse will be substantiated may be diminished unless other evidence exists. If a child has disclosed abuse to a parent but not to an investigator trained to interview children, an age-appropriate counseling referral may be helpful; the child may disclose more in the course of therapy.

Examination Findings

Parents may ask questions pertaining to the examination:

1. Will normal examination findings prevent prosecution?

2. Is my daughter still a virgin?

Normal medical evaluation findings alone should never prohibit prosecution.[22,23] However, it is likely that supporting evidence, such as a child who is able to provide credible testimony in court, another eyewitness, or a perpetrator's confession, will be needed. Most prosecutors are aware that child victims of sexual abuse commonly have normal examination findings, which the medical report should also state. The medical provider will be able to provide this information in court if needed. It should be emphasized that the priority at the time of the conference is protection of the child and emotional healing of the child and family.

The question regarding virginity is more difficult to answer. It is open to interpretation, depending on the beliefs and culture of parents and other participants in the postconference. If the hymen is normal, the examiner can reassure the parents that physical evidence of sexual intercourse is absent (although a normal hymen does not rule out the occurrence of hymenal penetration). An explanation of the anatomy may help parents understand the difference between labial and hymenal penetration.

In addition to identifying and alleviating sources of confusion, concerns, and stress, another psychosocial goal of the postexamination conference is to *identify those children and parents who need referral for mental health services*. This goal requires the assessment of the intensity of the effects of the sexual abuse and related events on the child. Other factors also influence the child's need for counseling. Preexisting psychosocial circumstances determine, at least in part, the functional outcome.[24,25] These include the family's preexisting mental state, beliefs, and attitudes, as well as the beliefs, attitudes, and judgments of those close to the child and family and those with whom they must interact.[2]

The multifaceted psychological needs of the child must be identified and managed, because sexual abuse is associated with negative outcomes in childhood and adulthood. Treatment may be needed to prevent these outcomes. These negative outcomes include the following:

— High-risk sexual behaviors[26,27]

— Suicidality[28,29]

— Depression[30]

— Occurrence of other adverse childhood experiences[31]

— Teen pregnancy[32]

— Sexually transmitted diseases later in life[33]

— Early initiation of illicit drug use and later addiction[34]

— Eating disorders[35]

— Regular smoking and drinking in adolescence[36]

— Poor adult physical and mental health outcomes[37-40]

Evaluation of Child's Psychological Distress

Although sexually abused children commonly have fears, behavior problems, sexualized behaviors, poor self-esteem, depression, and posttraumatic stress disorder, parents sometimes underestimate mental health issues in their children until asked about specific symptoms. It is not common for children to self-report significant levels of emotional distress.[11] Approximately one third of sexually abused children have been reported to have no symptoms.[41] Counseling needs should be suspected, identified if possible, and met. Many tools are available to assess the presence of stress-related behaviors in children, including the Children's Depression Inventory,[42] Mood and Feelings Questionnaire,[43] Pediatric Symptom Checklist,[44] Trauma Symptom Checklist for Young Children,[45] and others (**Table 4-2**).[8,46] Most of these validated screening instruments are time-consuming for the child, parents, and interviewer.

Table 4-2. Screening Tools for Behaviors in Children	
CHECKLIST	LOCATION
Child Sexual Behavior Inventory Children's Depression Inventory Trauma Symptom Checklist for Children Trauma Symptom Checklist for Young Children	Available for purchase from Psychological Assessment Resources, Inc. (copyrighted materials) 1-800-331-8378 http://www.parinc.com
Mood and Feelings Questionnaire	Available for download with registration at http://devepi.duhs.duke.edu/mfq.html
Pediatric Symptom Checklist	Available for download from http://www.brightfutures.org/ mentalhealth/pdf/tools.html

A formal psychological screening evaluation is usually unnecessary at the level of the postexamination conference. Child victims of sexual abuse should be referred to an appropriate mental health professional regardless of the presence or absence of reported symptoms. A self-report questionnaire that includes symptoms such as suicidal ideations may assist in separating those requiring emergent referral versus a scheduled appointment. These questions may include:

— Have you (has your child) talked about or caused harm to self?

— Have you (has your child) talked about or attempted suicide?

A self-report questionnaire may also reinforce a referral for counseling. The ability of a caregiver to understand the need for counseling for a child who has been sexually abused has been shown to be an important factor in the child successfully entering therapy.[47]

Family Support Structure

Although addressing the child's mental health issues in a postexamination conference is important, an assessment of the stability of the family support structure is equally necessary. Negative reactions to a child's disclosure of abuse can have harmful effects on the adult's well-being.[12] Parents may not volunteer information regarding their own disturbing mental health symptoms, but they usually provide compelling information when asked how they are handling their stress. They commonly report symptoms of posttraumatic stress disorder, especially when told that parents who had bad experiences growing up often have difficulty with problems such as a recurrence of flashbacks when they learn their children have been sexually abused. Mothers who are still experiencing symptoms of trauma from their own past abuse are much more likely to have children with behavioral issues than mothers without a history of abuse.[48] A parent's unresolved mental health problems, including depression, may be exacerbated by a child's disclosure. Answering yes to the following 2 questions on a self-report questionnaire has been found to detect over 70% of women with depressive symptoms[49]:

1. Lately, do you feel down, depressed, or hopeless?

2. During the past month, have you felt very little interest or pleasure in the things you used to enjoy?

Adverse Childhood Experiences

Child sexual abuse has been defined as an *adverse childhood experience* (ACE). Other ACEs, including physical abuse and neglect, are also commonly found in the homes of sexually abused children.[31] ACEs involving the family support structure include intimate partner violence (IPV) and substance abuse. The examiner should ask about these issues during the postexamination conference and make appropriate referrals, if needed, as these issues can affect family functioning beyond parental health issues. All conference professionals should have information and be prepared to identify and manage IPV and substance abuse.

Intimate Partner Violence

IPV is commonly found in families where children are reported as victims of abuse or neglect.[50] Also, children have been found to be at higher risk for an ACE such as abuse or neglect if IPV is present in the home.[51,52] Children of mothers who have been victims of IPV are more likely to have behavioral problems than children of nonabused mothers.[53-55] Screening for IPV in the home at the time of the conference provides an opportunity for intervention to improve the child's support structure. Three brief screening questions have been found reliable for detecting IPV in an emergency department, and they can be adapted for use in a self-report questionnaire.[56]

1. Have you been hit, kicked, punched, or otherwise hurt by someone within the past year? If so, by whom?

2. Do you feel safe in your current relationship?

3. Is there a partner from a previous relationship who is making you feel unsafe now?

Care must be taken when exploring the possibility of IPV. The parent's safety may be jeopardized if the offender finds shelter or hotline information in the written clinic support material.

Substance Abuse

Parental substance abuse is often associated with poor parenting, physical abuse, psychological abuse, and neglect, and often results in ACEs.[57,58] Substance abuse and IPV are often intertwined.[59] Parents may be asked if there is a personal or family history of illegal drug use. Screening questions such as the CAGE and CAGE Adapted to Include Drugs may be useful for inclusion on a self-report questionnaire.[60] A positive response to 1 or more of the following questions can be used as a positive screen.

— Have you ever felt you should cut down on your drinking or drug use?

— Have people annoyed you by criticizing your drinking or drug use?

— Have you ever felt bad or guilty about your drinking or drug use?

— Have you ever had a drink or used drugs first thing in the morning to steady your nerves or to get rid of a hangover?

Children may be psychologically or developmentally affected whether a parent's drug use is current or in the past.

ENDING THE CONFERENCE

The stress of a child's disclosure and ensuing investigation may impede the family's ability to recall information from the conference. Written information should be available for the family to take home. The information should address follow-up, such as repeat blood tests, prescriptions, order of protection, examinations of siblings, or counseling. Other support information that may be provided, depending on issues identified during the conference, includes brochures, Internet sites, and telephone numbers for legal services, victim advocates, domestic violence shelters, and support groups such as Alcoholics Anonymous, Narcotics Anonymous, and parent and child sexual abuse support groups. The sexual abuse examiner should be prepared to provide resources and referral numbers to caregivers and iterate the importance of following through with the referrals.

The conference should be concluded with a verbal summary of information and recommendations. Parents should be commended for any actions warranting praise, and the examiner should offer to be available for questions that may arise later. The examiner should also close the visit with a handshake, a highly important gesture for many parents.

PREVENTION OF CONFERENCE PROBLEMS

Postexamination conferences are often more difficult than expected. Child sexual abuse medicine is a relatively new field requiring training and continuing education, and some questions are not easily answered. Peer review, consultations, and referral resources should be available to the examiner. Although the psychosocial aspects of sexual abuse have been more researched than the physical aspects, gaps in information remain.

A family's dysfunction can create a sense of chaos or futility, which is compounded by the flagging efforts of overburdened agencies. It is not surprising that new challenges regularly arise in these conferences. Perhaps the most troubling to professional participants is their vulnerability to questions and family issues for which they are not prepared. The most emergent may be the child who is at risk for suicide. Conference participants should establish a relationship with an appropriate mental health provider to deal with such cases promptly. Other issues such as the child's safety may require consultation with investigators, prosecutors, child protective services, or attorneys ad litem. Such resources should be established before problems arise.

FOLLOW-UP

A telephone call to the family within a few days after the conference can be beneficial. Parents often do not understand or recall information provided at medical visits, and this is likely a greater problem for emotionally charged families dealing with sexual abuse. Many parents are in denial or have difficulty focusing on meeting their needs and those of their children. Almost all families need additional encouragement or the opportunity to reaffirm the information and recommendations given in the post-examination conference.

Depending on the issues that need to be addressed, a social worker, family advocate, or other professional who was present at the initial conference can make this follow-up call instead of the medical provider. The caller should ask how the parents and children are handling stressors identified in the conference and ask about symptoms of anxiety, stress, and depression. The caller should also ask the parents if there are new concerns regarding themselves, their children, and the agency investigation. Prior recommend-ations should be reinforced. Parents should be given the results of tests that were performed at the initial visit. If the family members appear to be doing well, they should be encouraged to call if future concerns develop. Generally, no additional follow-up should be initiated unless requested, since it may appear intrusive.

RESEARCH NEEDS

Published studies regarding crisis intervention have primarily involved psychiatric and critical incident situations. Rigorous evaluations of postsexual abuse examination conferences appear to be absent in the published literature, and little has been written on the subject. Areas in need of research include the usefulness of screening measures for child and family stressors, the effectiveness of crisis intervention, parental understanding of information provided, and compliance with recommendations and referrals. Use of control groups is confounded by possible ethical issues, difficulty in matching subjects, and the potential availability of other sources of information and intervention.

CONCLUSION

The medical evaluation of a child victim of sexual abuse should encompass more than a forensic examination and provision of results to a family and agencies. Medical needs should be identified. A parent-completed report that includes the child's behavior symptoms and the parent's stress, depression, past physical and sexual abuse, neglect, IPV, and substance abuse can be a helpful adjunct to the postexamination conference. The examiner should determine that the child likely will be safe, supported, and provided needed medical and mental health treatment. Family members should receive support, intervention, and referrals for their stress, as well as enhancement of their ability to help their child. They should leave the medical evaluation process functioning more confidently and effectively than when they entered.

REFERENCES

1. Finkel MA. Initial medical management of the sexually abused child. In: Reece RM, ed. *Treatment of Child Abuse: Common Ground for Mental Health, Medical and Legal Practioners*. Baltimore, MD: Johns Hopkins University Press; 2000:3-6.

2. Renner KE, Keith A. The establishment of a crisis intervention service for victims of sexual assault. *Can J Comm Mental Health*. 1985;4:113-123.

3. Mitchell JT. Characteristics of successful early intervention programs. *Int J Emerg Ment Health*. 2004;6(4):175-184.

4. Rosenthal S, Feiring C, Taska L. Emotional support and adjustment over a year's time following sexual abuse discovery. *Child Abuse Negl*. 2003;27(6):641-661.

5. Paradise JE. The medical evaluation of the sexually abused child. *Pediatr Clin North Am*. 1990;37(4):839-862.

6. Dubowitz H. Children's responses to the medical evaluation for child sexual abuse. *Child Abuse Negl*. 1998;22(6):581-584

7. Negrao C, Bonanno GA, Noll JG, Putnam FW, Trickett PK. Shame, humiliation, and childhood sexual abuse: distinct contributions and emotional coherence. *Child Malteat*. 2005;10(4):350-363.

8. Wenninger K, Heiman JR. Relating body image to psychological and sexual functioning in child sexual abuse survivors. *J Trauma Stress*. 1998;11(3):543-562.

9. Kearney-Cooke A, Ackard DM. The effects of sexual abuse on body image, self-image, and sexual activity of women. *Percept Mot Skills*. 2006;102:485-497.

10. Goodman-Brown TB, Edelstein RS, Goodman GS, Jones DP, Gordon DS. Why children tell: a model of children's disclosure of sexual abuse. *Child Abuse Negl*. 2003;27(5):525-540.

11. Berliner L, Elliott DM. Sexual abuse of children. In: Myers JE, Berliner L, Briere JN, Hendrix CT, Reid TA, Jenny CA, eds. *APSAC Handbook on Child Maltreatment*. 2nd ed. Thousand Oaks, CA: Sage; 2002:55-60.

12. Ullman SE. Social reactions to child sexual abuse disclosures: a critical review. *J Child Sex Abus*. 2003;12(1):89-121.

13. Plunkett A, O'Toole B, Swanston H, Oates RK, Shrimpton S, Parkinson P. Suicide risk following child sexual abuse. *Ambul Pediatr*. 2001;1(5):262-266.

14. Leifer M, Kilbane T, Grossman G. A three-generational study comparing the families of supportive and unsupportive mothers of sexually abused children. *Child Maltreat*. 2001;6(4):353-364.

15. Pullins LG, Jones JD. Parental knowledge of child sexual abuse symptoms. *J Child Sex Abus*. 2006;15(4):1-18.

16. Thomas D, Flaherty E, Binns H. Parent expectations and comfort with discussion of normal childhood sexuality and sexual abuse prevention during office visits. *Ambul Pediatr*. 2004;4(3):232-236.

17. Friedrich WN, Fisher JL, Dittner CA, et al. Child Sexual Behavior Inventory: normative, psychiatric, and sexual abuse comparisons. *Child Maltreat*. 2001;6(1):37-49.

18. Friedrich WN, Grambsch P, Broughton D, Kuiper J, Beilke RL. Normative sexual behavior in children. *Pediatrics*. 1991;88(3):456-464.

19. Jones L. Findings from the UNH multi-site evaluation of children's advocacy centers (CACs). Crimes against Children Research Center. May 2006. Available at: http://www.unh.edu/ccrc/pdf/CAC_eval_executive_summary.pdf. Accessed June 15, 2007.

20. Joa D, Edelson MG. Legal outcomes for children who have been sexually abused: the impact of child abuse assessment center evaluations. *Child Maltreat*. 2004;9(3):263-276.

21. Smith DW, Witte TH, Fricker-Elhai AE. Service outcomes in physical and sexual abuse cases: a comparison of child advocacy center-based and standard services. *Child Maltreat*. 2006;11(4):354-360.

22. DeJong AR, Rose M. Frequency and significance of physical evidence in legally proven cases of child sexual abuse. *Pediatrics*. 1989;84(6):1022-1026

23. Frasier LD, Makoroff KL. Medical evidence and expert testimony in child sexual abuse. *Juvenile Fam Court J*. 2006;57(1):41-50.

24. Mannarino AP, Cohen JA, Berman SR. The relationship between preabuse factors and psychological symptomatology in sexually abused girls. *Child Abuse Negl*. 1994;18(1):63-71.

25. Paradise JE, Rose L, Sleeper LA, Nathanson M. Behavior, family function, school performance, and predictors of persistent disturbance in sexually abused children. *Pediatrics*. 1994;93(3):1452-1459.

26. Hillis SD, Anda RF, Felitti VJ, Marchbanks PA. Adverse childhood experiences and sexual risk behaviors in women: a retrospective cohort study. *Fam Plann Perspect*. 2001;33(5):206-211.

27. Bensley LS, Van Eenwyk J, Simmons KW. Self-reported childhood sexual and physical abuse and adult HIV-risk behaviors and heavy drinking. *Am J Prev Med*. 2000;18(2):151-158.

28. Bergen HA, Martin G, Richardson AS, Allison S, Roeger L. Sexual abuse and suicidal behavior: a model constructed from a large community sample of adolescents. *J Am Acad Child Adolesc Psychiatry*. 2003;42(11):1301-1309.

29. Dube SR, Anda RF, Felitti VJ, Chapman DP, Williamson DF, Giles WH. Childhood abuse, household dysfunction, and the risk of attempted suicide throughout the life span: findings from the Adverse Childhood Experiences Study. *JAMA*. 2001;286(24):3089-3096.

30. Chapman DP, Whitfield CL, Felitti VJ, Dube SR, Edwards VJ, Anda RF. Adverse childhood experiences and the risk of depressive disorders in adulthood. *J Affect Disord*. 2004;82(2):217-225.

31. Dong M, Anda RF, Dube SR, Giles WH, Felitti VJ. The relationship of exposure to child sexual abuse to other forms of abuse, neglect, and household dysfunction during childhood. *Child Abuse Negl*. 2003;27(6):625-639.

32. Hillis SD, Anda RF, Dube SR, Felitti VJ, Marchbanks PA, Marks JS. The association between adverse childhood experiences and adolescent pregnancy, long-term psychosocial consequences and fetal death. *Pediatrics*. 2004;113(2):320-327.

33. Hillis SD, Anda RF, Felitti VJ, Nordenberg D, Marchbanks PA. Adverse childhood experiences and sexually transmitted diseases in men and women: a retrospective study. *Pediatrics*. 2000;106(1):e11.

34. Dube SR, Felitti VJ, Dong M, Giles WH, Anda RF. The impact of adverse childhood experiences on health problems: evidence from four birth cohorts dating back to 1900. *Prev Med*. 2003;37(3):268-277.

35. Ackard DM, Neumark-Sztainer D, Hannan PJ, French S, Story M. Binge and purge behavior among adolescents: associations with sexual and physical abuse in a nationally representative sample: the Commonwealth Fund survey. *Child Abuse Negl*. 2001;25(6):771-785.

36. Simantov E, Schoen C, Klein JD. Health-compromising behaviors: why do adolescents smoke or drink? Identifying underlying risk and protective factors. *Arch Pediatr Adolesc Med*. 2000;154(10):1025-1033.

37. Walker EA, Gelfand A, Katon WJ, et al. Adult health status of women with histories of childhood abuse and neglect. *Am J Med*. 1999;107(4):332-339.

38. Dong M, Giles WH, Felitti VJ, et al. Insights into causal pathways for ischemic heart disease: adverse childhood experiences study. *Circulation*. 2004;110(13): 1761-1766.

39. Felitti VJ, Anda RF, Nordenberg D, et al. Relationship of childhood abuse and household dysfunction to many of the leading causes of death in adults: the Adverse Childhood Experiences (ACE) Study. *Am J Prev Med*. 1998;14(4): 245-258.

40. Dube SR, Felitti VJ, Dong M, Chapman DP, Giles WH, Anda RF. Childhood abuse, neglect and household dysfunction and the risk of illicit drug use: the adverse childhood experiences study. *Pediatrics*. 2003;111(3):564-572.

41. Kendall-Tackett KA, Williams LM, Finkelhor D. Impact of sexual abuse on children. *Psychol Bulletin*. 1993;113:164-180.

42. Timbermont B, Braet C, Dreesen L. Assessing depression in youth: relation between the Children's Depression Inventory and a structured interview. *J Clin Child Adolesc Psychol*. 2004;33(1):149-157.

43. Daviss WB, Birmaher B, Melhem NA, Axelson DA, Michaels SM, Brent DA. Criterion validity of the Mood and Feelings Questonnaire for depressive episodes in clinic and non-clinic subjects. *J Child Psychol Psychiatry*. 2006;47(9):927-934.

44. Reijneveld SA, Vogels AG, Hoekstra F, Crone MR. Use of the Pediatric Symptom Checklist for the detection of psychosocial problems in preventive child healthcare. *BMC Public Health*. 2006; 6:197.

45. Briere J, Johnson K, Bissada A, et al. The Trauma Symptom Checklist for Young Children (TSCYC): reliability and association with abuse exposure in a multi-site study. *Child Abuse Negl*. 2001;25(8):1001-1014.

46. Revah-Levy A, Birmaher B, Gasquet I, Falissard B. The Adolescent Depression Rating Scale (ADRS): a validation study. *BMC Psychiatry*. 2007;7:2.

47. Haskett ME, Nowlan NP, Hutcheson JS, Whitworth JM. Factors associated with successful entry into therapy in child sexual abuse cases. *Child Abuse Negl*. 1991;15(4):467-476.

48. Paredes M, Leifer M, Kilbane T. Maternal variables related to sexually abused children's functioning. *Child Abuse Negl.* 2001;25(9):1159-1176.

49. Dubowitz H, Feigelman S, Lane W, et al. Screening for depression in an urban pediatric primary care clinic. *Pediatrics.* 2007;119(3):435-443.

50. Hazen AL, Connelly CD, Kelleher KJ, Landsverk JA, Barth R. Intimate partner violence among female caregivers of children reported for child maltreatment. *Child Abuse Negl.* 2004;28(3):301-319.

51. Dube SR, Anda RF, Felitti VJ, Edwards VJ, Williamson DF. Exposure to abuse, neglect, and household dysfunction among adults who witnessed intimate partner violence as children: implications for health and social services. *Violence Vict.* 2002;17(1):3-17.

52. Ernst AA, Weiss SJ, Enright-Smith S. Child witnesses and victims in homes with adult intimate partner violence. *Acad Emerg Med.* 2006;13(6):696-699.

53. McFarlane JM, Groff JY, O'Brien JA, Watson K. Behaviors of children who are exposed and not exposed to intimate partner violence: an analysis of 330 black, white and Hispanic children. *Pediatrics.* 2003;112(3 pt 1):e202-e207.

54. Kernic MA, Wolf ME, Holt VL, McKnight B, Huebner CE, Rivara FP. Behavioral problems among children whose mothers are abused by an intimate partner. *Child Abuse Negl.* 2003;27(11):1231-1246.

55. Hazen AL, Connelly CD, Kelleher KJ, Barth RP, Landsverk JA. Female caregivers' experiences with intimate partner violence and behavior problems in children investigated as victims of maltreatment. *Pediatrics.* 2006;117(1):99-109.

56. Feldhaus KM, Koziol-McLain J, Armsbury HL, Norton IM, Lowenstein SR, Abbott JT. Accuracy of 3 brief screening questions for detecting partner violence in the emergency department. *JAMA.* 1997;277(17):1357-1361.

57. Barnard M, McKeganey N. The impact of parental problem drug use on children: what is the problem and what can be done to help? *Addiction.* 2004;99(5):552-559.

58. Walsh C, MacMillan HL, Jamieson E. The relationship between parental substance abuse and child maltreatment: findings from the Ontario Health Supplement. *Child Abuse Negl.* 2003;27(12):1409-1425.

59. Cohen JB, Dickow A, Horner K, et al; Methamphetamine Treatment Project. Abuse and violence history of men and women in treatment for methamphetamine dependence. *Am J Addict.* 2003;12(5):377-385.

60. Brown RL, Leonard T, Saunders LA, Papasouliotis O. The prevalence and detection of substance use disorders among inpatients ages 18-49: an opportunity for intervention. *Prev Med.* 1998;27(1):101-110.

Chapter 5

NON-EMERGENT MEDICAL EXAMINATION PROCEDURES AND TECHNIQUES

Nancy D. Kellogg, MD

When sexual abuse is first reported, medical staff should determine when and where the medical evaluation should be conducted. Some communities have a single program or facility that provides evaluations for all victims regardless of when the abuse occurred, whereas other communities have one program for victims with recent or acute injuries and another for victims who were abused several days or more prior to their clinical presentation. Victims of recent abuse are likely to require forensic evidence collection, photodocumentation, or treatment for injuries. Victims of chronic or remote abuse usually do not have emergent medical or forensic needs and their medical evaluations can occur in an outpatient setting. Child advocacy centers and outpatient facilities often provide a child-friendly, calm, safe, and supportive setting for non-emergent medical evaluations, victim assistance, counseling, and other services.

INDICATIONS FOR A MEDICAL ASSESSMENT

Because the majority of examinations for sexual abuse result in normal findings, some experts are questioning the need for a medical examination, especially when the last incident of abuse may have occurred some time previously. There are several reasons why the medical assessment is recommended.

— The child may not provide a full disclosure of the abusive acts and the examination may reveal evidence of penetrative trauma.

— The child and family are often concerned about whether the child's body is normal, and more specifically, whether the hymen is undamaged.

— Reassuring the child and family that the examination findings are normal may reduce anxiety and make the child feel less stigmatized by the abuse. Some cultures place value on the virginity of young females, and may even deny certain celebrations (eg, the Quinceañera) if virginity is in question.

— In court proceedings, jurors and judges may perceive the lack of a medical assessment as an incomplete investigation, negating the importance of the victim's statement.

— Some children are victims of repeated sexual abuse. Examinations with photo-documentation allow for detection and comparison of changes that can occur over time.

— The presence of a previously undiagnosed sexually transmitted infection (STI) such as venereal warts may be detected.

The need for an emergent examination is not solely dependent on the time frame of the last sexual abuse. Following are situations that may require an emergent examination more than 72 hours from the time of the abuse:

— Anal or genital pain or bleeding.

— Penetrative trauma occurring within the prior 7 days. In general, forensic evidence is not collected later than 72 hours in adolescents and adults after abuse or assault (depending on state guidelines); however, more severe acute injuries may be visible for several days following the abuse. These injuries are likely to resolve completely within days, so it is important to photodocument the injuries for legal purposes. In prepubertal children, forensic evidence is generally not found after 24 hours, and the best chance of finding transfer evidence is in clothing or bedding.

— Submission of items, such as clothing and linens, for forensic analysis. These items can be collected and packaged in accordance with chain-of-custody procedures at either a hospital equipped and trained in forensic collection or by law enforcement.

— Family/child request. Parents have common concerns when they learn their child has been sexually abused, even when the last episode of abuse occurred months earlier. A medical assessment conducted in the hospital can provide answers to questions such as, "Is my child okay?" and "Was my child penetrated?" and alleviate parents' fears expeditiously.

THE MEDICAL EXAMINATION: SETTING THE SCENE

The medical examination of a suspected victim of sexual abuse should not cause the victim additional psychological or physical trauma. The keys to a successful genital examination of a child or teenager are

— Adequate preparation of the child (and often the parent) for the examination.

— Familiarity and dexterity with utilizing various examination positions and techniques.

— A confident yet sensitive approach.

Overall, the clinician should prioritize the patient's need for respect, privacy, and control, especially if the patient is an adolescent. The goal of preparation is to reduce anxiety and to promote the child's sense of control. The child or teenager should be shown the examination room and equipment prior to the medical evaluation. This preparation is ideally done by a nurse or other support personnel. It may be helpful to show the patient a cotton-tipped applicator used for sample collection and let the patient touch the cotton tip to appreciate how soft it feels. Preparation can be done in the presence of parents to reduce their anxiety as well. With adequate preparation, most examinations can be done without sedation.

When an examiner is nervous and anxious, the child or teenager is more likely to be nervous and anxious. The child's privacy and need for control should be respected. The examiner should explain everything that is about to occur. Raising the head of the examination table allows the child to see the examiner and the examiner to gauge the child's reaction and anxiety during the examination. Children should be allowed to change into the examining gown in private and keep all other areas of their bodies that are not being examined draped. Children should choose whether they want a support person to be with them during the examination; many adolescents prefer not to exercise this option. The examiner should avoid "shop talk" and move quickly and gently through the examination. When using any of the examination techniques, constant, even, gentle pressure should be applied to avoid groping movements. It is sometimes a more effective distraction to have the child talk during the examination rather than have an adult talk to the child (J. McCann, personal communication, 1990). Some photocolposcopes utilize a digital system that captures and displays images on a computer. The child and family should be informed ahead of time that genital images will appear on the computer screen, which they may or may not wish to view.

A knowledgeable medical assistant or nurse can greatly facilitate the examination. The assistant can show the child the examination room and orient the child to the various positions and equipment used during the examination. The assistant can also help position the child and provide distractions that may assist in relaxing younger children during the examination. By handing the examiner the speculum or swabs needed to examine the child and collect specimens, ensuring that the child is adequately draped at all times, and capturing the images on the computer, the assistant can ensure that the examination is more comfortable and efficient.

It is a challenge for the clinician when an adolescent or older child adamantly refuses an examination. Unless there are immediate medical or forensic needs, the examination may be delayed. In this situation, the clinician should clarify examination procedures and what information the examination may provide to allow the adolescent to make a more informed decision about whether or not to undergo the examination. Following are common reasons that adolescents refuse examinations and the appropriate clinician responses:

— **Concern that a speculum will be used.** In most instances, a speculum examination is not required. Vaginal swabs may provide adequate samples when the patient is reluctant to undergo a speculum examination. The physician should strive to minimize the trauma of the sexual abuse examination by utilizing less traumatic sampling techniques, such as using smaller swabs and using urine samples to test for STIs in lieu of vaginal samples for adolescents who cannot tolerate vaginal sampling.

— **"I don't feel comfortable with anyone looking down there."** The physician can clarify the examination techniques and use of draping to reassure the adolescent that only one area of the body will be uncovered at a time. In addition, the benefits of ensuring patient health should be stressed.

— **"I know I am okay."** The physician should explain that the only way to make sure someone is okay is through examination. Many, if not most individuals with STIs have no noticeable symptoms. This is especially true for venereal warts, which are the most common sexually transmitted infection.

Speculum examinations should not be conducted on the prepubertal child unless there is a need to establish and/or treat a source of bleeding or to identify a vaginal foreign body, and this should only be done under anesthesia. Digital examinations of the rectum are not informative and therefore not necessary.

Because children and adolescents are often victims of more than one type of abuse, suspected victims of sexual abuse should be examined carefully for any signs of physical abuse and neglect. A head-to-toe examination with careful and thorough inspection of all body surfaces may reveal inflicted injuries that occurred either during the sexual abuse or because of the sexual abuse. For example, some adolescents who are sexually abused by strangers or peers are blamed for their assault and beaten by their parents.

EXAMINATION POSITIONS AND TECHNIQUES

The practitioner should become familiar with the appropriate uses of the various examination *positions* (patient placement) to ensure adequate and complete visualization of anogenital anatomy and the *techniques* (examiner manipulation) required to perform a comfortable and thorough examination. These skills can be achieved through numerous examinations on nonvictimized children and adolescents.

EXAMINATION POSITIONS

There are 5 positions that may be helpful during the medical examination. Most examinations require only 2 of these positions—either the supine frog-leg position or the supine lithotomy position (depending on the child's age and size) and the prone knee-chest position. For males, the genitalia may be examined while the patient is lying supine on the examination table. Although the legs need to be parted during the testicular examination, a frog-leg position is not necessary. The prone knee-chest position is still recommended for males, as this position provides the best visualization of the perianal structures.

Supine Frog-leg Position

This position is used for smaller prepubertal female children. The child places the soles of the feet together with knees flexed laterally (**Figure 5-1-a**). If the feet can be placed on a pull-out shelf at the base of the examination table, this may allow for better manipulation and visualization of the genitals, especially if the shelf is slightly below the level of the table. Some clinicians allow the child to adopt a modified version of this position while sitting in the mother's lap (**Figure 5-1-b**). This position usually provides an adequate view of the vulva, hymen, and vestibule. If abnormalities of the hymen are seen in this position, examination in the prone knee-chest position is essential to confirm these findings (**Figure 5-2**). In the supine position, the normal hymen may

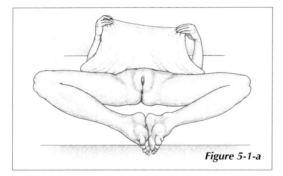

Figure 5-1-a

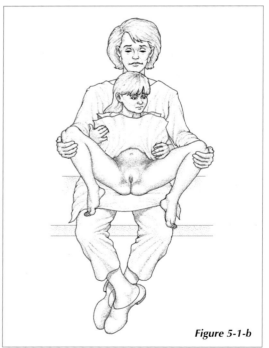

Figure 5-1-b

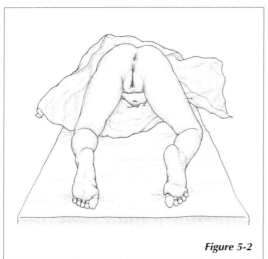

Figure 5-2

Figure 5-1-a. *Child in the supine frog-leg position.*

Figure 5-1-b. *Child in the supine knee-chest position while sitting on the caregiver's lap.*

Figure 5-2. *Child in the prone knee-chest position.*

sometimes fold on itself, creating an artificial abnormality (thickening or irregularity) that unfolds or normalizes in the prone knee-chest position. In addition, hymenal hemorrhages may intensify and become more apparent in the prone knee-chest position.

Supine Lithotomy Position

This position is used for larger female prepubertal children and all female adolescents. The feet are first placed in the examination table stirrups. The child then moves or slides the hips and buttocks to the end of the table and flexes the knees outward. This position provides an adequate view of the vulva, hymen, and vestibule.

Prone Knee-chest Position

This position provides the best view of the perianal area. The child's shoulders, elbows, and forearms are placed on the table in order to make the lower back lordotic and to extend the hips upward. The knees are placed about 18 inches apart. The angle of the knee should approximate 90 degrees. This position is important for confirming irregularities of the hymen that are seen in the supine position. In the prone knee-chest position, it is possible to visualize the vaginal walls and cervix without inserting a speculum.

Supine Knee-chest Position

This position is generally used to examine the anus of infants and small toddlers. The knees are drawn up onto the chest to visualize perianal structures. The lateral decubitus position may be used instead of the supine knee-chest position.

Lateral Decubitus Position

This position can be used for all age groups to examine the anus. The knees should be together and drawn up on the chest such that the anus can be visualized with minimal gluteal separation or distortion of the tissue. This position does not provide the optimal visualization accomplished with the prone knee-chest position, but it is a good transition position between the supine and prone knee-chest placements and is preferable to the knee-chest position for gathering samples for evidence or sexually transmitted infection testing.

EXAMINATION TECHNIQUES

For female patients, the examiner should begin with labial separation with the patient in the supine position, moving the labia majora laterally and inferiorly using the ventral/distal aspects of 2 to 3 fingers placed just below the inferior margins of each labia minora (**Figure 5-3**). As the examiner proceeds to labial traction, the labia majora are grasped just above the posterior commissure, using the ventral aspects of the thumb placed medially and the lateral aspect of the first digit, which should be flexed at both joints. The labia are then pulled gently in the anterior direction, toward the examiner. This technique often causes the folds of the hymen to separate and the opening of the hymen to become apparent (**Figures 5-4-a** and **b**). Moving the fingers anteriorly and posteriorly will afford the examiner several views of the vestibule and hymen.

Figure 5-3.
Appearance of the hymen and vestibule using labial separation in the supine lithotomy position.

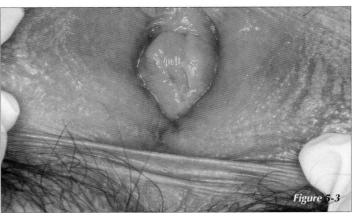

Figure 5-3

The lateral decubitus position should follow the supine position. The buttocks are gently separated, allowing some visualization of the anal folds. There is potential for distortion of the anatomy if the pressure of the examiner's hands is uneven. This position is primarily utilized when there is little or no concern for sexual contact involving the anus or for collecting samples for forensic and infectious disease testing prior to examination in the prone knee-chest position.

The final position is the prone knee-chest position. This position can be particularly embarrassing for the child so the examiner should work quickly, keeping the child draped appropriately throughout this portion of the examination. The examination sheet should be draped over the child's hips and waist, and the edges brought down and together to form a small circular drape that uncovers first the anus and then the genitalia. An assistant or support person should hold the drape so it does not fall and cause undue embarrassment to the child. After the child is properly positioned, the examiner should visualize the anus and perianal tissues without tissue traction, then gently apply traction to the anal folds to reveal any excoriations, fissures, or scars. Significant anal findings are usually, but not always, visible without examiner traction on the tissues. After moving the drape downward to expose the genitalia, the examiner places the dorsal aspects of each thumb at the 2 and 10 o'clock positions of the posterior labial commissure (**Figure 5-5**), lifting the gluteus muscles upward while keeping fingers firmly placed on the buttocks superior to the thumbs, exposing the rim of the hymen. Complete visualization of the posterior rim of the hymen may require viewing each posterior third in sequence by lifting first to the left,

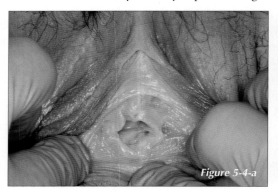

Figure 5-4-a

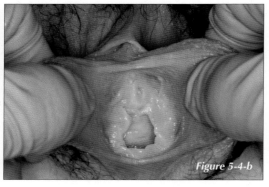

Figure 5-4-b

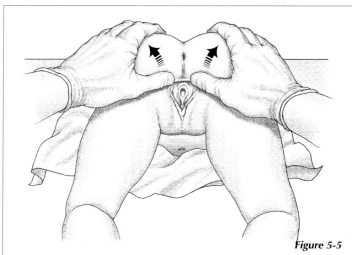

Figure 5-5

Figure 5-4-a. Labial separation in an adolescent who is in the supine lithotomy position.

Figure 5-4-b. Same adolescent where the examiner is using the labial traction technique in the supine lithotomy position.

Figure 5-5. Child in the prone knee-chest position.

leading with the left thumb, then straight up with both thumbs, and finally, lifting to the right, leading with the right thumb. Apparent hymenal notches and clefts seen and/or demonstrated with cotton-tipped applicators should be confirmed in the prone knee-chest position. See **Figures 5-6** through **5-9**.

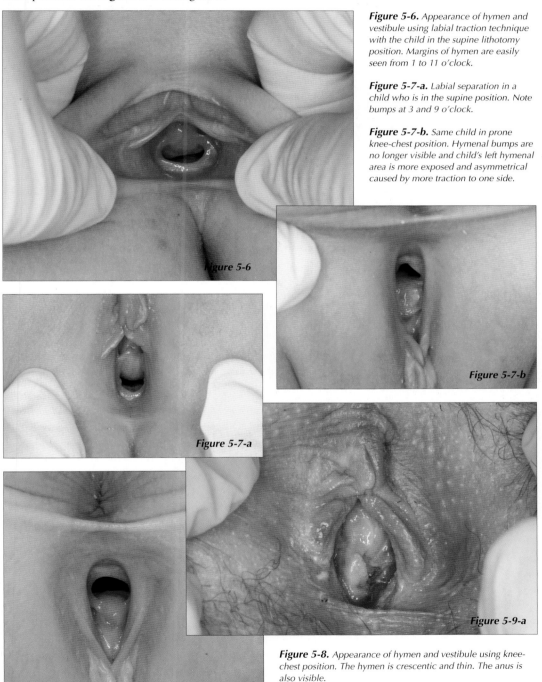

Figure 5-6. *Appearance of hymen and vestibule using labial traction technique with the child in the supine lithotomy position. Margins of hymen are easily seen from 1 to 11 o'clock.*

Figure 5-7-a. *Labial separation in a child who is in the supine position. Note bumps at 3 and 9 o'clock.*

Figure 5-7-b. *Same child in prone knee-chest position. Hymenal bumps are no longer visible and child's left hymenal area is more exposed and asymmetrical caused by more traction to one side.*

Figure 5-6

Figure 5-7-b

Figure 5-7-a

Figure 5-9-a

Figure 5-8

Figure 5-8. *Appearance of hymen and vestibule using knee-chest position. The hymen is crescentic and thin. The anus is also visible.*

Figure 5-9-a. *Demonstration of labial separation showing hymenal injury in supine lithotomy position.*

Figure 5-9-b.
Demonstration of labial traction showing hymenal injury in supine lithotomy position.

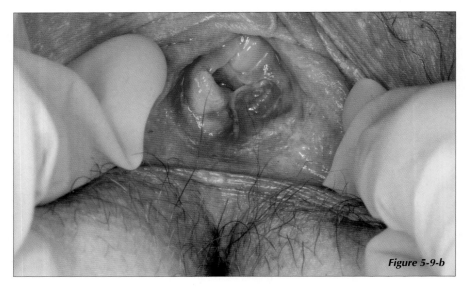

Figure 5-9-b

Common examination position and technique errors include

— Insufficient labial traction to adequately visualize the hymenal margins and vestibule.

— Inadequate lower back lordosis while in the prone knee-chest position.

— Inadequate lifting of the gluteus muscles with the examiner's thumbs during examination of the child in the prone knee-chest position.

Additional techniques that enhance visualization of genital structures include

— Moistening the hymen with water or nonbacteriostatic saline so that redundant folds that adhere to the vestibule or vaginal structures are straightened and freed.

— Manipulation of the hymenal edges with a Foley catheter filled with water[1] or air,[2] a balloon-covered large cervical swab,[3] or a moistened cotton-tipped applicator may demonstrate clefts that are obscured by overlapping hymenal folds (**Figure 5-10**). The Foley catheter is inserted into the vaginal canal, inflated with a small amount of water, and then pulled gently in an external direction so that the edges of the hymen are splayed over the inflated catheter balloon. The balloon-covered swab is placed just inside the vaginal opening and then used to stretch out the hymen. Problems with this technique are considerable and include discomfort to the patient and the potential to misinterpret the hymen as missing or the hymenal rim as too narrow when the Foley catheter balloon flattens the hymen during extraction.

— Demonstration of the hymenal rim integrity can also be accomplished utilizing a cotton-tipped applicator (**Figure 5-11**). The applicator can be used to reflect the folds of the hymen both externally and internally to allow for complete inspection of all surfaces. This is particularly useful to reveal occult hymenal hemorrhages. The examiner should attempt to stretch out the hymenal rim from 6 to 9 o'clock by placing the applicator internal to the hymen at 9 o'clock and gently pulling the hymen upward. The applicator should then be placed just inside the hymenal rim at 6 o'clock, then at 3 o'clock, stretching outward then upward, respectively. The disadvantage of this technique is occasional patient discomfort and the potential to artificially create a defect or obscure a defect in the hymen because of incorrect placement of the applicator.

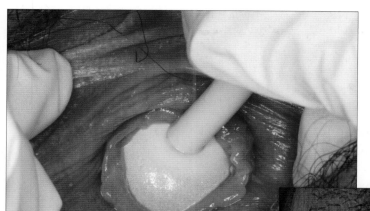

Figure 5-10. *This picture shows the Foley catheter balloon technique (using air). The examiner placed the catheter into the vaginal vault and then inflated the balloon with air. Firm but gentle pressure was placed close to the inflated balloon, and the catheter was pulled upward to allow for the display of the hymen's edges around the balloon in this adolescent in a supine lithotomy position.*

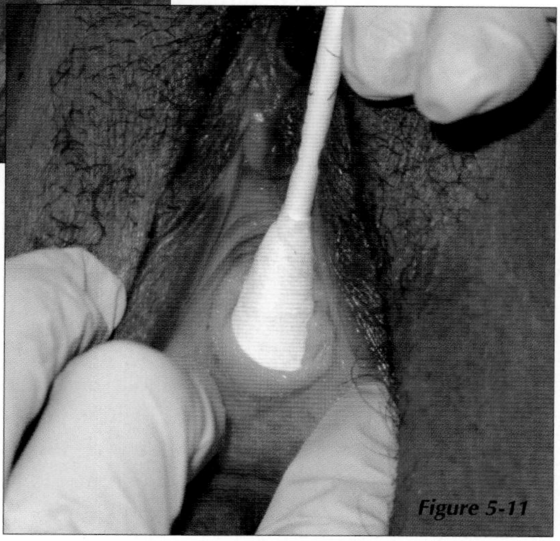

PHOTODOCUMENTATION

Photodocumentation of anal and genital examination findings, regardless of whether such findings are interpreted as normal or abnormal, is an accepted standard of care in the medical assessment of suspected sexual abuse. In addition, equipment that magnifies and illuminates the genitalia and perianal tissues should be utilized during the examination.[4,5] Photodocumentation has become integral to peer review and quality assurance as the range of knowledge and expertise has broadened,[6] and it has provided a valuable adjunct for many studies of abnormal and normal anogenital findings. There are several additional advantages to photodocumentation:

— Photographs, videotape clips, and slides are valuable teaching aids.

— Changes in the examination findings over time may be accurately documented in some cases of repeat victimization.

— Images of trauma may be effectively presented in legal proceedings.

— Images of examination findings may obviate the need for repeated examinations when there is clinician difference in opinion.

— Photodocumentation allows for peer review and, when needed, mentoring.

Figure 5-11. *Demonstration of hymenal rim from 3 to 10 o'clock in an adolescent using a large cotton-tipped applicator. There are no defects or transections present in the hymen.*

METHODS OF PHOTODOCUMENTATION

There are a variety of methods for photodocumentation. Examination findings can be documented with a digital camera or with a photocolposcope with a video or still camera attachment. Photocolposcope systems provide additional features that facilitate the examination, such as a foot-pedal shutter release and hands-free visualization, a system that incorporates patient record information with image capture, and encryption features, but are considerably more expensive than a camera-only system. During the examination, the photocolposcope or camera is placed between the examiner and the patient, at a right angle to the plane of the anatomy being examined. In a study of 122 experienced (average of 1700 examinations) clinicians, 85% used photocolposcopes.

Photocolposcope use was significantly associated with a greater number of correct interpretations of anal and genital findings in this study.[3]

Images taken during a sexual abuse evaluation can be scanned into the computer or captured directly during the examination. Software programs are available to archive such data and create patient files. Images can then be encrypted and sent (or received) through electronic mail.

DISCUSSION OF FINDINGS WITH CHILD AND PARENT(S)

After completing the examination, the child should sit up and be adequately draped or changed into clothing before discussing the results of the examination. In a brief, age-appropriate way, the child should be addressed first about the examination findings. Children should be reassured that they are normal and healthy, and that even if minor injuries are found, they will heal quickly and completely. After discussing the examination with the child, a separate and more comprehensive discussion can be held with the caretaker(s).

CONCLUSION

A medical assessment is recommended for all children who may be victims of sexual abuse. The medical evaluation may reveal evidence of events that the child did not disclose, can reassure the child and family that the child is normal, and may be useful in court proceedings. The medical evaluation should be conducted with confidence and sensitivity, and should not cause additional psychological or physical trauma to the child. Various examination positions and techniques are used, and photodocumentation should be used whenever possible. The results should be discussed with children and caretakers, and children should be reassured that they are normal and healthy.

REFERENCES

1. Persaud DI, Squires JL, Rubin-Remer D. Use of Foley catheter to examine estrogenized hymens for evidence of sexual abuse. *J Pediatr Adolesc Gynecol*. 1997;10(2):83-85.

2. Jones JS, Dunnuck C, Rossman L, Wynn BN, Genco M. *Acad Emerg Med*. 2003;10(9):1001-1004.

3. Kellogg ND, Adams, J. The role of clinician expertise and training in the interpretation of examination findings in suspected victims of child sexual abuse. *SCAN*. 2003;15(4):1-2.

4. Jones JG, Lawson L, Rickert CP. Use of optical glass binocular magnifiers in the examination of sexually abused children. *Adolesc Pediatr Gynecol*. 1990;3:146-148.

5. Bays J, Chadwick D. Medical diagnosis of the sexually abused child. *Child Abuse Negl*. 1993;17(1):91-110.

6. Adams JA. The role of photo documentation of genital findings in medical evaluations of suspected child sexual abuse. *Child Maltreatment*. 1997;2(4):341-347.

Chapter 6

ADOLESCENT ISSUES IN SEXUAL ABUSE AND ASSAULT

Nancy D. Kellogg, MD
Michelle Clayton, MD, MPH, FAAP

The medical care of adolescents who are suspected victims of sexual abuse or assault presents unique challenges for the health care provider. When sexual abuse is first suspected, there is often some confusion as to where the adolescent should go for a medical assessment. Pediatricians typically provide care for children and teenagers up to at least age 17; menarcheal adolescents are often referred to adult sexual assault programs for forensic examinations. An adolescent may achieve adulthood in terms of physical and sexual maturity by age 13, and some may reach menarche as early as 10 years old; however, an adolescent's cognitive development—including comprehension of complex and abstract concepts—is still incomplete. In addition to the incomplete cognitive development of adolescents, the psychological responses and needs of sexually victimized adolescents are distinctly different from those of adult victims.

The clinical approach to the adolescent is further complicated by issues of confidentiality and consent. What if an adolescent does not want her parent to know she was a victim of date rape? What if the patient does not consider his sexual relationship with a 23-year-old abusive, but the parent of that 23-year-old does? Under what circumstances should a clinician report sexual experiences involving an adolescent as abuse? Establishing an approach to the examination also raises questions: Are speculum exams always indicated or appropriate for female adolescents who are suspected victims of abuse? If the adolescent is sexually active, should testing for sexually transmitted infections (STIs) be done? If so, what kinds of tests for STIs should be used?

What is known is that adolescent victims of sexual abuse or assault face a greater likelihood of health-risky behaviors that include running away, delinquency, drug and alcohol use, unprotected or early sexual activity, and teenage pregnancy. Prevention of these deleterious sequelae and behaviors begins with the medical assessment. It is incumbent upon medical providers to address not only the emergent issues of medical needs and forensic collection, but also the long-term outcomes that may compromise the adolescent's development into a healthy adult.

Sexual abuse is a clinical diagnosis with legal, cultural, and health implications. The definition of sexual abuse is variable and encompasses a spectrum of circumstances including "date rape," incest, sexual activity that is consensual but illegal, sexual harassment, and on-line solicitation of a minor for sex. The diagnosis of sexual abuse in a clinical setting is frequently made based upon the medical history, because injuries, forensic evidence, and STIs are uncommonly present or unhelpful in determining whether sexual abuse or assault has occurred. Nonetheless, addressing the adolescent's medical and mental health concerns is critical in the management and prevention of short- and long-term deleterious effects of sexually abusive experiences.

DEFINITIONS AND VICTIM PERCEPTIONS OF ABUSIVE EXPERIENCES

While most clinicians understand their legal obligation to report suspected abuse, issues surrounding "the age of consent" and rights to confidential health care obfuscate the physician's role in providing for the health and well-being of their adolescent patients. All states have laws that mandate reporting of suspected child abuse and generally individuals are immune from liability as long as the report is made in good faith. However, the legal definition of which sexual acts are considered criminal and prosecutable varies somewhat from state to state. For example, if an adult fondles the buttocks of a child, this may be considered sexually abusive in some locales, but in other states such contact is not considered "indecency with a child" unless the anus is also touched. Most states utilize age parameters to define a "minor," and most states clearly indicate that any sexual activity between a minor and an adult is abusive and reportable. With regard to sexual activity between 2 consenting adolescents, some states require the clinician to make a report if it is their professional judgment that the contact is abusive (eg, lack of consent, drug-facilitated sexual assault), while other states require reporting based solely on age criteria. Still, other states provide age criteria for reporting sexual assault, but alter legal definitions for sexual assault among adolescents. For example, in one state, any sexual contact involving at least one minor under age 17 may be illegal and reportable, but if the adolescents are mutually consenting and both are between 14 and 17 years old, these conditions could be claimed as a defense during criminal proceedings. The clinician, however, is responsible for following reporting laws, not penal code laws that define the parameters of a crime.

In states where sexual acts involving 2 consenting adolescents are reportable because of age-defined criteria, such cases are generally not prosecuted. Recently, some states are attempting to reinterpret or reinstate child abuse reporting laws to require that clinicians report sexual abuse based on age criteria only. Proponents of this approach reason that minors do not have the knowledge necessary to consent to health-risky behavior such as sexual activity, and opine that mandated reporting will deter adolescents from engaging in sexual activity because of the threats of parental notification, humiliation, and criminal prosecution. It is not clear, though, which of the 2 (if not both) consenting adolescents would be prosecuted. Others, however, consider such laws significant deterrents to adolescent health care. Reporting all sexual activity involving minors would breach the adolescent's right to confidential health care and make them reluctant to seek or maintain health care. The care of adolescents who are sexually active and in need of health maintenance and prevention for pregnancy and STIs could be significantly compromised. There are no current data to support that age-based reporting laws would deter sexual activity among adolescents, but there is evidence that such laws would negatively affect an adolescent's willingness to share sexual health information with their health care provider.[1,2] The long-term effects of such laws could be detrimental to the health of adolescents if they do not seek health care and STIs and pregnancies are undetected and untreated. In Kansas, for example, physicians filed suit and successfully opposed the attorney general's attempt to reinterpret child abuse laws based solely on age criteria.[3]

In a clinical setting, sexual abuse may encompass a variety of contact and non-contact sexual encounters that affect the health and well-being of the patient. For example, sexual harassment may result in significant anxiety and school refusal in some adolescents, yet is not defined as a reportable act or crime. Teens may fabricate symptoms to avoid going to school. Such harassment now extends to the Internet as students may receive sexually explicit or insulting material from others. In one study, 20% of adolescents were solicited for sex by strangers through the Internet.[4]

Although medical and mental health consequences are commonly associated with sexual abuse or assault, symptoms and severity vary considerably. Adolescents are often embarrassed and ashamed, but some present clinically behind a veneer of apparent nonchalance in speaking about their abuse, consistent with feelings of invincibility common to mid-adolescence. The clinician should not allow a cavalier or obstinate demeanor in an adolescent who is a suspected victim of sexual abuse to dissuade her or him from this diagnosis.

The victim's perception is yet another facet of how abuse is defined and identified. For example, many adolescents feel that rape must include a beating or bodily injury and that the absence of such means the act was not abusive, and therefore not reportable. Many do not realize that a verbal refusal is sufficient to establish the parameters of a rape. About one third of all sexual abuse victims blame themselves to some degree for the assault or abuse.[5] Self-blame can, in turn, influence whether a victim labels a sexual assault as abuse. Self-blame can derive from illogical ideas such as "if I weren't there, it would not have happened." In a study of 5829 ninth graders in Denmark, 1.3% of boys and 4.5% of girls had sexual experiences with a person at least 5 years older but did not perceive the experiences as abusive.[6] Clinicians can play a key role in helping victims appropriately recognize sexually abusive experiences.

CLINICAL PRESENTATIONS

About 90% of sexual assault or abuse is first detected when a victim discloses the abuse to a third party.[7] Sexual abuse is uncommonly diagnosed when a patient presents to a clinical setting with symptoms or signs of anogenital trauma or infection; fewer than 10% of children and adolescents with a history of sexual abuse or assault will have injuries or infections indicative of abuse.[8] In addition, the presence of visible anogenital trauma does not necessarily differentiate consensual and abusive causes. The severity or number of anogenital injuries may not correlate with the likelihood that the assault was non-consensual; the injuries should be interpreted within the context of a medical history. Bodily injury—such as ligature marks or bruises on the victim's forearms sustained during an attempt to protect his or her face from an attacker's blows—may provide more specific evidence of assault. In addition, adolescents who present to clinical settings with signs of alcohol or drug toxicity should be questioned carefully about the possibility of sexual assault. Many state laws include provisions for drug-facilitated sexual assault when a person is unable to consent because of impairment from such substances. The clinician should be especially concerned by the possibility of sexual assault if the patient gives a history of drinking small amounts of alcohol or another drink followed by a rapid onset of altered mental status or brief alternating periods of impairment and lucidity; such symptoms suggest drink spiking with intent to facilitate sexual assault.

Victims occasionally present with STIs; these infections are rare in adolescents who are not sexually active, but common among sexually active adolescents and young adults. The presence of an STI in a patient who is sexually active and also sexually assaulted has no forensic significance as the origin of the STI cannot be reliably determined. However, sexual abuse in childhood is correlated with earlier and unprotected sexual activity in adolescence. The presence of an STI should prompt the clinician to ask the adolescent about the type and nature of all previous sexual contact, including non-consensual and abusive encounters. It is important to remember that the presence of an

STI does not always imply sexual contact as the only mode of transmission. Familiarity with different modes of transmission will assist the clinician in the appropriate interpretation of results of laboratory tests for STIs.

Adolescent victims of sexual assault are rarely detected based on an assessment of behavioral symptoms, although it is widely acknowledged that many adolescents do have behavioral symptoms caused by sexual abuse and may not disclose their abuse even when queried directly. Many victims are also asymptomatic, accommodating to the abuse and effectively hiding their symptoms of anxiety, depression, and post traumatic dissociation. Mood swings typical of adolescence may mask or conceal symptoms attributable to victimization. As with detection of an STI, behavioral changes and problems should prompt the clinician to ask screening questions regarding abuse and violence, including sexual assault.

If a patient presents with a history of sexual abuse or assault, or the patient reveals sexual abuse during the course of a medical assessment, the clinician should be aware of the options and resources available in deciding the best course of action. When the assault has occurred within the previous 72 hours, the patient should be referred immediately for forensic evidence collection. These examinations are usually conducted at regional hospitals by sexual assault nurse examiners (SANEs) or physicians. Very rarely, a victim may present with genital injuries that require hemostasis and laceration repair; these patients should also be referred at once to a hospital setting, preferably one with an established sexual assault program.

Most adolescent victims of sexual assault, however, do not require immediate medical attention and many present for examinations more than 72 hours after sexual contact, obviating the need for forensic evidence collection. The urgency of the medical assessment for these patients depends primarily upon emotional and physical symptoms, as well as the need for establishing a safety plan to protect the victim from further abuse. There are many well-established programs that provide medical evaluations, victim assistance, and crisis counseling for victims of sexual abuse. In the US, medical evaluations of children and adolescents are usually conducted by experienced and trained pediatricians or nurses as well as gynecologists, emergency medicine physicians, and family practitioners. In regions where such programs are available, the clinician should refer the patient for complete medical assessment and treatment. A report to child protective services or law enforcement should be made immediately; referral to a specialty program does not preclude the clinician's legal obligation to report.

Programs that specialize in the assessment and treatment of pediatric sexual assault or abuse victims can provide valuable guidance to clinicians. Many parents present to clinicians with the concern that their teen has been sexually abused based on an observed physical or behavioral symptom. The TEAMHEALTH approach (**Table 6-1**) provides some general approaches for the medical history that can also be utilized in situations when abuse is suspected but the adolescent has not disclosed it.

CLINICAL EVALUATION

The TEAMHEALTH approach (**Table 6-1**) outlines the scope of clinical care for adolescents who are suspected victims of sexual abuse or assault and encompasses the medical history, clinical assessment, treatment, and follow-up care. The components are not presented as an inclusive protocol or in a suggested sequence; while some adolescents may benefit from a rapport-building introduction to the medical history that includes discussion of less embarrassing or intrusive topics, other adolescents may respond better to a direct approach, beginning with the reason for the office visit. In the

---

Table 6-1. The TEAMHEALTH Approach

MEDICAL HISTORY

T	**T**ell them your agenda
E	**E**arn trust
A	**A**ssure safety
	— Family history, support by non-abusive parent, protection of abuser or concern for integrity of family
	— Health-risky behaviors, including drug and alcohol use, runaway tendencies, self-harm behaviors, and unsafe sexual activity
M	**M**edical history
	— Past medical and gynecologic history
	— Physical and emotional symptoms
	— Sexual/physical victimization
	— Behavioral symptoms

MEDICAL EXAMINATION

H	**H**ead-to-toe examination
E	**E**vidence collection: clothing/linens, foreign debris, orifice swabs, serology
A	**A**ssess for bodily, oral, anal, and genital injury
L	**L**essen embarrassment and anxiety (keep parts of body not being examined draped)
T	**T**est
	— Sexually transmitted diseases
	— Pregnancy
	— Toxicology for drugs, alcohol
H	**H**ealing
	— Referral for counseling, mental health assessments, crisis support
	— Treatment of injuries, STIs, intoxication
	— Prophylaxis for STIs, pregnancy
	— Follow-up to ensure healing, complete assessment for STIs with prolonged incubation periods

---

latter situation, the clinician may gather a brief past medical history prior to asking what the adolescent's understanding of the purpose of the visit is. After gathering information about the abuse, the remainder of the medical history, including behavioral and emotional responses to the abuse, can be gathered.

As most adolescents do not have injuries, forensic evidence, or an STI that provides specific evidence of sexual assault or abuse, medical diagnosis and treatment often rely on the patient's history. The extent to which a medical history is gathered depends on clinician expertise and comfort level, the local investigative procedures for interviewing victims, the victim's willingness to talk, and the context within which the victim first discloses. For example, if an adolescent discloses sexual abuse for the first time within a clinical setting, the clinician may encourage and support the patient by allowing him or her to share any information, but may defer the complete assessment to an experienced sexual abuse unit. The clinician still needs to gather information necessary to assess the patient's immediate medical, psychological, and safety needs. Such information is best gathered from the patient directly, out of the presence of family members. Family members may be supportive, distraught, unsupportive, or disbelieving—all of which can impact the victim's willingness to disclose information to the clinician.

MEDICAL HISTORY
Tell Them Your Agenda
The clinician should begin the interview by stating his or her role in the adolescent's health care and what is known about the reason for the adolescent's visit ("As your doctor, it's my job to find ways to help you keep healthy and safe. I understand something sexual or physical may have happened to you. I'd like to ask some questions so we can come up with a plan that can help you.") If abuse has not been disclosed, the clinician might instead say, "I am going to ask you some questions about how your body is doing, how your feelings are doing, how your life is going, and about any hurtful or uncomfortable things that may have happened to you. The reason I am asking these questions is so I can figure out what I need to check you for, what tests I might need to do, and how I can best help you with your health." In addition, it is important for the clinician to explain the limits of confidentiality to the adolescent: "If we talk about something that places you or someone else in danger, I may have to share this with your parents or someone else who can make sure people are safe."

Earn Trust
Because a victim's trust is often violated during abuse, it is important for the clinician to establish rather than expect trust. Truthfully disclosing the clinical agenda (see above) is the first step, as is providing an explanation of the procedures and of the purpose of the various components of the medical assessment. The cooperative nature of the medical evaluation should be stressed, as some adolescents may view the process as something they are undergoing for their parents, the police, the authorities, or the physician, rather than for themselves. A nonjudgmental, clinically focused approach reduces anxiety in the patient and facilitates information sharing.

When the adolescent confides his or her feelings and reactions to abuse, the clinician should acknowledge these feelings. Adolescents may describe shame, guilt, fear, or embarrassment about their victimization, family life, criminal behavior, and health-risky lifestyle. They will be sensitive to the responses of health professionals as they disclose and share feelings about these circumstances. Clinicians should maintain a nonjudgmental demeanor, restate their reasons for asking such questions, and acknowledge that such feelings are normal among children in similar circumstances: "I know this is hard for you to talk about. I have talked with other teens about this, and it is hard for them, too. These questions will help me decide whether I should check you for sexually transmitted infections. If you feel more comfortable, you can write down or whisper your answers instead of saying them out loud. I really need your help before I can decide how to best help you."

Assure Safety
Family History, Support by Non-Abusive Parent, Protection of Abuser, or Concern for Integrity of Family
In one study, more than half of the children and teens evaluated in a sexual abuse clinic reported past or present domestic violence in their home.[7] Risk of serious injury and

death may arise if an adult victim of violence leaves the abuser when it is discovered that the abuser has also sexually assaulted one or more of the children in the home. In addition, up to 40% of mothers of sexual abuse victims either don't believe their child or are unsure that abuse occurred[7]; in these circumstances, teens may recant their abuse history to avoid jeopardizing the parent-child relationship and to preserve the integrity of the family. Similarly, one-third of victims feel ambivalent toward their abuser, and may withdraw their statements of abuse to protect the abuser or the integrity of the family. Clinicians may uncover these concerns by asking adolescents how much they think their non-abusive parent believes or supports them and by asking what outcome or outcomes they would prefer for their family and the abuser. If victims appear protective of their abuser and disclose only low-risk types of sexual contact, the clinician may wish to test for STIs anyway in the event that not all abuse details have been disclosed. In addition, clinicians should explicitly ask whether victims are afraid of their parents or of going home.

Another area that adolescents may have concerns about is the effect of their abuse on siblings. The clinician may ask how siblings are responding to recent family changes or how they are responding to the abuse (if they are aware it took place).

Health-Risky Behaviors
Adolescent victims of abuse may suffer suicidal thoughts and may engage in unhealthy activities, including cutting, overdosing on medications or recreational drugs, unprotected sex, sexual activity with multiple partners, runaway behavior, criminal activity, and drug or alcohol abuse. Substance use and sexual assault are strongly associated; in one large study sample, drug abuse and alcohol intoxication among adolescents were associated with a risk of sexual assault 1.5 to 4.7 times greater than that among adolescents who did not abuse drugs or alcohol.[9] Substance abuse tends to be a peer group activity, and it is not uncommon for such a peer group to engage in other health-risky behaviors, including unprotected sexual activity and sexual assault. **Table 6-2** provides a useful screening tool for adolescent substance abuse.

Table 6-2. CRAFFT Screening Test for Adolescent Substance Abuse

C	— Have you ever ridden in a **CAR** driven by someone (including yourself) who was "high" or had been using alcohol or drugs?
R	— Do you ever use alcohol or drugs to **RELAX**, feel better about yourself, or fit in?
A	— Do you ever use alcohol/drugs while you are by yourself, **ALONE**?
F	— Do your family or **FRIENDS** ever tell you that you should cut down on your drinking or drug use?
F	— Do you ever **FORGET** things you did while using alcohol or drugs?
T	— Have you gotten into **TROUBLE** while you were using alcohol or drugs?

Reprinted from CeASAR: The Center for Adolescent Substance Abuse Research. The CRAFFT questions. Available at: http://www.slp3d2.com/rwj_1027/webcast/docs/screentest.html. Accessed October 19, 2010.

Medical Issues

The components of the medical history that are pertinent to sexual assault are not significantly different from any other medical care and include the following:

— *Past medical history* includes chronic medical conditions that may affect the anogenital examination findings. Examples include neurologic conditions that affect anorectal or pubic muscle laxity, labial adhesions, and Crohn's disease.

— *Gynecologic history* begins with menarche (years of menstruation correlates with regularity of cycles) and addresses last menstrual period (need for pregnancy testing), regularity of cycles and menstrual volume (need for pregnancy testing), and prior gynecologic exam/tampon use (may be better prepared to tolerate sexual abuse/assault examination; painful tampon insertion has been associated with hymenal findings).[10]

— *Sexual history* details types of prior sexual contact with male or female partners, last consensual and last abusive contact (STI risk; interpretation of exam findings with regards to abuse/assault—acute findings may be specific to assault only if consensual contact is remote), and use of barrier contraception (STI risk). When gathering a sexual history, it is important to acknowledge the possibility of alternative sexual identity or orientation in the adolescent. For example, the clinician may inquire whether the adolescent has ever had or thought about having sexual experiences with males, females, or both, and what questions or concerns the adolescent might have about those thoughts.

— *Current and past sexual victimization* includes the type or types of sexual contact (sites for STI and forensic evidence collection), the time since the last sexual contact (timing of STI testing), the frequency of intervals between sexual contact (STI risk), the number of abusers (STI risk, interpretation of exam results), the penetrative types of sexual contact (pain or bleeding may be associated with penetration but not necessarily signs of physical injury), the use of lubricant (may decrease likelihood of injury), the use of condoms (may decrease STI risk), and any abuser risk factors if known (IV drug user, multiple sexual partners of same or different gender, gang member: more extensive STI testing recommended).

— *Physical symptoms and concerns* include conditions that may obscure exam findings (eg, encopresis and obesity may make it more difficult to visualize the hymen and vestibule), conditions that may be sequelae of abuse (eg, dysuria after genital contact, pain or bleeding after penetration, painful defecation, and vaginal or anal discharge as signifiers of a potential STI), and symptoms reported by patients that may reflect anxiety/concerns related to abuse rather than medical causes (eg, genital pain, discharge, enlarging stomach, and nausea as potential indicators of pregnancy). Although exam findings often do not reflect reported symptoms, the clinician needs to provide appropriate reassurance.

— *Behavioral symptoms* are also a cause for concern; more commonly reported symptoms include sleeping difficulties such as nightmares, trouble falling or staying asleep (symptoms of anxiety, intrusive memories), and school or work difficulties that may include trouble concentrating or staying on task because of intrusive thoughts of abuse. Adolescents should also be screened for anxiety, depression, self-injurious behaviors, eating disorders, and dissociative symptoms.

MEDICAL EXAMINATION

While it is preferable to conduct the interview out of the presence of family members and friends, the patient should be allowed to have a support person present during the examination portion. Many adolescents prefer not to include a parent but may opt for the presence of a sibling or friend.

Head-to-Toe Examination

It is important for the clinician to not focus solely on the genitals during the sexual assault examination. Many adolescents have some degree of anxiety regarding the examination because it is embarrassing or because they expect discomfort, and may have been told that a speculum examination would be done. In many cases, the adolescent has not had a health maintenance examination for years, and the clinician may use this opportunity to perform needed health screening, including immunizations. Performing the general and more familiar pediatric examination may also facilitate cooperation and lower anxiety as the exam progresses to include the abdomen, genitals, and anus.

Evidence Collection

Most states provide standardized evidence collection kits with detailed instructions for collecting, processing, packaging, and maintaining the chain of forensic evidence. If the clinician determines that sexual assault likely occurred within the previous 72 hours, a prompt referral to a specialized program with trained sexual assault examiners is strongly urged. Evidence collection requires not only adherence to state protocols and expert examiners, but also specialized equipment and sufficient space to ensure appropriate processing and maintenance of a chain of custody for forensic materials. Clinicians that opt to collect evidence must familiarize themselves with all necessary procedures and protocols prior to conducting any part of the examination. Forensic material is time-sensitive, so collection must occur as soon as feasible.

In general, evidence collection should be done prior to other exam procedures. Most protocols require the victim to unclothe over paper or a sheet, which is submitted for debris analysis. Then, samples are taken from the oral cavity, head hair, pubic hair, fingernails, genitals, genital orifices, anus, and any areas potentially containing apparent dried secretions or bite marks are swabbed. The areas sampled depend upon the specific protocol instructions, the history of assault, and prior examination findings.

Samples are air-dried, sealed, and signed in accordance with chain of custody procedures. Typically, the sealed kit is retained in a locked, secured freezer until it is retrieved by law enforcement. State forensic labs process the contents for DNA and genetic markers; some labs process the samples with less sensitive or specific tests such as acid phosphatase and P30 protein. Forensic analysis of samples continues to evolve and improve, and will likely affect the procedures and time frame for forensic evidence collection in the future.

Assess for Bodily, Oral, Genital, and Anal Injuries

Victims of acute assault should be examined carefully for bruises, especially involving the face, neck, and head (more common sites for blows) as well as the forearms and lower extremities (more common sites for defensive injuries). While areas of tenderness may be noted, the clinician should be cautious in attributing such findings to trauma without accompanying erythema, ecchymoses, or edema; muscle strain and anxiety are other possible causes. **Table 6-3** provides examples of bodily injuries that have been associated with sexual assault. See **Figures 6-1** through **6-9** for examples of genital and anal injuries.

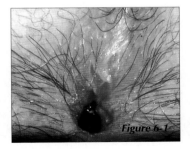

Figure 6-1. Adolescent who denied anal penetration and denied any pain or bleeding in her anal area. In the prone knee-chest position, 2 tears are seen at 12 and 1 o'clock.

Forced oral-penile penetration may result in intra-oral injuries, possibly accompanied by grasp marks or bruises to the cheeks or

Table 6-3. Nongenital Injuries in Assault Victims	
TYPE	POSSIBLE MECHANISIM
Perioral or intraoral injuries, especially erythema/petechiae near junction of hard/soft palate	Hand restraint (voice muffling) Forced penile-oral penetration
Neck bruises, "hickies"	Choke by hand or ligature Suction/bite
Oval or semicircular bruises to neck, chest, breasts, extremities	Bite
Impact bruises to face, body, especially lips and eyes; intra-abdominal hematomas or organ rupture	Penetrating blow with fist
Impact bruises to extensor surfaces of upper/lower arms, knuckles	Defense injuries (victim tries to protect head with arms)
Traumatic alopecia, subgaleal hematoma	Hair-pulling
Numerous small (2-3 cm) bruises on shoulders, arms, thighs, face	Hand restraint bruises or grab marks
Ligature marks to wrists/ankles	Restraint with rope or wire
Abrasions, friction injuries to bony prominences of back	Victim struggle while restrained in supine position on firm surface

neck. Petecchial hemorrhages associated with forced penetration generally occur at the junction of the soft and hard palate, near the uvula.

Genital injuries from sexual assault are uncommon. While erythema and superficial excoriations of the vestibule and vulva are frequently noted, such findings are non-specific for trauma. Acute injuries of sexual assault most frequently occur in the posterior vestibule, between the posterior attachment of the hymen and the posterior commissure. Other acute injuries include lacerations of the hymen, bruising of the hymen, and abrasions and bruising of the vestibule or inner labia minora folds (**Figure 6-5**). Findings that indicate healed penetrative trauma of the hymen include lateral and posterior clefts (defects in the hymen between the 3 and 9 o'clock positions that extend the entire width of the hymen at a discrete point), and scarring in the posterior vestibule (scarring that is palpable or causes contraction of surrounding tissue) (**Figures 6-6, 6-7,** and **6-8**). An evidence-based classification system indicates that deep notches extending more than 50% of the width of the hymen located in the posterior half of the hymen are indeterminate findings for healed penetrative trauma although they have been described in sexually abused females.[11] The majority of acute injuries heal without sequelae or scarring in a matter of a few days (**Figures 6-4-a** and **b**). In one large patient series of children and adolescents who were examined for acute and non-acute sexual assault, 96% had normal or nonspecific findings of penetrative trauma.[8] While "it's normal to be normal," "normal" does not mean "nothing happened"[12]; in a study of 36 adolescents undergoing sexual abuse examinations while pregnant, 82% had normal "intact" hymens and no scarring.[13]

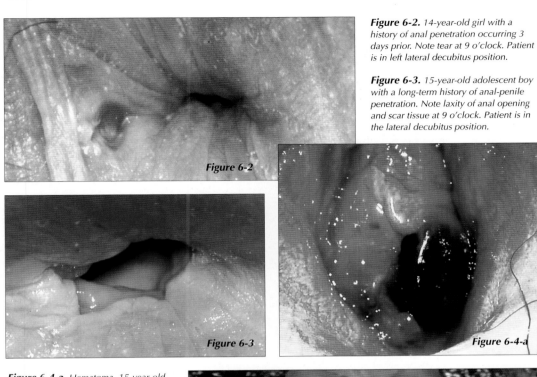

Figure 6-2. *14-year-old girl with a history of anal penetration occurring 3 days prior. Note tear at 9 o'clock. Patient is in left lateral decubitus position.*

Figure 6-3. *15-year-old adolescent boy with a long-term history of anal-penile penetration. Note laxity of anal opening and scar tissue at 9 o'clock. Patient is in the lateral decubitus position.*

Figure 6-4-a. *Hematoma. 15-year-old victim of vaginal-penile penetration 36 hours previously.*

Figure 6-4-b. *Same patient, 5 days after initial exam.*

Figure 6-5. *5-year-old girl victim of vaginal-penile penetration occurring 36 hours earlier. Complete hymenal tear at 6 o'clock, and posterior vestibule tear with bruising.*

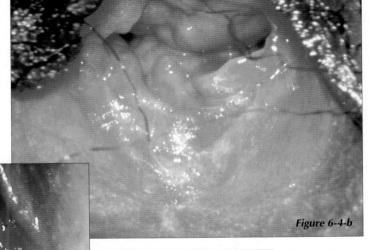

Figure 6-6. *Adolescent female with several hymenal clefts, resulting in isolated "clumps" of hymen (caruncles). There is no visible hymenal tissue from 4 to 8 o'clock.*

Figure 6-7.
Healed tear, or cleft, from 5 to 7 o'clock.

Figure 6-8.
Posterior vestibule scar and large area from 4 to 8 o'clock of no visible hymenal tissue.

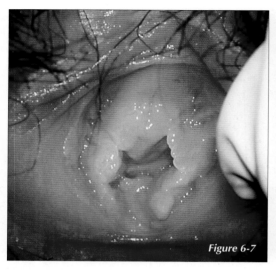

Figure 6-7

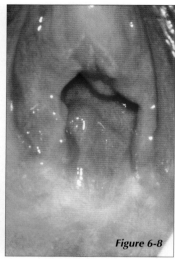

Figure 6-8

Anal findings of acute or healed penetrative trauma are rarer than genital findings. Acute findings include deep anal tears, usually in a stellate pattern close to the 12 and 6 o'clock midline, and hematomas, which should not be confused with hemorrhoids or venous pooling (**Figures 6-1, 6-2,** and **6-3**). Healed penetrative trauma of the anus is exceedingly rare; any scarring should be confirmed by palpation or observed contraction of the tissue (**Figure 6-9**). Anal dilatation, once thought to be an indicator of acute or chronic penetration, is a non-specific finding for sexual abuse and can be attributable to a number of non-traumatic and physiologic causes.

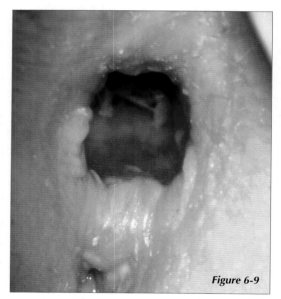

Figure 6-9

Figure 6-9. *13-year-old female victim of repeated anal-penile penetration by 2 individuals over a period of 3-4 years. Extensive perianal scarring and immediate anal sphincter dilatation is noted (patient is in the prone knee-chest position). The absence of stool in the anal vault and the presence of other traumatic findings supports trauma as the cause of this dilatation. The child also reported some difficulty with fecal incontinence over the past year.*

Lessen Embarrassment and Anxiety by Keeping Parts of Body Not Being Examined Draped

Adolescents are self-conscious and embarrassed about various features of their bodies. Most have considerable reluctance and, in some cases, resistance to having their genitals, anus, or breasts examined. Such concerns can be partly assuaged by ensuring that these private areas of the body are uncovered for as little time as possible.

The examination positions and techniques can be difficult to master effectively. The ability of the clinician to see the often subtle signs of trauma depends on their technical and judicious use of exam techniques as well as the ability of the patient to relax the pelvic and gluteal muscles during the anogenital component of the examination. Chapter 5 describes the examination techniques in more detail.

Testing for STIs, Pregnancy, Drugs and Alcohol

When an adolescent presents within 72 hours of a sexual assault, forensic evidence, including swabs of orifices, should be collected prior to conducting tests for STIs. Appropriate testing for STIs requires consideration of the time since the assault, symptoms, risk factors, the purpose of the test, availability of the test, and the cooperation of the adolescent. The optimal time to test for STIs depends on the incubation period of the STI in question. For example, most initial medical assessments for sexual assault involve testing for gonorrhea, chlamydia, and sometimes trichomonas, as these are the more common STIs and because infected individuals are often asymptomatic. Based on the incubation periods of these infections, an optimal time to test is at least 10-14 days after the sexual assault; if the sexual contact has occurred over several weeks or months, adolescents can be tested at the time of their evaluation even if the most recent sexual abuse occurred within 10 days. Variable testing schedules reflect variable incubation periods. Chapter 10 discusses STIs in more depth.

A sexually assaulted adolescent who presents with symptoms or signs such as dysuria, genital discharge, ulcers, or verruceous lesions may require more extensive testing for STIs. Adolescents with symptoms often presume the worst and a negative test may provide reassurance. Similarly, adolescents may worry that they have an infection even when they are asymptomatic, especially if the assailant is a stranger or if the teen has heard that the assailant has an STI. It is important for the clinician to address these concerns, and testing may be the most effective way to provide reassurance.

The primary role of the clinician is to provide for the health and well-being of the patient, although each procedure and test can be subjected to legal scrutiny in a court of law. These dual roles of clinical and forensic assessment present some controversy, particularly when selecting diagnostic tests for gonorrhea and chlamydia. This choice is most difficult when testing for chlamydia. While the culture is considered the legal "gold standard," its sensitivity is low, averaging 60-70%. Nucleic acid amplification tests are more sensitive, but the Centers for Disease Control and Prevention requires 2 of these tests, targeting different genomes of the organism, to equate the result to a gold standard, an approach that is costly and requires that the child be retested. In a significant majority of cases, the diagnosis of sexual abuse is based on the victim's history, not the exam findings. If the clinician feels confident in the diagnosis prior to conducting the exam, then the clinician may wish to use the STI tests to optimize the management of the patient rather than to diagnose sexual abuse; in which case, the clinician should become familiar with the test used so that the rationale for choosing the test can be adequately explained if court testimony is required. If the clinician wishes to legally confirm the diagnosis of sexual abuse, then the gold standard may be the appropriate test. In victims with prior sexual contact with another abuser or with a partner, testing for STIs no longer has forensic significance to the abuse, so the most sensitive and specific test is appropriate.

Prior to selecting the type of STI diagnostic test, the clinician should become familiar with the equipment and materials needed at the clinical site to conduct the test, the capability of local laboratories to process the test, and the expertise of laboratory personnel in processing and interpreting such tests. In some hospitals, for example, chlamydia culture is no longer available, while other regions lack the capability to process nucleic acid amplification tests.

Finally, it is important to consider the adolescent's ability and willingness to cooperate with the examination. Adolescents may deny penetration that has, in fact, occurred, and refuse the exam because they think the doctor will be able to determine from the examination that they've had sex. Others refuse the exam because of extreme embarrassment and shame. Some may become distraught during the genital portion of the exam. If the patient cannot cooperate, the clinician may opt to defer the tests until later, not test, or send a urine nucleic acid amplification test for gonorrhea and chlamydia (if available). Similarly, vaginal swabs can be obtained instead of cervical samples if the adolescent is anxious and has not had a speculum exam prior to the sexual assault examination.

Other Diagnostic Tests

The clinician should evaluate the need for pregnancy and drug testing, depending on the history and clinical presentation of the victim. If the adolescent is menarcheal, a pregnancy test should be conducted and confirmed as negative prior to giving post-coital contraception. Because adolescents do not always report their menstrual history with accuracy, the clinician should test for pregnancy whenever there is a concern. A drug test (urine or serum or both, depending on the time frame and symptoms) or an electrolyte panel should be submitted whenever the victim reports ingestion of a substance that altered his or her mental status or there are signs of intoxication on examination. Drug-facilitated sexual assault is a recognized entity, and while alcohol remains the single most commonly used substance in such cases, drugs such as Xanax, ketamine, Rohypnol, gamma hydroxybutyric acid, and even insulin have been employed by assailants.

Serologic tests for syphilis, AIDS, and hepatitis should be done when risk factors in the abuser are present or unknown, if the patient or family requests it, or if the patient is found to have at least one STI. As most adolescents have been immunized for Hepatitis B, serology is rarely needed, but if immunization status is unknown, adolescents can be given one dose of the vaccine as prophylaxis. HIV prophylaxis remains controversial, but can be given when the assailant is known to be HIV-positive and the victim presents within 72 hours of the assault; baseline tests for renal and bone marrow function are also required at the time of the initial medical evaluation.

Healing

Healing for the adolescent victim of sexual abuse or assault is the most comprehensive phase of the TEAMHEALTH approach. While the focus tends to be on the components that take minutes to gather—injuries, STI, and forensic materials—the health harms of sexual abuse can extend for years. For example, once the abuse has been reported and the initial medical assessment completed, it can take up to 3 years or longer for the criminal trial to occur. During this time, the adolescent and his or her family receive numerous subpoenas and trial reset notices, constant reminders of the abuse, and potential triggers for emotional distress. During this period, the clinician can provide reassurance and be a resource for the adolescent and his or her family.

Comprehensive, long-term management of the sexual abuse or assault survivor must encompass the medical, mental health, and safety needs of the victim. Immediate medical needs include surgical or medical management of acute injuries, STI prophylaxis (**Table 6-4**), and postcoital contraception in cases where the sexual assault involves penile contact or penetration occurring within 5 days of the examination and the pregnancy test is negative. Plan B, Ovral, and LoOvral are approved options as of early 2009 and may be available over-the-counter in some regions. Victims of acute sexual assault may also be candidates for STI prophylaxis against Chlamydia, gonorrhea, and, in some cases, trichomonas and HIV. Prophylaxis for HIV is costly and requires several weeks of antiviral medication with significant side effects; the efficacy of this prophylaxis is currently unknown.

It is important to provide appropriate medical follow-up, especially for victims of acute sexual assault, given the prolonged incubation period of some STIs, such as human papillomavirus (HPV). **Table 6-5** provides guidelines for medical follow-up evaluations. Because HPV is one of the more prevalent STIs, a follow-up exam 2-3 weeks after the initial evaluation and, in some cases, again several months later is recommended to optimize detection of this disease, which carries risk of cancer later in life. Although there is no formal recommendation at this time, female victims of acute sexual assault may benefit from treatment with the HPV vaccine. Follow-up examinations also provide opportunities for the clinician to reassure the victim of injury resolution and to assess any need for further mental health services. The adolescent should be screened for depression and self-injurious thoughts and behaviors during follow-up appointments.

The clinician can play a key role in the emotional recovery of the victim and the family. Victims and family members may have a number of fears and anxieties, some of which can be alleviated by the clinician. For example, victims and family members may be wondering whether the victim is still a "virgin," or may believe the abuse did not occur when they are told the exam is "normal." Clinicians may clarify such terms, and provide reassurance that "normal" does not mean "nothing happened." Some victims feel guilty

Table 6-4. Management of Uncomplicated Sexually Transmitted Diseases in Adolescent* Victims of Sexual Abuse

Organism	Prophylactic Treatment	Treatment of Confirmed Disease
Gonorrhea	Cefixime 400 mg PO† x 1 or ceftriaxone 125 mg IM x 1 PLUS treatment for chlamydia	Same as for prophylaxis
Chlamydia	Azithromycin 1 g PO x 1 PLUS treatment for gonorrhea	Azithromycin 1 g PO x 1 or Doxycycline 200 mg/d (BID) x 7 days
Hepatitis	Begin or complete hepatitis A and B immunization	None
Trichomonas, bacterial vaginosis	Metronidazole 2 g PO x 1	Metronidazole 2 g PO x 1 or 250 mg TID x 7 days
Syphilis‡	(Gonorrhea prophylaxis has efficacy against incubating syphilis)	Benzathine penicillin G 2.4 million U IM x 1 or doxycycline 200 mg/d (BID) PO x 14 days
Herpes simplex virus type 2	None	Acyclovir 1000-1200 mg/d (3-5 x /d) PO x 7-10 d
Human papillomavirus	None	Patient administered: Podofilox .5% solution or gel or Imiquimod 5% cream Clinician administered: Podophyllin, trichloracetic acid, cryotherapy, or surgical excision
Human immuno-deficiency virus	Consider if high-risk contact occurs: zidovudine 150 mg (BID) x 4 weeks	Consult with infectious disease specialist

*Includes preadolescents weighing > 100 lbs.
†Abbreviations: PO=orally, IM=intramuscularly, BID=2 times daily, TID=3 times daily.
‡CSF examination is recommended for those with central nervous system symptoms.
Adapted from American Academy of Pediatrics. 2000 Red Book: Report of the Committee on Infectious Diseases. 25th ed. Elk Grove Village, Il: American Academy of Pediatrics; 2000.

Table 6-5. Follow-up Considerations for Victims of Sexual Trauma

2 WEEKS

1. Healing of injuries

2. Type 2 herpes simplex virus: 3-10 days incubation

3. Trichomoniasis, bacterial vaginosis, chlamydia, gonorrhea: 10-14 days incubation (if no initial prophylaxis given)

4. Pregnancy (if oral contraception is not provided at initial evaluation)

5. Psychological support/reassurance of patient and family

6. Drug/alcohol monitoring/treatment (if coordinated with specialist)

2-3 MONTHS

1. HIV testing: repeat at 6 weeks, 3 months, 6 months, 1 year

2. Syphilis and hepatitis: 6-8 weeks incubation

3. Human papillomavirus: 2-3 months average incubation; up to 20 months incubation in rare cases

4. Psychological support of patient and family

5. Drug/alcohol monitoring (if coordinated with specialist)

Adapted from Kellogg ND, Sugarek NJ. Sexual trauma. Atlas of Office Procedures. 1998;1(1):181-197.

because they delayed their disclosure; the clinician can reassure them that most victims delay their disclosure because of a variety of valid fears. The clinician can also provide encouragement that recovery from sexual assault and return to normalcy is possible.

It is critically important for the clinician to encourage and facilitate the use of community supports and services for victims and their families. Children's Advocacy Centers and regional rape crisis organizations often provide crisis services or referrals to victims of sexual abuse or assault, which can be of significant benefit to victims and family members immediately following the assault and in the difficult weeks and months that follow. Therapists trained and skilled in treating adolescent sexual assault victims are another valuable resource

DOCUMENTATION

Documentation during all phases of the TEAMHEALTH approach is essential, especially because any of the information gathered may become significant in court proceedings. To the extent that it is possible, the clinician should document the questions asked and the patient's answers as direct quotations. This is particularly important if the victim is disclosing abuse for the first time, as the circumstances of the "first outcry" are critical to the investigation and legal proceedings that follow. Examination findings should be carefully documented, with extensive details of any visible injuries supported by high-quality photographs. Location, size, color, and characteristics such as bleeding and abrasions should be noted on bodily or anogenital findings. The clinician should provide a meaningful interpretation of the findings for non-medical professionals involved in investigation. If the medical diagnosis of sexual abuse is based primarily on the patient's history, the clinician should document this, adding that most examinations of sexually abused adolescents are normal or nonspecific.

CONCLUSION

The medical assessment of an adolescent who is a suspected victim of sexual abuse or assault presents challenges that are distinctly different from evaluations of prepubertal children or adults. The TEAMHEALTH approach provides a framework for gathering the medical history, conducting a thorough examination for injuries, utilizing the appropriate diagnostic tests, and providing for the physical and emotional healing of the adolescent victim. In meeting these challenges of clinical care, the clinician is also presented with an opportunity to facilitate recovery and to promote a transition into healthy adulthood. TEAMHEALTH is a reminder that restoring health after sexual assault or abuse is achieved through a cooperative bond between the physician and his or her adolescent patient.

REFERENCES

1. Miller CA, Tebb KP, Williams JK, Neuhaus JM and Shafer M. Chlamydial screening in urgent care visits. *Arch Pediatr Adol Med.* 2007;161(8):777-782.

2. Klein JD, Wilson K. Delivering quality care: adolescents' discussion of health risks with their providers. *J Adolesc Health.* 2002;30(3):190-195.

3. Aid for Women et al v. Nola Foulston et al. Case No 6: 03-cv-01353-JTM-DWB, 2005.

4. Mitchell KJ, Finkelhor D, Wolak J. Risk factors for and impact of online sexual solicitation of youth. *JAMA.* 2001;285:3011-3014.

5. Kellogg ND, Hoffman TJ. Unwanted and illegal sexual experiences in childhood and adolescence. *Child Abuse Negl.* 1995;19(12):1457-1468.

6. Helweg-Larsen K, Larsen HB. The prevalence of unwanted and unlawful sexual experiences reported by Danish adolescents: Results from a national youth survey in 2002. *Acta Paediat.* 2006;95:1270-1276.

7. Kellogg ND, Menard SW. Violence among family members of children and adolescents evaluated for sexual abuse. *Child Abuse Negl.* 2003;27(12):1367-1376.

8. Heger A, Ticson L, Velasquez O, Bernier R. Children referred for possible sexual abuse: medical findings in 2384 children. *Child Abuse Negl.* 2002;26:645-659.

9. Raghavan R, Bogart LM, Elliott MN, Vestal KD, Schuster MA. Sexual victimization among a national probability sample of adolescent women. *Perspect Sex Reprod Health.* 2004;36(6):225-232.

10. Adams, J., Botash, A., Kellogg ND. Differences in hymeneal morphology between adolescent girls with and without a history of consensual sexual intercourse. *Archives of Pediatrics and Adolescent Medicine.* 2004;158:280-285.

11. Adams JA, Kaplan RA, Starling SP, Mehta NH, Finkel MA, Botash AS, Kellogg ND, Shapiro RA. Guidelines for medical care of children who may have been sexually abused. *J Pediatr Adolesc Gynecol.* 2007;20:163-172.

12. Adams JA, Harper K, Knudson S, Revilla J. Examination findings in legally confirmed child sexual abuse: it's normal to be normal. *Pediatrics.* 1994;94:310-317.

13. Kellogg ND, Menard SW, Santos A. Genital anatomy in pregnant adolescents: "normal" does not mean "nothing happened." *Pediatrics*. 2004;113(1). Available at: www.pediatrics.org/cgi/content/full/113/1/e67.

Chapter 7

EVIDENCE-BASED APPROACH TO CHILD SEXUAL ABUSE EXAMINATION FINDINGS

Robert A. Shapiro, MD
Anthony C. Leonard, PhD
Kathi L. Makoroff, MD

Competent clinical decision-making and treatment require knowledge of the published literature that is specific to the field in which one practices and the skills to critically assess the methodology behind these studies. Original studies must be carefully reviewed so that limitations, methodological errors, and unrecognized biases are identified before determining whether the stated conclusions are justified and whether the studies provide strong evidence that can be incorporated into patient diagnoses and care. Evidence-based medicine (EBM) stresses the examination of evidence from clinical research and from other sources by giving the practitioner a set of guidelines for use in interpreting available medical literature. Patient values, benefits, and risks must also be factored into the clinical decision-making process. There are many good references available on the use of EBM and critically assessing the literature.[1-3] This chapter provides a background on and examples of EBM relating to the diagnosis of children who have been sexually abused.

EBM uses the best combination of research evidence and clinical experience to optimize clinical diagnoses. In full, EBM consists of 5 steps: (1) formulating an answerable question, (2) finding the best evidence to answer the question, (3) critically appraising the evidence for validity, (4) integrating the critical appraisal with clinical experience and other patient circumstances, and (5) evaluating steps 1-4 to continually improve the process.[3] In part, the remainder of this chapter will address step 3, critically appraising the evidence for validity, by presenting the classic "properties of diagnostic tests"; properties that can also be applied to issues that are not generally thought of as diagnostic tests, but that involve the prevalence of some trait across a group with or without a diagnosis. When assessing original research that pertains to interpreting diagnostic test results, it is useful to consider these 3 considerations: (1) is the methodology sound and are the results valid, (2) does this test enable differentiation between patients with and without the condition, and (3) how can the study results be applied to patient care?

METHODOLOGY SOUNDNESS AND RESULT VALIDITY

The diagnostic validity of examination findings and laboratory test results must be determined through the study of subjects whose test results (ie, examination findings) and true disease statuses (ie, condition) are known. The most appropriate study designs used to assess the diagnostic validity of examination and test findings are case-control studies and cross-sectional studies. Case reports or case series can be informative or suggestive, but the information derived from them cannot be used to rigorously establish the rates and proportions associated with a test. Although the double-blinded, randomized, controlled study is often listed as the design producing the "strongest" evidence, it is not typically used to answer questions concerning the accuracy and usefulness of examination findings or tests because neither the test results nor the conditions for which they test are under experimenter control. Well-designed and well-executed case-control and cross-sectional studies can provide valid and useful information by preventing or minimizing methodological errors that can cause bias and unjustified conclusions. Understanding the strengths and limitations of different study designs is necessary to critically assess methodology and results.

CASE-CONTROL STUDIES

The case-control study typically compares 2 groups to each other; cases and controls. The 2 groups compared in many child abuse studies are children who have been abused (ie, "cases") and children who have not been abused (ie, "controls," or "control subjects"). Cause and effect cannot be determined from the case-control study, and caution is always in order when conclusions are extrapolated beyond the population and conditions for observation from which the data were sampled. A limitation of case-control studies is that they cannot establish population rates for a condition because the researcher sets the rate of sampled cases. A related strength of these studies is that they often require far fewer subjects than do cross-sectional studies, especially when the conditions or diseases studied are rare.

A common cause of bias in case-control studies is the failure to accurately select which patients should be considered cases and which controls. This type of bias is particularly prevalent in child abuse literature, because there is no gold standard available to accurately differentiate controls from cases. Without a gold standard, study designers must use a methodology that will minimize this type of error. If serious methodological limitations or errors exist, the resulting bias may lead to unjustified or incorrect study conclusions. Poor study design may also fail to remove the examination finding(s), test finding(s), or other study variables from case or control determination. For example, a study that is designed to identify examination findings in children who were abused but that also uses specific examination findings in selecting cases versus controls introduces this type of error. A less obvious design flaw that introduces the same error results when outcome data, such as court proceedings, are used to determine which patients are cases (ie, in the abuse group). The study variable, such as an examination or test finding, would likely have influenced the court's decision, thus causing this circular type of error. These methodological errors can invalidate the study's results.

Bias can also be introduced into a case-control study if the researchers who are measuring or assessing the study findings are not blinded to which patients are cases and which are controls. This type of bias, although unintentional, is not uncommon. Blinding will strengthen the conclusions of a case-control study.

CROSS-SECTIONAL STUDIES

A cross-sectional study examines a specific group of patients at a single point in time. This study design is applicable when asking questions such as "what is the normal configuration of the newborn hymen" or "what is the appearance of the pregnant adolescent hymen?" The prevalence of disease or examination findings can be determined through the cross-sectional study. As in case-control studies, effective patient selection is critical to the study methodology and must be clearly understood before applying study conclusions to clinical scenarios. Cause and effect cannot be determined from the cross-sectional study, but this kind of study can provide information regarding findings in a specific population (eg, abused or not). For example, a cross-sectional study that examines the hymenal findings of pregnant adolescents may demonstrate that a certain percentage of adolescent girls have no hymen transections. It would be reasonable to conclude, therefore, that transections are not always found in the hymenal examination following vaginal penetration. The same study may find that a certain percentage of teens have transections of the hymen. A cause-and-effect relationship should not be assumed from this study, however, and it would not be reasonable to conclude that transections are caused by vaginal penetration.

CASE REPORTS AND CASE SERIES

A case report is a descriptive study of a single patient's clinical course, history, and findings. A case series is a descriptive report of more than one patient. Case series are useful when reporting rare events or events that have clear causation. A case report is typically published when it will provide new information or supportive evidence that will help professionals in the field. Examples of case reports include children who have sustained known genital trauma and how their injuries heal or reports of unusual events that result in mimics of abuse.

REVIEW ARTICLES AND SUMMARY REPORTS

Review articles summarize the available original research for the reader. The authors take responsibility for finding and critically assessing the research relevant to the topic. Although some summary reports provide more supportive documentation regarding research methodologies than others, reading and critiquing the original research will often provide the reader with a better understanding of the literature.

A meta-analysis is a specific type of summary report analyzing the mathematical data from numerous original studies. The meta-analysis combines studies that use quantitative methods to summarize results and, by combining data, the meta-analysis may be able to demonstrate a level of certainty increased beyond that of any of the individual studies. Meta-analyses are limited by the quality of the original research as well as issues that arise when combining studies that may use different patient populations.

ASSESSING STUDY VALIDITY

Regardless of the type of study design, an assessment of the study population and the research methods is required to determine the validity of the study results. Research findings may be invalid because of bias in the study design, which can be introduced by poor patient selection (ie, selection bias) or lack of researcher blinding to patient characteristics (ie, measurement bias), as discussed in the previous sections. The following questions should be considered when assessing the validity of original research:

— Regarding Study Population

    — Who comprised the study population?

    — How were they recruited?

    — Was the selection of control subjects and cases appropriate?

    — What bias may have been introduced by this selection and exclusion?

    — Were patients who may have similar findings included in the study?

    — Was an appropriate standard used to identify cases?

— Does this study population represent a general group of patients or only a small subset?

— Was the study population large enough to allow for the discovery of meaningful differences?

— Regarding Study Methodology

— Were the study methods appropriate for addressing the stated hypothesis?

— Was circular reasoning excluded (ie, was the outcome made independent of any study variables)?

— Were measurement error and differences between examiners prevented? If not, were these factors assessed and accounted for in the statistical analyses?

— Was examiner bias reduced by including blinding in the methodology?

— Are examination findings well defined and reproducible by other examiners in different settings?

— Have the study results been independently confirmed by another study?

USEFUL PATIENT DIFFERENTIATION

Often, a thorough understanding of research findings requires knowledge of the statistical processes through which those findings are expressed. One particular set of statistical processes, those used to generate the properties of a diagnostic test, are sometimes especially relevant to studies of sexual abuse. The diagnostic test situation, in which a test with a dichotomous (ie, yes and no) outcome is used to predict a likewise dichotomous disease state, parallels the situation in which a dichotomous clinical finding is used to ascertain whether sexual abuse has occurred; the clinical finding acting as a diagnostic test for the condition of having been sexually abused is shown in the study by Berenson et al, which is further discussed later in this chapter. A number of important numerical qualities of such a test can be calculated by using **Table 7-1** and the following formulae. The value of a is the number of patients who have the disease and test positive (ie, the number of children who have been abused and who have a specific examination or test finding). The value of b is the number of patients who do not have the disease and test positive. The value of c is the number of patients who do have the disease and test negative. The value of d is the number of patients who do not have the disease and test negative.

Table 7-1. Possible Relationships Between a Diagnostic Test Result and the Condition for Which It Tests

STATUS OF TEST	POSITIVE FOR DISEASE/CONDITION	NEGATIVE FOR DISEASE/CONDITION
Positive Test Result/Finding	a (true-positive)	b (false-positive)
Negative Test Result/Finding	c (false-negative)	d (true-negative)

— ***Disease prevalence*** *(ie, pretest probability)* = $(a + c)/(a + b + c + d)$. Defined as the proportion of people who have the disease or condition and is sometimes simply referred to as prevalence. The posttest probability will be affected by the disease prevalence in the tested population. The posttest probability of a test is discussed later in this chapter.

— ***Odds ratio*** = $(ad)/(bc)$. Defined as the measure of the overall strength of the relationship between the test and the condition for which it tests. An odds ratio of 1 indicates that the test and the condition are unrelated (ie, the probability of having the condition is the same for those whose test results are positive as for those whose test results are negative). The odds ratio increases as the test and condition become more strongly linked, whereas an odds ratio between 0 and 1 would indicate that a negative test result was more predictive of the condition than was a positive test result. A useful property of the odds ratio is that it remains constant if the prevalence is artificially changed or specified, as occurs in a case-control study. In such a study the research design dictates the prevalence of the disease, often requiring one case (ie, a patient with the disease condition) for every one control (ie, a control subject without the disease being studied). The odds ratio from the resulting table will match the odds ratio from the population as a whole, in whom the disease is far less prevalent than in the research sample. Note that when rows or columns of the table are reversed, the odds ratio becomes its own multiplicative inverse (bc/ad), indicating the odds in favor of negative test results. For this reason, a clear statement about the odds ratio takes the following form: "the odds ratio in favor of positive test results and existence of the disease condition is X," where an X greater than 1 indicates an association of positive test results and the condition or disease, and an X less than 1 indicates that a negative test result is associated with the condition or disease."

A shortcoming of the odds ratio as a summary statistic is that it does not enable differentiation between the two types of errors from the diagnostic test (ie, a positive test result in a study subject without the condition or a negative test result in a patient in whom the condition is actually present). These two errors may have very different consequences, so it is important to consider statistics that focus on one or the other.

— ***Sensitivity*** = $a/(a + c)$. Defined as the proportion of patients with the target disorder or condition who have a positive test result or examination finding. A test with a high sensitivity will have few false-negative results (ie, negative test results for patients who actually have the condition), so that a negative test result should indicate with high probability that the condition is absent.

— ***Specificity*** = $d/(b + d)$. Defined as the proportion of patients without the target disorder or condition who have a negative test result or examination finding. A test with a high specificity has few false-positive results (ie, positive test results for study subjects who do not actually have the condition), so that a positive test result should indicate with high probability that the condition is present.

It is assumed for the remainder of this discussion that sensitivity and specificity are fixed qualities of a test, invariant to changes in prevalence or to use of the test in different populations. In the real-life use of diagnostic tests, this is generally a reasonable assumption. There are situations, however, when the sensitivity or specificity, or both, of a real-life test may change when applied to a different population.[4]

— ***Positive predictive value*** *(ie, PPV, or posttest probability)* = $a/(a + b)$. Defined as the proportion of patients with a positive test result or examination finding who have the target disorder/condition. A complementary value is the false-positive rate (FP), the proportion of patients with positive test results who do not actually have the condition: FP = $b/(a + b)$. The sum of these two values is 1; PPV + FP = 1. Given a particular sensitivity and specificity of a test, PPV and FP are dependent on the prevalence of the condition. It is very important to keep in mind that, for rare conditions, a test with excellent (ie, very high) sensitivity and specificity can still have a high rate of false-positives, even to the point that most of the patients with positive test results do not actually have the condition. The dependence of FP rates and false-negative rates on prevalence means that, unless a test enables flawless prediction, its usefulness is always dependent upon properties of the population in which it will be used.

— **Negative predictive value** *(NPV)* = $d/(c + d)$. Defined as the proportion of patients with a negative test result or examination finding who do not have the target disorder/condition. A complementary value is the false-negative rate (FN), the proportion of patients with negative test results who actually have the condition; FN = $c/(c + d)$. The sum of these two values is 1; NPV + FN = 1. As with PPV and FP, given a particular sensitivity and specificity of a test, NPV and FN are dependent on the prevalence of the condition.

The PPV and NPV are both dependent on prevalence, also referred to as pretest probability. If the prevalence of a condition is low, PPV becomes lower, and therefore less useful, but the NPV becomes higher. This becomes an important factor when critiquing the literature and applying it to clinical child abuse decision-making. For example, when reviewing an article regarding the use of a new laboratory test designed to diagnose a sexually transmitted infection (STI), if the values given for PPV and NPV pertain to a population with a high incidence of disease such as an adolescent population, the PPV and NPV must be recalculated to take into account the low prevalence of STI in the child abuse population. In a description of the qualities of a test, independent of any population to which it might be applied, it is informative to cite the likelihood ratios (LR) of the test.

— **Positive likelihood ratio** *(LR+)* = sensitivity/(1 − specificity) = $[a/(a + c)] / [b/(b + d)]$. The positive likelihood ratio (LR+) represents the probability that someone with the condition will have a positive test result, divided by the probability that someone without the condition will have a positive test result. The LR+ is sometimes simply referred to as the likelihood ratio of the test, and it is obviously desirable that a test have a high positive likelihood ratio. Because LR+ is dependent solely upon a test's sensitivity and specificity, as long as they are unchanging from one population to another, the LR+ does not change when the population or prevalence changes; that is, LR+ is a property of the test—and the test alone.

— **Negative likelihood ratio** *(LR−)* = (1 − sensitivity)/specificity = $[c/(a + c)] / [d/(b + d)]$. The negative likelihood ratio (LR−) represents the probability that someone with the condition will have a negative test result, divided by the probability that someone without the condition will have a negative test result. It is desirable that this be a small number, much less than 1. It is, like LR+, a property of the test, independent of the prevalence or population, as long as the sensitivity and specificity are independent of the prevalence or population.

The LR+ of a test can be used to determine the relationship between the pretest probability (ie, prevalence) and the posttest probability (ie, PPV, or the proportion of patients testing positive who actually have the condition). The relationship makes use of the concept of odds, where the odds of something happening is equal to its probability divided by 1 minus that probability. For example, something that happens 4 times out of 5 has a probability of 0.8 and odds of 4 divided by 1, or 4. The pretest odds of having a condition (ie, prevalence divided by 1 minus the prevalence) multiplied by LR+ is equal to the posttest odds, or the odds that someone has the condition given that they tested positive. Those odds can be reverse-transformed into the posttest probability by the following transformation: probability = odds/(odds + 1). A likelihood ratio of 1.0 means that the posttest and pretest probabilities are exactly the same and that the positive test result is uninformative. In other words, having a positive test result does not make one any more likely to have the condition than that person was before taking the test (ie, the population prevalence). Two aids to making this transformation from pretest to posttest probabilities using odds and LR+ are the nomogram, a slide rule–like chart that has the intervening calculations built in (see **Figure 7-1**), and a table linking possible pretest and posttest probabilities (**Table 7-2**).

— ***P values, hypothesis testing, and confidence intervals.*** The reporting of many statistics includes reporting of their associated *P* values, but evaluations of diagnostic tests are sometimes reported without *P* values. This is because *P* values usually address a null hypothesis of "no difference" or "no relationship." In the diagnostic test situation, this is a hypothesis that the test is worthless; stated another way, it is that patients with positive test results will have the same probability of having the condition as those with negative test results.

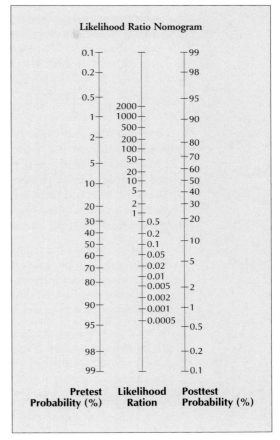

Figure 7-1. A Likelihood Ratio Nomogram. Reproduced with permission from Sackett DL, Straus SE, Richardson WS, Rosenberg W, Haynes RB. Evidence-based medicine: how to practice and teach EBM. *London: Churchill-Livingstone, 2000.*

Table 7-2. Posttest Probabilities for Pairs of Likelihood Ratios and Pretest Probabilities

LIKELIHOOD RATIO	PRETEST PROBABILITY					
	1%	**2%**	**10%**	**25%**	**50%**	**70%**
50	34%	51%	85%	94%	98%	99%
10	9%	17%	53%	77%	91%	96%
5	5%	9%	36%	63%	83%	92%
1	1%	2%	10%	25%	50%	70%
0.5	1%	1%	5%	14%	33%	54%
0.1	0%	0%	1%	3%	9%	19%
0.05	0%	0%	1%	2%	5%	10%

Rejecting that null hypothesis and establishing that the test is probably not worthless meets a very low standard; the evaluators of the test are usually interested in establishing how good the test is, not whether it is any good at all. A different null hypothesis could be tested (eg, that the odds ratio is 3), but the selection of what odds ratio or other measure of the strength of the test/condition relationship to test tends to be arbitrary. For these reasons, statistics associated with test properties are often reported with confidence intervals (CI) rather than with P values. The confidence interval quantifies the precision or uncertainty of a study result. A 95% is the range of values within which we can be 95% certain that the true value for the whole population lies. Another way of thinking about a CI is that 95% of such intervals will contain the true population value. As with P values, a larger sample size allows for more precision in the estimates, shrinking the size of the CI.

The computation and use of many of the statistics just discussed can be illuminated through examination of a particular example. Data provided by the study performed by Berenson and colleagues[5] show the association between female children who have been abused sexually and the putative indicators of sexual abuse. In this study, a sample of 192 children who had been abused was compared to a similar sample of 200 children believed not to have been abused. Vaginal discharge was evaluated as an indicator of previous sexual abuse; the raw numbers from the study are presented in **Table 7-3**.

In the sample populations represented in **Table 7-3**, the prevalence of the condition of having been sexually abused is 192/392 = 0.49, or 49%. This prevalence is, of course, set by the researchers and is not informative concerning the prevalence of sexual abuse in the population at large. Most of the statistics derived from the table, however, are invariant across changes in population prevalence.

The table has an odds ratio of $(21 \cdot 192)/(8 \cdot 171) = 2.95$, and an associated P value of 0.01 the derivation of the P value not being shown. The odds ratio indicates that the odds of experiencing discharge is almost 3 times as high in children who were abused as in children who were not abused.

The sensitivity of the test is 21/192 = 0.109, or 10.9%, meaning that only 10.9% of children who were abused exhibit the indicator of vaginal discharge. The specificity is 192/200 = 0.96, or 96%, meaning that for children who were not abused, only 4% display the indicator.

The PPV is 21/29 = 0.724, or 72.4%, meaning that a positive test result (ie, the presence of vaginal discharge) indicates, for this sample, a 72.4% probability of having been abused. The complement of this is the false-positive rate of $1 - 0.724 = 0.276$, or 27.6%, meaning that if one assumes that a positive test result (ie, discharge) indicates

Table 7-3. Vaginal Discharge As an Indicator of Previous Sexual Abuse			
PRESENCE/ABSENCE OF DISCHARGE	ABUSED PATIENT POPULATION	NONABUSED PATIENT POPULATION	ABUSED PLUS NONABUSED
Discharge Present (+)	21	8	29
No Discharge Present (-)	171	192	363
Total	192	200	392

previous abuse, that assumption would be wrong 27.6% of the time. These numbers are obviously dependent upon the overall prevalence of child abuse in the sample (eg, the population at large), where abuse is much less frequent, most cases of vaginal discharge would occur in girls who had not been previously abused.

The NPV is 192/363 = 0.529, or 52.9%, meaning that among girls with no vaginal discharge, 52.9% had not been abused. The complementary false-positive rate of 47.1% indicates that, if one assumes that the lack of discharge indicates that no abuse had occurred, that assumption would be wrong 47.1% of the time. Again, these numbers are dependent upon the prevalence of abuse in the sample under consideration, which is a sample intentionally rich in abuse cases. These numbers would be far better (ie, with a higher NPV and lower false-negative rate) if figured from the prevalence of abuse in the population at large, not only from the sample of sexually abused girls.

The positive likelihood ratio, or LR+, is 0.109/(1 − 0.96) = 2.7, meaning that abused girls had almost 2 times the probability of discharge as did the girls believed not to have been abused.

The negative likelihood ratio, or LR−, is (1 − 0.109)/0.96 = 0.93, meaning that the abused girls had a probability of not showing discharge that was just 7% lower (1 − 0.93) than that of girls believed not to have been abused.

APPLYING STUDY RESULTS TO PATIENT CARE

The numbers reported above reveal many things about the use of vaginal discharge as a sign that sexual abuse has occurred. The odds ratio of 2.95 and its associated *P* value of 0.01 indicate that vaginal discharge is almost certainly associated with earlier abuse, but that the association is far from perfect. Only 10.9% of abused girls have discharge, meaning that one would not want to interpret a lack of discharge as indicating the nonexistence of abuse. The specificity of 96% means that among girls believed not to have been abused, only 4% will have discharge, indicating that perhaps discharge is a strong indicator of earlier abuse, because so few girls who have not been abused have it. It is also true, however, that because only 10.9% of the abused girls have discharge, a fair portion of girls with discharge have not been abused. That portion (ie, the false-positive rate) goes up as the prevalence of abuse goes down, to the point that if only 5% of a population of girls had been abused, 7 out of 8 girls with positive test results actually would not have been abused. Thus, vaginal discharge should never be used as forensic evidence of abuse, and even in a clinical setting discharge should be viewed as a very weak indicator of possible abuse and, conversely, a lack of discharge as a weak indicator of the absence of abuse.

REVIEWING THE LITERATURE REGARDING CHILD SEXUAL ABUSE EXAMINATION FINDINGS

The following sections contain a review of 3 original research articles to assess the research methodology and validity (ie, methods); to discern the usefulness of a diagnosis of child sexual abuse (ie, results); and to analyze the application of the research results to patient care.

REVIEW OF CROSS-SECTIONAL STUDY[6]

Methods

This is a cross-sectional study describing the hymenal examination findings in adolescent patients who were pregnant. Three examiners retrospectively reviewed examination photographs and patient files to determine examination findings. The examiners reviewed the images together and were blinded to history except for the patient's pregnancy status. Examination findings were classified as nonspecific, suggestive of penetration, or definitive evidence of penetration. The examination findings used to define each of these criteria were listed in the article. If consensus was not reached, the examination findings were included in an inconclusive group. This study addresses only adolescents who had no recent sexual contact; at the time of examination, the last sexual encounter was an average of 3 months earlier.

Methods Discussion

The authors designed this study to address a specific question encountered by many child abuse physicians: Can the hymenal examination yield normal results or fail to demonstrate signs specific for penetration even if vaginal penetration is reported? This population, adolescents who were pregnant, is suitable to answer this question because pregnancy typically indicates that vaginal penetration has occurred. Bias caused by population selection is not an issue, and as this was a cross-sectional study, there were no control subjects. The selection of study population is appropriate to answer the study hypothesis.

A significant limitation to this study, as stated by the authors, was that the case reviewers were not blinded to pregnancy status. This may have introduced unintended bias in the form of lowered rates of observing signs of trauma, stemming from the researchers' desire to demonstrate that vaginal penetration does not necessarily cause recognizable trauma to the hymen. It could have also introduced the opposite bias, observing heightened rates of observing signs of trauma stemming from the researchers' knowledge that a possible cause for such trauma exists. In addition, the examiners were together when they reviewed the photographic documentation, which may have limited independent interpretations.

Results

Examination documentation from 36 adolescents was reviewed. Normal or nonspecific exams were noted in 64%, inconclusive examination findings in 22%, 8% had suggestive findings, and 6% had definitive findings of penetration. These data demonstrate that the hymenal examination may not reveal vaginal penetration using examination criteria defined in this study. The authors conclude that the hymenal examination of pregnant adolescent girls may not indicate penetration.

In regard to using this data in clinical practice, this study provides good evidence that the hymenal examination may not indicate vaginal penetration. Future studies should attempt to eliminate potential bias caused by the failure to blind the investigators to pregnancy status. The authors used a classification scale to define the examination finding categories of "nonspecific," "suggestive," and "definitive." Readers should be familiar with this classification system and might need to consider how this study's findings would change should another classification system be used.

REVIEW OF CASE-CONTROL STUDY[5]

Methods

This study was designed to identify vulvar and hymenal characteristics among girls who were sexually abused between 3 and 8 years old. Case subjects were recruited from a child protective health clinic, and control subjects (ie, children who were not abused) were recruited from the waiting rooms of a pediatric clinic at a different location. Inclusion criteria for both groups were equal with regard to gender, age, breast development (ie, all Tanner 1), and ethnicity. Potential subjects in the control (ie, children who were not abused) group were excluded if there was confirmed or suspected child sexual abuse, current genitourinary (GU) complaints, prior vaginal speculum insertion, or a history of trauma that caused bruising or bleeding of the genitalia. Children in the control group were recruited to match the age and ethnicity of the children who were abused. Each child in the control group was screened for possible sexual abuse by using a 4 step process and excluded from the study if any of the 4 steps revealed possible sexual abuse. The 4 processes consisted of the following: (1) a parent interview about concerns that abuse may have occurred, (2) the completion of the Child Sexual Behavior Inventory by the child's parent, (3) an interview of the child by a trained worker, and (4) a review of the child's medical record for any signs, concerns, or indications that abuse may have occurred. If patients completed the study, they received $25 compensation.

Case subjects were screened for vaginal penetration by means of a Digital/Penile Vulvar Penetration Rating Scale, a previously untested rating scale created by the authors that was designed to increase the likelihood that children enrolled as case subjects were more likely to have had vaginal penetration compared with those in the general population of children who visited the child abuse center. Only children with a rating above an arbitrary cut-off were included as case subjects for the study.

Children in both the control and case groups were examined and photographed using similar and standardized methods so that the study authors would be blind to cases or controls when photographs of examination findings were later reviewed and scored. The reviewers later tried to guess which recruitment site obtained the photographs of particular children. Analysis revealed that they could not identify control from case patients more often than chance would predict.

Two of the authors reviewed all of the study photographs. The two reviewers first coded their observations independently, then they discussed their findings and reached a consensus, where differences existed. To assess reliability in examination interpretation, 10% of the examinations were reviewed a second time and matched to the original interpretation. Consensus was reported to have ranged from 93% to 100% for all but one finding. Those findings that were documented both during the examination and seen on photographic review were included in the data analysis.

Methods Discussion
The methods for this cross-sectional study were carefully designed to minimize bias. Although no gold standard exists to exclude child sexual abuse, the authors made a significant effort to differentiate cases from control subjects. Their decision to include as cases only those children whose history of sexual abuse included indicators of probable penetration likely increased the power of the study. Even though their penetration rating scale was untested, its use should not have introduced any negative bias. Without penetration, vulvar and hymenal changes would be unlikely. The authors also worked to reduce any interpretation bias by making certain that the reviewers were blinded to cases and controls. Their methods seemed to be sufficient regarding the collection of study material (ie, diagnostic-quality photographic documentation and the review of examination findings); therefore, this study seems well designed and should provide valid results.

Results
Because of space limitations, only a few results will be discussed. The study was conducted over a 3-year period. A total of 192 children were enrolled as cases; 40% were white, 38% were Hispanic, and 22% were black. The control group consisted of 200 children with a similar ethnic distribution.

The authors demonstrated that there were very few differences in the examination findings between the case and control groups. Two examination findings (ie, vaginal discharge and septate hymens) showed *P* value differences between the 2 groups that reached the statistically significant level of 0.05; however, the positive likelihood ratios for vaginal discharge and septate hymen are 2.73 and 4.17, respectively (refer to **Table 7-2**). Neither of these factors is very high, indicating that neither of the physical findings acts as a persuasive indicator of penetration.

The authors also noted that, although not statistically significant, certain findings were found only in the group of children who were abused. These findings included deep notches, transections, and perforations of the hymen; this evidence led the authors to note in the comments section that "[a] deep notch, transection, or perforation on the inferior portion of the hymen may be considered as a definitive sign of sexual abuse or other trauma." This may be too strong a statement. To illustrate this issue, consider another finding from this study; increased pigmentation was found in 4 of the children who were not abused and in none of the children who were abused. Intuitively, we know not to conclude that a finding of increased hymenal pigmentation excludes abuse even if the finding was present only in the control subjects. For much the same reason, we should probably not conclude that deep notches, transections, or hymenal perforations are diagnostic of penetration unless other evidence is available to show that these findings can be caused only by trauma.

The authors looked at a subpopulation of children who had been abused and who had been examined within 7 days of an assault (ie, 17 children). The positive likelihood ratio for vaginal discharge in this group was only slightly higher, 5.88, than it was in the larger group and 6% (ie, 1 child) of this subpopulation of children also had a deep notch, compared to 0% of the control group (ie, a *P* value of 0.01). Although the authors reported statistical significance, the numbers are too small to make this a clinically useful finding and to allow for exclusion of the possibility of chance.

It is tempting to claim certainty when a finding is seen in the cases and is not found in the control group; however, the possibility that chance may account for the lack of findings in one group must be considered. For example, if we were to sample a random population of 200 in which a dichotomous (ie, yes and no) trait has a rate of 2/200 (ie, 1%), the chance that we would find no cases in this sample is 13.4%. If the rate of occurrence is only 1 in 200, as seen in the some of the results of this study, the chance of finding no cases in this random population is 36.7%.

In regard to using this data in clinical practice, this study contributes significantly to the literature, providing strong evidence that the physical examination is typically not sufficient to enable differentiation between those prepubertal children who probably experienced abuse and vaginal penetration and those children who were not abused. This study incorporated strong methodology to minimize patient bias and interpretation bias. Other studies, including a meta-analysis, may support these findings. The conclusions reached by the authors regarding those findings seen only in the abuse population may not be statistically correct and should be reexamined by other authors.

REVIEW OF CASE SERIES[7]

Methods

This is a case series of well-documented motor vehicle crashes involving pedestrians who were children. The case histories of four children who had anal or genital injuries suggestive of sexual abuse after being run over by slow-moving vehicles are described. The authors provide detailed descriptions of the presenting histories, the examination findings, and an intensive investigation to exclude sexual abuse. Diagnostic-quality photographs of the genital and anal injuries are reproduced in the article.

Methods Discussion

There is no apparent bias in this study, and the investigators present sufficient data about each of the four cases to allow the reader to determine whether these case reports are valid.

This data is useful for clinical practice because, although this is a case series involving only four patients, this study provides clinicians with a report of an unusual, but important, traumatic finding that may be seen in children who have been run over by a motor vehicle.

CONCLUSION

Understanding medical literature requires study using informed methodologies. Medical professionals who are involved in the medicolegal outcomes that often follow reports of child sexual abuse should be familiar with the original research that supports or refutes accusations of abuse. Detailed analysis of the original research is needed before making conclusions about a study's utility and applicability for a specific clinical question.

REFERENCES

1. What is EBM? Centre for Evidence-Based Medicine Web site. http://www.cebm.net/ ?o=1014. Accessed August 12, 2009.

2. Cochrane AL. *Effectiveness and Efficiency: Random Reflections on Health Services*. London: Nuffield Provincial Hospitals Trust; 1972.

3. Sackett DL, Straus SE, Richardson WS, Rosenberg W, Haynes RB. *Evidence-based medicine: How to practice and teach EBM*. London: Churchill-Livingstone; 2000.

4. Eckman MH, Erban JK, Singh SK, Kao GS. Screening for the risk of bleeding or thrombosis. *Ann Inter Med*. 2003;138(3):W15-W24.

5. Berenson AB, Chacko MR, Wiemann CM, et al. A case-control study of anatomic changes resulting from sexual abuse. *Am J O Gynecol*. 2000;182(4):820-834.

6. Kellogg ND, Menard SW, Santos A. Genital anatomy in pregnant adolescents: "normal" does not mean "nothing happened." *Pediatrics*. 2004;113:e67-e69.

7. Boos SC, Rosasa AJ, Boyle C, McCann J. Anogenital injuries in child pedestrians run over by low-speed motor vehicles: four cases with findings that mimic child sexual abuse. *Pediatrics*. 2003;112:e77-e84.

Chapter 8

INTERPRETATION OF GENITAL AND ANAL FINDINGS IN CHILDREN AND ADOLESCENTS WITH SUSPECTED SEXUAL ABUSE: STATE OF THE SCIENCE

Joyce A. Adams, MD

The identification and interpretation of medical and laboratory findings in children with possible sexual abuse require an evaluation by a health care provider who has a high level of knowledge, clinical expertise, and familiarity with the research studies describing findings in nonabused and abused children.

This chapter will review the changes in interpretation of medical and laboratory findings with respect to sexual abuse that have resulted from the publication, between 1989 and 2005, of cross-sectional, case-control, and longitudinal studies of abused and nonabused children. An approach to the interpretation of findings in children with suspected abuse will be presented. This approach was developed as a collaborative project by a group of physician specialists who met to update and revise a classification system first proposed by Adams and colleagues in 1992.[1]

HISTORY

In the early 1980s, as the magnitude of the problem of child sexual abuse was becoming apparent, child protection and law enforcement agencies began to refer more children for medical examinations as part of the investigation of abuse allegations. The physicians who performed these examinations were handicapped, however, by a lack of data concerning normal anatomical variations in the appearance of the genital and anal tissues in children of different ages. As most children were not examined within hours or days of an episode of violent sexual assault, but weeks or months after the most recent molestation, signs of acute injury, such as bleeding or bruising, were often absent. Because most of the physicians who examined these children had not previously used magnification and specialized techniques to study the detailed appearance of children's genitalia findings, such as a hymenal opening appearing "too big" or dilation of the child's anus during the examination, among many others, such findings were taken to be signs of abuse.

STUDIES IN GENITAL AND ANAL FINDINGS IN CHILDREN AND ADOLESCENTS WITH SUSPECTED SEXUAL ABUSE

Between 1989 and 1991, three studies that describe genital or anal findings in non-abused children were published. McCann and colleagues described anal findings in 267 prepubertal children who were carefully screened and found to have no suspicion of abuse[2]; of these 267 children, they also obtained genital findings in 93 girls between 10 months and 10 years of age from the same study who were examined using a colposcope.[3] Another study, which describes the appearance of the hymen in newborn infants, provided additional important normative data.[4] Data from these studies, along with recommendations from the American Academy of Pediatrics,[5] were used to develop an approach to classifying anogenital and laboratory findings in children with suspected sexual abuse.[1]

This approach was not presented as a consensus document, but as a tool that might be helpful in descriptive studies looking at the frequency of genital findings in studies of abused children. Many findings that had previously been interpreted as being due to abuse, but were commonly documented in the studies of newborn infants and nonabused children, were listed as "normal" or "nonspecific." In the "suspicious" and "suggestive" categories, findings were listed that had been described in a small percentage of nonabused children but were also described in children giving a history of abuse. Findings in the "clear evidence of penetrating injury" category were all characteristic of trauma or the residua of trauma.

The table listing the different categories of physical findings has been revised several times since 1992. As additional cross-sectional studies reporting genital findings in nonabused prepubertal girls and healing of injuries have been published, findings have been added or reclassified.[6-10] **Table 8-1** is modified from the version that appeared in an article by Adams,[11] and it lists the results of a collaborative process involving a group of physician experts and other health care providers who have met over several years to revise the listing of findings using the best research data available. As additional studies are published, there may be further changes to this document.

Several changes in the listing of findings were made after Berenson et al published, in 2000, the first case-control study of genital findings in nonabused girls between 3 and 8 years of age compared to girls who described digital or penile-vaginal penetration.[12] This study was important because the subjects in the nonabused group had the most complete screening available to ensure their nonabused status, including interviews of the child and parents, record review, and completion of behavioral surveys by the parents.

Table 8-1. Interpretation of Physical and Laboratory Findings in Children with Suspected Sexual Abuse

FINDINGS DOCUMENTED IN NEWBORNS OR COMMONLY SEEN IN NONABUSED CHILDREN*

Normal Variants

1. Periurethral or vestibular bands

2. Intravaginal ridges or columns

3. Hymenal bumps or mounds

4. Hymenal tags or septal remnants

5. Linea vestibularis (midline avascular area)

6. Hymenal notch/cleft in the anterior (superior) half of the hymenal rim (prepubertal girls), on or above the 3 o'clock–9 o'clock line, patient supine

(continued)

Table 8-1. *(continued)*

7. Shallow/superficial notch or cleft in inferior rim of hymen (below 3 o'clock–9 o'clock line)

8. External hymenal ridge

9. Congenital variants in appearance of hymen, including the following: crescentic, annular, redundant, septate cribiform, microperforate, and imperforate

10. Diastasis ani (smooth area)

11. Perianal skin tag

12. Hyperpigmentation of the skin of labia minora or perianal tissues in children of color, such as Mexican-American and African-American children

13. Dilation of the urethral opening with application of labial traction

14. "Thickened" hymen (may be due to estrogen effect, folded edge of hymen, swelling from infection, or swelling from trauma. The latter is difficult to assess unless follow-up examination is done.)

Findings Commonly Caused by Other Medical Conditions

15. Erythema (redness) of the vestibule, penis, scrotum, or perianal tissues (may be due to irritants, infection, or trauma†)

16. Increased vascularity (dilatation of existing blood vessels) of vestibule and hymen (may be due to local irritants, or normal pattern in the non-estrogenized state)

17. Labial adhesion (may be due to irritation or rubbing)

18. Vaginal discharge (many infectious and non-infectious causes, cultures must be taken to confirm if it is caused by sexually transmitted organisms or other infections)

19. Friability of the posterior fourchette or commisure (may be due to irritation, infection, or may be caused by examiner's traction on the labia majora)

20. Excoriations/bleeding/vascular lesions (these findings can be due to conditions such as lichen sclerosus, eczema or seborrhea, vaginal/perianal Group A Streptococcus, urethral prolapse, or hemangiomas)

21. Failure of midline fusion (also called perineal groove)

22. Anal fissures (usually due to constipation, perianal irritation)

23. Venous congestion, or venous pooling in the perianal area (usually due to positioning of child, also seen with constipation)

24. Flattened anal folds (may be due to relaxation of the external sphincter or to swelling of the perianal tissues because of infection or trauma†)

25. Partial or complete anal dilatation to fewer than 2 cm (anterior-posterior dimension), with or without stool visible.

Indeterminate Findings: Insufficient or conflicting data from research studies: (May require additional studies/evaluation to determine significance. These physical/laboratory findings may support a child's clear disclosure of sexual abuse, if one is given, but should be interpreted with caution if the child gives no disclosure. A report to child protective services may be indicated in some cases.)

(continued)

Table 8-1. Interpretation of Physical and Laboratory Findings in Children with Suspected Sexual Abuse *(continued)*

Physical Examination Findings

26. Deep notches or clefts in the posterior/inferior rim of hymen, between 4 and 8 o'clock, in contrast to transections (see 41)

27. Deep notches or complete clefts in the hymen at 3 or 9 o'clock in adolescent girls

28. Smooth, non-interrupted rim of hymen between 4 and 8 o'clock, which appears to be less than 1 mm wide, when examined in the prone knee-chest position or using water to "float" the edge of the hymen when the child is in the supine position.

29. Wart-like lesions in the genital or anal area (biopsy and viral typing may be indicated in some cases)

30. Vesicular lesions or ulcers in the genital or anal area (infectious and non-infectious causes; cultures, serology, or nucleic acid amplification tests should be done)

31. Marked, immediate anal dilation to an anterior-posterior diameter of 2 cm or more in the absence of other predisposing factors such as chronic constipation, sedation, anesthesia, neuromuscular conditions

Lesions with Etiology Confirmed: Indeterminate Specificity for Sexual Transmission

32. Genital or anal *Condyloma accuminata* in child, in the absence of other indicators of abuse

33. Herpes type 1 or 2 in the genital or anal area in a child with no other indicators of sexual abuse

Findings Diagnostic of Trauma and/or Sexual Contact: The following findings support a disclosure of sexual abuse, if one is given, and are highly suggestive of abuse even in the absence of a disclosure, unless a clear, timely, plausible description of accidental injury is provided by the child and/or caretaker.

Acute Trauma to External Genital/Anal Tissues

34. Acute lacerations or extensive bruising of labia, penis, scrotum, perianal tissues, or perineum (may be from unwitnessed accidental trauma, or from physical or sexual abuse)

35. Fresh laceration of the posterior fourchette, not involving the hymen (must be differentiated from dehisced labial adhesion or failure of midline fusion; [see 21]. Posterior fourchette lacerations may also be caused by accidental injury or consensual sexual intercourse in adolescents.)

Residual (Healing) Injuries‡

36. Perianal scar (rare, may be due to other medical conditions such as Crohn's disease, accidental injuries, or previous medical procedures)

37. Scar of posterior fourchette or fossa (pale areas in the midline may also be due to linea vestibularis or labial adhesions)

Injuries Indicative of Blunt Force Penetrating Trauma (or from Abdominal/Pelvic Compression Injury If Such History Is Given)

38. Laceration (tear, partial or complete) of the hymen, acute

39. Ecchymosis (bruising) on the hymen (in the absence of a known infectious process or coagulopathy)

(continued)

Table 8-1. *(continued)*

40. Perianal lacerations extending deep to the external anal sphincter (not to be confused with partial failure of midline fusion)

41. Hymenal transection (healed). An area between 4 and 8 o'clock on the rim of the hymen where it appears to have been torn through, to or nearly to the base, so there appears to be virtually no hymenal tissue remaining at that location. This finding has also been referred to as a "complete cleft" in sexually active adolescents and young adult women.

42. Missing segment of hymenal tissue. Area in the posterior (inferior) half of the hymen, wider than a transection, with an absence of hymenal tissue extending to the base of the hymen, which is confirmed using additional positions/methods.

Presence of Infection Confirms Mucosal Contact with Infected and Infective Bodily Secretions, Contact Most Likely to Have Been Sexual in Nature:

43. Positive confirmed culture for gonorrhea from genital area, anus, or throat in a child outside the neonatal period

44. Confirmed diagnosis of syphilis, if perinatal transmission is ruled out

45. *Trichomonas vaginalis* infection in a child older than 1 year of age, with organisms identified by culture or in vaginal secretions by wet-mount examination

46. Positive culture from genital or anal tissues for chlamydia, if child is older than 3 years at time of diagnosis, and specimen was tested using cell culture or comparable method approved by the Centers for Disease Control

47. Positive serology for HIV, if perinatal transmission, transmission from blood products, and needle contamination has been ruled out

Diagnostic of Sexual Contact

48. Pregnancy

49. Sperm identified in specimens taken directly from a child's body

---

* *The numbering of the following findings is for convenience of reference only; there is no implication of increasing significance.*

† *(Follow-up examination is necessary before attributing these findings to trauma.)*

‡ *These findings are difficult to assess unless an acute injury was previously documented at the same location*

Reprinted from Adams JA, Kaplan RA, Starling SP, et al. Guidelines for medical care of children who may have been sexually abused. J Pediatr Adolesc Gynecol. *2007;20:163-172, with permission from Elsevier.*

RESEARCH

The "gold standard" for research design in a study that tries to determine cause and effect is a randomized, double-blind control study in which subjects are randomly selected to receive or not receive the treatment or intervention; neither the subjects nor the researchers know who is receiving the treatment or intervention. This is obviously not an option when trying to study the changes in genital and anal anatomy caused by sexual abuse. The next best method is the case-control study. The selection of subjects in the Berenson, et al study[12] was not random—for each child evaluated for suspected sexual abuse at one center who agreed to participate in the research study, a child of the same age and ethnicity was recruited from a population of children receiving well-child examinations at another site. The researchers were blinded as much as possible by using the same examination methods, photographic equipment, and number and type of photographs taken, so that when blindly reviewing the photographs, the site where the child had been examined could not be determined.

Details in the appearance of the genital tissues were carefully recorded and then compared between the 2 groups: those who described having experienced vaginal penetration and those who were determined to be nonabused after careful screening.

There were very few significant differences between the 2 groups. Vaginal discharge was more common in the abused group, although no cultures were taken to determine the cause of the discharge. Labial adhesions were more common in Caucasian girls who had been abused compared to their nonabused controls, but that was not the case for Mexican-American or African-American girls.

HYMENAL DATA

Superficial notches in the hymen (arbitrarily defined as extending through up to 50% of the width of the hymen) located below the 3 o'clock–9 o'clock line were equally common in abused and nonabused girls, which threw doubt on the connection between this finding and trauma to the hymen. It is important to note that when a mound or bump was noted on the edge of the hymen, the area next to the bump, even if it gave the impression of being an indentation, was not counted as a notch.

The authors identified notches through more than 50% of the width of the posterior hymen (deep notches) only in girls who described digital or penile-vaginal penetration; however, this was seen in only 2 out of 192 girls between the ages of 3 and 8 years alleging penetration. Distinguishing between superficial notches (through 50% or less of the width of the hymen) and deep notches (through more than 50% of the width of the hymen) can be extremely difficult.

Myhre and associates[7] found that only 1 of 175 nonabused girls age 5 to 7 years in their study had a superficial notch in the hymen, and none were found to have a deep notch, using the same definitions as Berenson et al.[12] However, they described bumps (mounds) on the hymen in 21% to 23% of subjects, depending on the examination position. The researchers in the Myhre study followed the same convention as described in the Berenson case-control study, and did not identify a narrowing in the hymen next to a bump as a notch.

In a study of the appearance of the hymen in adolescent girls admitting consensual intercourse compared to girls who denied such contact, there was no statistically significant difference in the frequency of deep notches in the posterior rim of hymen below 3 to 9 o'clock.[13] However, deep notches and complete clefts in the hymen in a lateral location—3 and 9 o'clock—were both significantly more common in girls admitting vaginal intercourse than in girls who denied intercourse (26% v. 5%, p<.01 for each). The fact that these features were identified in 5 out of 58 adolescent girls denying intercourse suggests that notches or clefts at the 3 or 9 o'clock position might represent normal variants, but they could also be the result of previous penetration.

The finding of a posterior rim of hymen that measures less than 1 mm in width was not reported in prepubertal girls selected for nonabuse in 4 separate studies in which measurements were taken from magnified photographs using a calibration method.[3,6,7,12] In another study, a posterior rim of hymen estimated to be less than 1-2 mm wide was found in 22% of the girls referred for gynecologic examination for other reasons and had no history or suspicion of abuse.[14] Most experts acknowledge that it is very difficult to measure the width of the posterior rim of hymen in many cases, and that estimates of rim width are often inaccurate.

If magnified photographs are taken using a camera attached to a colposcope, and a photograph is taken of a millimeter ruler at the same magnification and same focal length, the printed photograph of the ruler can be held next to the printed photograph of the hymen in order to take measurements. The problem arises in deciding where to start measuring the width of the posterior hymenal rim, as it is difficult to determine where the hymen attaches to the muscular portion of the introitus from a 2-dimensional image.

The hymen may appear very narrow in the posterior/inferior rim in children when it has folded out or folded inward. This phenomenon was documented in Myhre's study of nonabused girls in Norway,[7] in which the use of water instilled during the examination of the child in the supine position caused the rim to "float" up and be seen more clearly. In the longitudinal follow-up study by Berenson et al, girls examined at age 3 years were reexamined at 5, 7, and 9 years of age.[15] Measurements of the width of the hymen at the 6 o'clock position, with the patient supine, showed a significant decrease in hymenal width as the child aged and a significant increase in the width of the hymenal opening.

SEXUALLY TRANSMITTED INFECTIONS

Warts, vesicles, and ulcers in the genital or anal area may cause concern for the possible sexual transmission of infections such as *Condyloma accuminata*, Herpes simplex, or syphilis. Wart-like lesions in the genital or anal area may be skin tags or warts not of the genital type, or they may be *Condyloma accuminata* that was acquired from perinatal transmission or other non-sexual transmission. While genital warts can also be transmitted by sexual contact, it is difficult to determine whether or not sexual abuse should be suspected in a child who is too young to give a history or who has denied that he or she has experienced any type of sexual abuse. As more studies are published that demonstrate the widespread prevalence of human papilloma virus (HPV) on the skin of children and adults using DNA analysis, the finding of *Condyloma accuminata* in a child will likely be considered less specific for sexual transmission. This is discussed in more detail in Chapter 10.

Vesicular lesions or ulcers in the genital or anal area can have infectious and non-infectious causes. These include herpes, syphilis, varicella, or other viruses; Behçet's disease; Crohn's disease; as well as idiopathic causes. Viral cultures or PCR analysis are needed to diagnose Herpes infections, and serologic tests must be done to diagnose syphilis. It is recommended that these tests be performed and the results received before reporting possible sexual abuse unless a child has given a disclosure of abuse.

MIMICS

The most common medical findings that are mistaken for signs of sexual abuse include the following: redness of the genital or anal tissues (many causes, see Chapter 9); the appearance of a "dilated" hymen, urethra, or anal opening felt by caretakers to be "too big"; a concern for an "absent" hymen because of a relatively narrow posterior rim of hymen when labial traction is applied in a well-relaxed child; mistaking the presence of labial adhesions as "scars" in the genital area; mistaking the iatrogenic breakdown of a labial adhesion as a tear of the posterior fourchette caused by abuse; mistaking the irregular appearance of the Pectinate line as scars or tears of the anus; and mistaking the blue coloration around the anus caused by venous congestion for anal bruising. Other rarer conditions—such as the congenital failure of midline fusion, or perineal groove, hemangiomas of the hymen or labia, urethral prolapse, lichen sclerosus, and lesions in the genital or anal area caused by conditions such as Crohn's disease or Behçet's disease—can also be confused with signs of sexual abuse trauma. Examples of normal variations in the appearance of the hymen and anus and other conditions that may be mistaken for abuse are shown in **Appendix Figures 8-1-a** to **8-43-b**.

ANAL DILATION

The finding of marked, immediate anal dilation to an anterior-posterior diameter of 2 cm or more, in the absence of other predisposing factors, is a rare finding in both abused[16] and nonabused[2,17] children. Anal dilation can be caused by chronic constipation, sedation, anesthesia, and neuromuscular conditions and can be seen during an autopsy.[18] No consensus currently exists among experts as to how this finding should be interpreted in the absence of a history of anal penetration given by the child; therefore, this finding is listed as being "indeterminate" for abuse.

INJURIES

As mentioned earlier, signs of acute trauma, such as bruising, abrasions, and lacerations, are rare in children who are examined for possible sexual abuse. In a review of findings in more than 2000 children presenting for examinations for suspected abuse to one large urban center, 96% of the children had normal or nonspecific findings on examination.[19] As several case reports have demonstrated, lacerations of the posterior fourchette, fossa, hymen, and anus can also be caused by accidental injuries.[20-22] The history from the child, as well as a thorough investigation of the setting in which the accident is alleged to have occurred, are essential to determine whether or not the injuries could have been caused by the described accident.

The limited number of studies that examined the healing of genital and anal injuries in children have shown that injuries heal very rapidly, within days or weeks, usually leaving no signs of residual injury such as scars.[8-10] The 17 cases of complete lacerations of the hymen reported in these studies, in which no surgery took place, all healed to leave a complete cleft or transection in the hymen at the location of the laceration. Two girls in the study by Heger et al had surgery to repair posterior fourchette and hymenal lacerations, and after healing, the rim of hymen was narrow but smooth, without a cleft or notch.[10]

A multicenter study of healing of genital injuries in prepubertal and adolescent girls provided new information on the rates of healing of injuries of different types.[23-25]

While the data indicate that complete lacerations of the hymen in prepubertal girls, if not repaired, usually heal to leave a deep notch or transection, the absence of a transection in an adolescent patient does not rule out the possibility that vaginal penetration occurred. Fewer than half of the adolescent girls describing consensual penile-vaginal intercourse in one study had complete clefts in the hymen.[13] In another study reviewing the appearance of the hymen in adolescent girls who were pregnant, only 2 of 36 girls had genital findings indicative of previous vaginal penetration.[26] These results are explained by the fact that the hymen in adolescent girls is fully estrogenized and can stretch to accommodate penile-vaginal penetration without tearing.

Lacerations or abrasions in the posterior fourchette can be caused by penetration, stretching of the skin, irritation of the skin, dermatitis, and infections such as those caused by *Candida albicans*.[27,28] Jones and colleagues reported that posterior fourchette lacerations, as highlighted by toluidine blue dye in adolescents brought for sexual abuse examinations, were not significantly more common in girls who said the intercourse was consensual than in girls who described forced intercourse.[27] Because the dye is taken up by nucleated cells and only the very top layer of the epidermis is made up of cells without nuclei, anything that disrupts the superficial epidermis will allow dye uptake by the cell layer just below. There have been no studies of prepubertal or adolescent girls with genital irritation, but without a history of recent sexual abuse or intercourse. It is therefore difficult to say with certainty that superficial abrasions or fissures in the skin of the vulva or anus are associated with sexual contact or may have other possible explanations.

CONCLUSION

The child or adolescent who is confirmed to have an infection caused by a sexually transmitted organism has most likely acquired that infection through sexual contact if perinatal transmission and auto-inoculation have been ruled out. Recommendations for testing for sexually transmitted infections, interpretation of the significance of positive tests, and treatment are discussed in detail in Chapter 10. Whether to offer prophylactic treatment is discussed in Chapter 11.

The photographs in the Appendix that follow are examples of some of the findings listed in **Table 8-1**. For examples of normal anatomic variants, see Chapter 2. Additional photographs can also be found on the CD-ROM accompanying this atlas.

Guidelines for medical care for children with suspected sexual abuse were published in 2007 in the *Journal of Pediatric and Adolescent Gynecology*.[29] These guidelines may be helpful to medical and non-medical professionals who are involved in the care of sexually abused children. A summary of research findings published since 2007 suggested some possible changes in these guidelines.[30]

APPENDIX 8-1: NORMAL VARIATIONS AND FORENSIC PHOTOGRAPHY

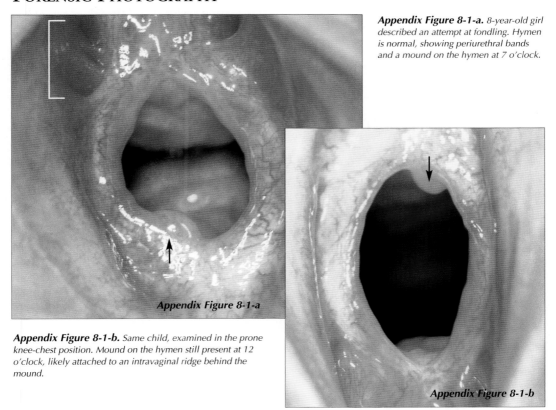

Appendix Figure 8-1-a. *8-year-old girl described an attempt at fondling. Hymen is normal, showing periurethral bands and a mound on the hymen at 7 o'clock.*

Appendix Figure 8-1-a

Appendix Figure 8-1-b. *Same child, examined in the prone knee-chest position. Mound on the hymen still present at 12 o'clock, likely attached to an intravaginal ridge behind the mound.*

Appendix Figure 8-1-b

125

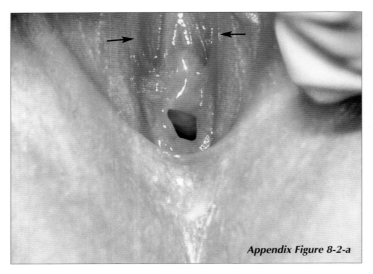

Appendix Figure 8-2-a

Appendix Figure 8-2-a. *6-year-old described fondling one week prior. This is a normal hymen, showing periurethral bands at 1 and 11 o'clock.*

Appendix Figure 8-2-b. *In the prone knee-chest position, the hymen is smooth, with a mound noted in the midline at 1 o'clock.*

Appendix Figure 8-3. *6-year-old girl examined using labial traction. The urethral opening is dilated, and there is an intravaginal column on the posterior vaginal wall in the midline at 7 o'clock. Both of these findings are normal.*

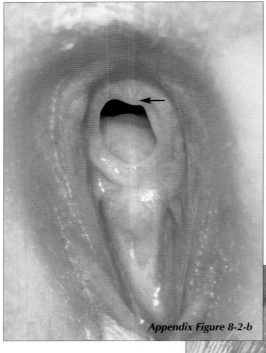

Appendix Figure 8-2-b

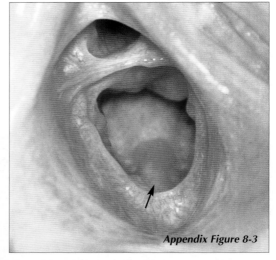

Appendix Figure 8-3

Appendix Figure 8-4. *This is a 7-year-old African-American girl, examined using separation. There are 2 mounds on the crescentic hymen, at 4 and 7 o'clock. Mounds are commonly seen in girls of this age and are not indicative of trauma.*

Appendix Figure 8-4

Appendix Figure 8-5. *6-year-old girl with normal hymen. There is a mound at 7 o'clock and a normal hypervascular appearance of the vestibular tissues in the sulci between the hymen and the inner labia minora bilaterally at 2 and 9 o'clock. The hymen on either side of a mound can appear relatively narrow, but should not be mistaken for a notch or cleft.*

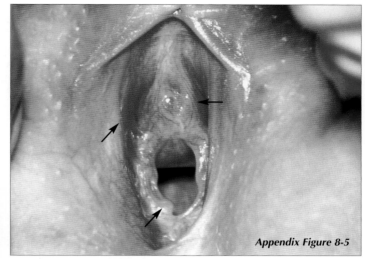

Appendix Figure 8-5

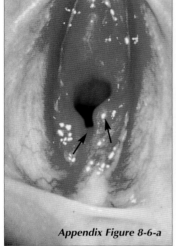

Appendix Figure 8-6-a

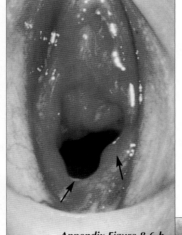

Appendix Figure 8-6-b

Appendix Figure 8-6-a. *This 5-year-old girl with vaginal discharge and increased vascularity of the vestibule and hymen has what appears in this photograph to be a notch at 6 o'clock, and a mound between 3 and 5 o'clock.*

Appendix Figure 8-6-b. *With additional labial traction, the posterior hymen smoothes out at 7 o'clock, and the mound is visible again at 3 to 5 o'clock. The "pseudo-notch" has disappeared. All cultures were negative. Even though this girl eventually gave a history of being molested, there is no sign of trauma to her hymen. Multiple examination techniques are needed if there appears to be an abnormality in one view.*

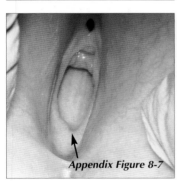

Appendix Figure 8-7

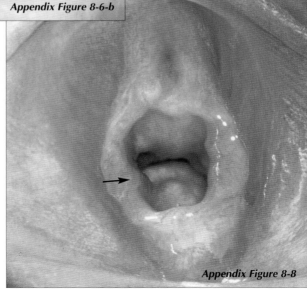

Appendix Figure 8-8

Appendix Figure 8-7. *8-year-old girl, developmentally delayed, obese, with an elongated hymenal opening and a very shallow indentation in the hymen at 5 o'clock. Another interpretation of this finding is that there is a mound on the hymen at 6 o'clock, and the area at 5 o'clock is only a "pseudo-notch." Neither finding is concerning for trauma, however, as both shallow notches and mounds are seen in nonabused children.*

Appendix Figure 8-8. *7-year-old girl, described fondling over clothes. The hymen is normal, with a mound at 9 o'clock and an intravaginal ridge behind the mound.*

Appendix Figure 8-9. *12-year-old girl, with a mound and ridge at 6 o'clock.*

Appendix Figure 8-10. *6-year-old girl with increased redness in the vestibule at 3 to 5 o'clock, a small follicle in the vestibule at 8 o'clock, and a midline avascular area at 6 o'clock. Follicles are probably mucosal inclusion cysts and are seen in both prepubertal and adolescent girls.*

Appendix Figure 8-11. *This 3-year-old girl has confluent, marked erythema in the vestibule and inner labia minora at 4 and 9 o'clock. Her cultures were positive for Group A beta hemolytic streptococci, a non–sexually transmitted infection.*

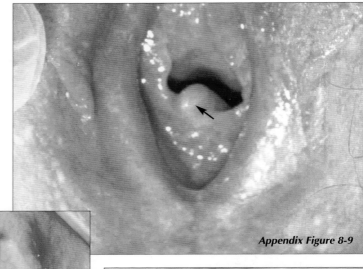

Appendix Figure 8-9

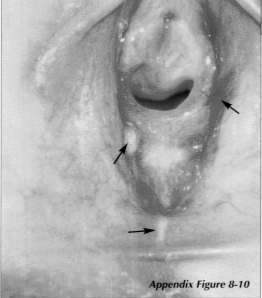

Appendix Figure 8-10

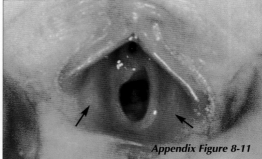

Appendix Figure 8-11

Appendix Figure 8-12. *Prepubertal girl with redness around the anus due to venous congestion, a common finding unrelated to trauma.*

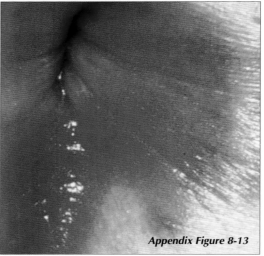

Appendix Figure 8-13

Appendix Figure 8-13. *This 4-year-old boy has marked erythema around the anus and complains of pain. The cultures were positive for Group A beta hemolytic streptococci, and he responded well to oral antibiotics.*

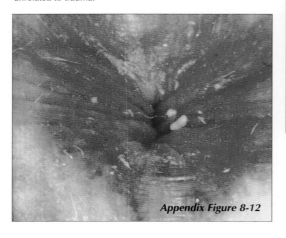

Appendix Figure 8-12

Appendix Figure 8-14. *This 3-year-old boy complained of pain due to inflammation of the perianal skin. This is also Streptococcal cellulitis. Children may complain of pain and even say that someone (often a caretaker) hurt their bottom, since wiping or cleaning such irritated tissue can be painful.*

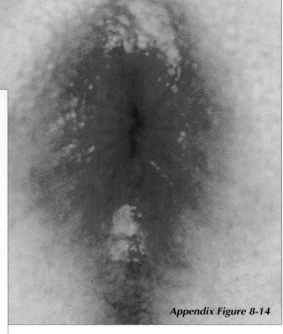

Appendix Figure 8-14

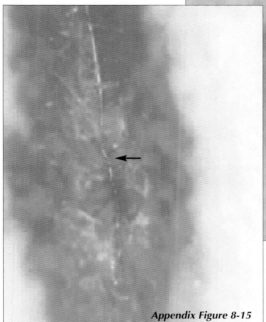

Appendix Figure 8-15

Appendix Figure 8-15. *This 3-year-old boy said "Big Momma hurt my cookie." His babysitter had wiped his bottom after having diarrhea, and he complained of pain. Cultures were positive for Streptococcus in this case.*

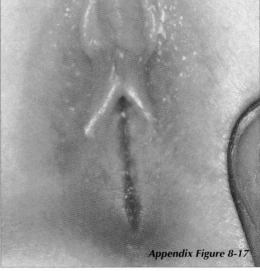

Appendix Figure 8-17

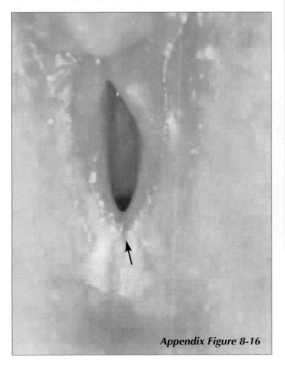

Appendix Figure 8-16

Appendix Figure 8-16. *4-year-old girl with posterior labial adhesion at 6 o'clock and no history of sexual abuse.*

Appendix Figure 8-17. *2-year-old in diapers had spot of blood on diaper causing concern. She has an almost total adhesion of her labia minora. The anterior opening is not visible on this photograph, but she was having normal passage of urine with no obvious discomfort.*

Appendix Figure 8-18. *30-month-old girl examined in prone knee-chest position. Posterior fusion of the labia is seen clearly in this photograph as a pale, midline avascular area. This can break down with labial separation, causing slight bleeding.*

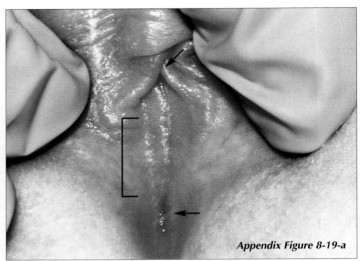

Appendix Figure 8-19-a

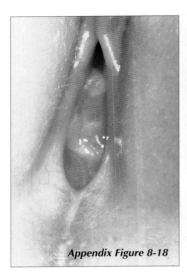

Appendix Figure 8-18

Appendix Figure 8-19-a. *6-year-old girl gave a history of one episode of genital fondling. There is a large labial adhesion, with a small opening just under the clitoral hood and another opening inferiorly. She was treated with estrogen cream.*

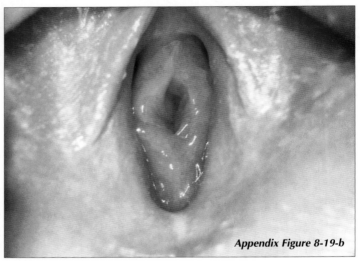

Appendix Figure 8-19-b

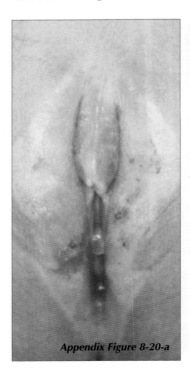

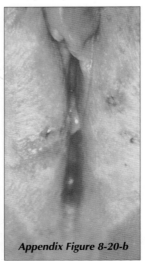

Appendix Figure 8-20-a

Appendix Figure 8-20-b

Appendix Figure 8-19-b. *One month later, after treatment with topical estrogen cream, the adhesion is almost completely resolved. The hymenal tissue is thickened and pale as a result of the effects of the estrogen cream.*

Appendix Figure 8-20-a. *7-year-old Mexican-American girl presented with genital itching and spots of blood on her underwear. There is hypopigmentation and thinning of the skin of the vulva, with small areas of excoriation. This is lichen sclerosus, a condition of unknown etiology that causes signs and symptoms that may be mistaken for trauma. Image reprinted with permission from eMedicine.com, 2010. Available at: http://emedicine.medscape.com/article/954024-overview.*

Appendix Figure 8-20-b. *A close-up view of the atrophic, hypopigmented skin. Note the very clear line of demarcation between the normal and affected skin.*

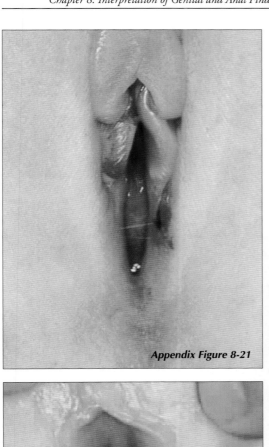

Appendix Figure 8-21

Appendix Figure 8-21. *This 7-year-old Caucasian girl also has lichen sclerosus. The hypopigmentation is a little harder to see, but the atrophic skin demonstrates the bleeding caused by minor rubbing or wiping. Using a red-free (green) filter on the colposcope can sometimes accentuate the hypopigmentation.*

Appendix Figure 8-22. *Lichen sclerosus affecting the perianal skin. The same pattern of hypopigmented, atrophic, easily abraded skin is evident in this photograph.*

Appendix Figure 8-23. *16-month-old girl referred for unusual appearance of the genital tissues. There was no history suggestive of injury or abuse. There is a mucosal defect extending from the fossa to the anus in the midline. This is failure of midline fusion, also called perineal groove. It did not change in appearance over a period of 6 months, ruling out trauma.*

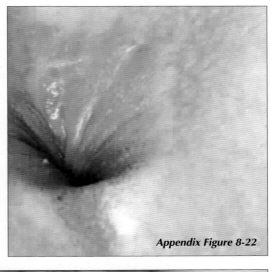

Appendix Figure 8-22

Appendix Figure 8-23

Appendix Figure 8-24. *This is a 4-month-old infant with the same condition. At the time she was evaluated, the condition of failure of fusion had not been recognized, and there was a concern for possible abuse. The child's family did not bring her back for a follow-up visit.*

Appendix Figure 8-24

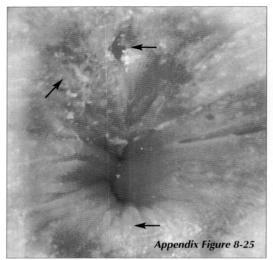

Appendix Figure 8-25

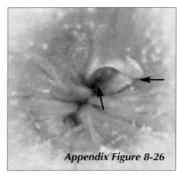

Appendix Figure 8-26

Appendix Figure 8-25. *6-year-old boy with a history of constipation who denied any anal trauma. There is an anal fissure at 12 o'clock and venous pooling at 1 o'clock. The area at 7 o'clock is called the anal verge.*

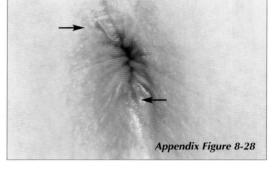

Appendix Figure 8-28

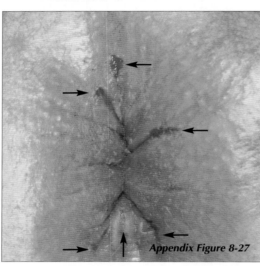

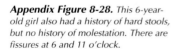
Appendix Figure 8-27

Appendix Figure 8-26. *8-month-old infant with an anal fissure at 12 o'clock and anal tag at about 1 o'clock. The most common cause of anal fissures is constipation, and tags may form at the site of the fissure.*

Appendix Figure 8-27. *This 9-month-old male was being cared for by an uncle. When mother came back, she found blood in the baby's diaper and became alarmed. When told that the baby had been screaming in pain while passing a stool, mother found the diaper with a large (4 centimeter diameter) rock-hard bowel movement in it and brought it along to the doctor. This baby has venous congestion and multiple small anal fissures caused by the passage of the large, hard stool.*

Appendix Figure 8-28. *This 6-year-old girl also had a history of hard stools, but no history of molestation. There are fissures at 6 and 11 o'clock.*

Appendix Figure 8-29. *This child had complained of anal itching. On examination, the anus is partially dilated at 1 o'clock, and there are two pinworms at 6 and 9 o'clock coming out of the opening.*

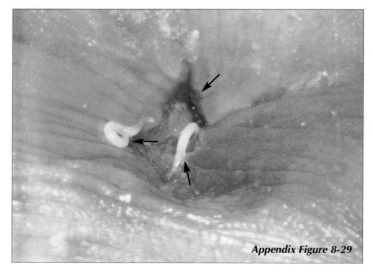

Appendix Figure 8-29

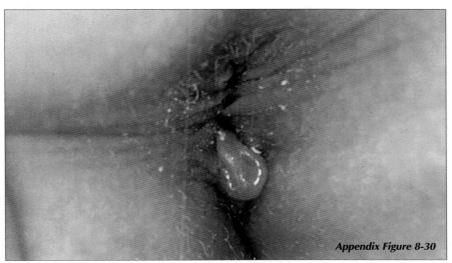

Appendix Figure 8-30. Anal polyp in an infant. These are large anal tags that sometimes also contain veins. They require no treatment.

Appendix Figure 8-30

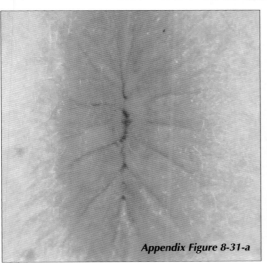

Appendix Figure 8-31-a

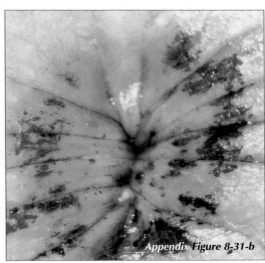

Appendix Figure 8-31-b

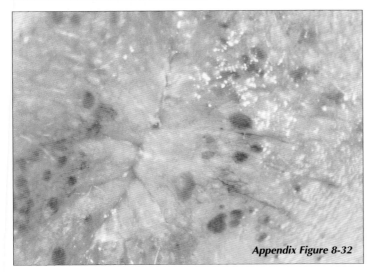

Appendix Figure 8-32

Appendix Figure 8-31-a. *2-year-old with red bottom after coming back from a visit with father. Parents are divorced and mother is always worried about the possibility of abuse.*

Appendix Figure 8-31-b. *After the application of Toluidine Blue dye, the superficial abrasions around the anus caused by diaper dermatitis are highlighted. Positive dye uptake is only indicative of disruption of the superficial layer of the epidermis, which can be caused by minor rubbing, scratching, or dermatitis.*

Appendix Figure 8-32. *4-month-old with diaper dermatitis, also after application of dye. The uptake pattern is not typical of lacerations.*

133

Appendix Figure 8-33. *Normal anal folds in an 11-year-old girl examined in the prone knee-chest position.*

Appendix Figure 8-34. *This 8-year-old girl, examined in the prone knee-chest position, has a partially relaxed anal sphincter, with a deep fold at 6 o'clock that should not be mistaken for a laceration. By allowing the child to further relax, the sphincter will usually dilate fully and the folds, including deep folds, will smooth out.*

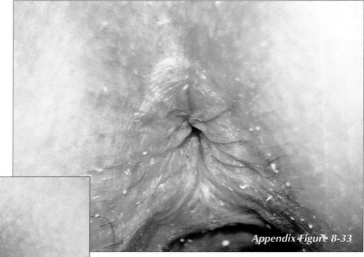

Appendix Figure 8-33

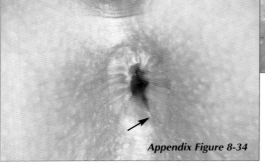

Appendix Figure 8-34

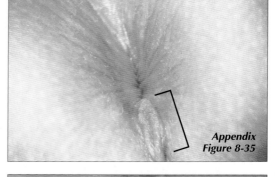

Appendix Figure 8-35

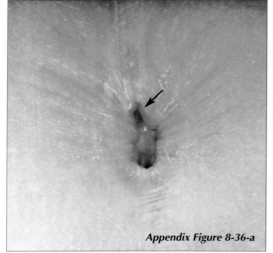

Appendix Figure 8-36-a

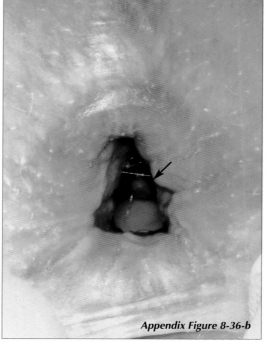

Appendix Figure 8-36-b

Appendix Figure 8-35. *This boy has a thick fold of skin in the median raphe, a normal finding.*

Appendix Figure 8-36-a. *Partial dilation of the anal sphincter with a very deep fold noted at the 12 o'clock location.*

Appendix Figure 8-36-b. *With more complete relaxation of the external and internal anal sphincters, stool is visible in the rectal vault at 2 o'clock, and the deep fold has disappeared.*

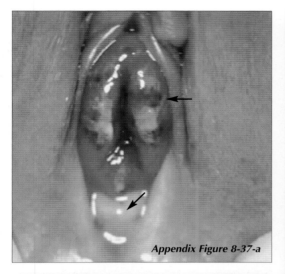

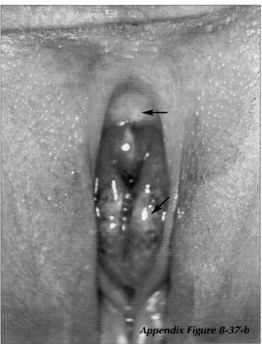

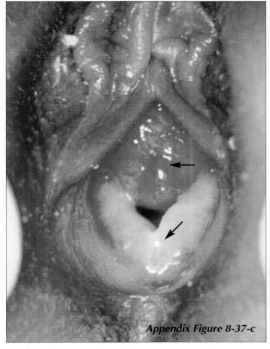

Appendix Figure 8-37-a. 3-year-old girl presented with blood in her underwear and a history of having pulled out a Foley catheter during a recent hospitalization. The bleeding is coming from a prolapsed urethra at 3 o'clock, which is showing some early signs of necrosis. The hymen at 6 o'clock is pale and smooth. Image reprinted with permission from eMedicine.com, 2010. Available at: http://emedicine.medscape.com/article/954024-overview.

Appendix Figure 8-37-b. In the prone knee-chest position, the prolapsed urethra is still occluding the hymenal opening. This condition can usually be successfully treated with warm soaks, oral antibiotics, and topical estrogen cream.

Appendix Figure 8-37-c. After 2 weeks, the prolapse at 3 o'clock has significantly improved. The hymen at 6 o'clock is now better visualized. Image reprinted with permission from eMedicine.com, 2010. Available at: http://emedicine.medscape.com/article/954024-overview.

Appendix Figure 8-38. 4-year-old African-American girl with urethral prolapse at 3 o'clock and normal, thick hymen at 6 o'clock.

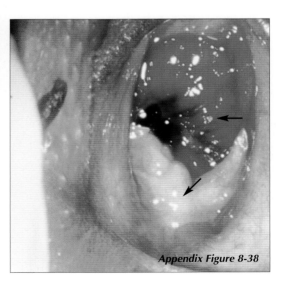

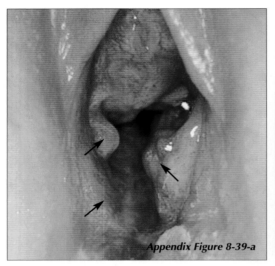

Appendix Figure 8-39-a

Appendix Figures 8-39-a through **8-39-g:** *9-year-old girl, sexually assaulted by her stepfather 6 days prior to presenting for evaluation. She was noted by the school nurse to be bleeding and told the nurse what had happened.*

Appendix Figure 8-39-a: *With minimal labial separation, a laceration of the posterior fourchette is seen at 6 o'clock and a loss of hymenal tissue between 3 and 9 o'clock. Reprinted with permission from "The Sexual Abuse CD ROM Teaching Set" published by the North American Society for Pediatric and Adolescent Gynecology, NASPAG.org.*

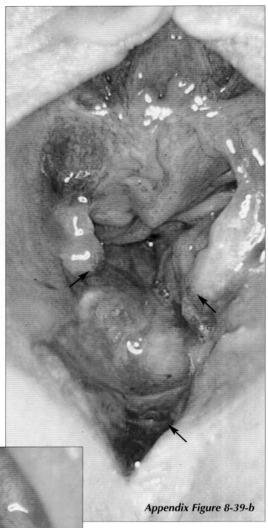

Appendix Figure 8-39-b

Appendix Figure 8-39-b: *With additional labial separation, the hymen is completely transected, with the torn edges indicated between 3 and 9 o'clock. The deep laceration of the fossa and posterior fourchette at 6 o'clock began to ooze blood when the labia were separated by the examiner. Image reprinted with permission from eMedicine.com, 2010. Available at: http://emedicine. medscape.com/article/954024-overview.*

Appendix Figure 8-39-c: *At 13 days after the assault, the posterier fourchette tear is beginning to heal. There is a loss of hymen tissue between 5 and 8 o'clock. Reprinted with permission from "The Sexual Abuse CD ROM Teaching Set" published by the North American Society for Pediatric and Adolescent Gynecology, NASPAG.org.*

Appendix Figure 8-39-c

Appendix Figure 8-39-d: *At 13 days post assault, in the knee-chest position, the loss of hymen in the midline between 2 and 11 o'clock is clearly evident. Reprinted with permission from "The Sexual Abuse CD ROM Teaching Set" published by the North American Society for Pediatric and Adolescent Gynecology, NASPAG.org.*

Appendix Figure 8-39-e: *One month post assault, the posterior fourchette tear has healed, leaving a midline scar shown at 6 o'clock. The 2 sections of hymen are again seen between 3 and 9 o'clock. An adhesion has developed anteriorly between the labia minora at 12 o'clock.*

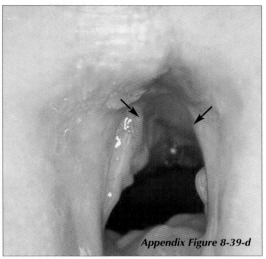

Appendix Figure 8-39-d

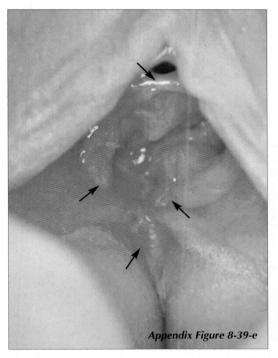

Appendix Figure 8-39-e

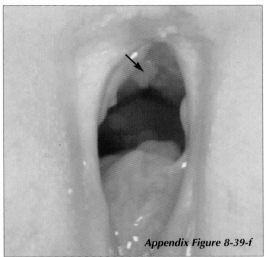

Appendix Figure 8-39-f

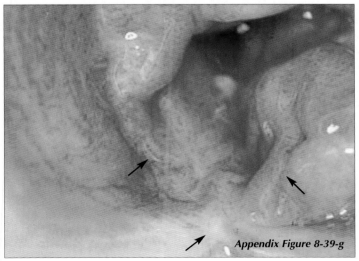

Appendix Figure 8-39-g

Appendix Figure 8-39-f: *In the knee-chest position at one month, reactive scar tissue appears to have developed within the vagina at 12 o'clock, on the posterior vaginal wall.*

Appendix Figure 8-39-g: *One year after the assault, the 2 edges of the hymen have not grown back together between 5 and 7 o'clock, and there is a midline scar of the posterior fourchette at the location of the laceration shown at 6 o'clock. Reprinted with permission from "The Sexual Abuse CD ROM Teaching Set" published by the North American Society for Pediatric and Adolescent Gynecology, NASPAG.org.*

Appendix Figures 8-40-a through **8-40-h:** *This 9-year-old girl was abducted and raped by a stranger. She was found walking along the highway and given a ride to the hospital when she told what had happened to her. She identified the truck of her assailant, and he was arrested, charged, and convicted.*

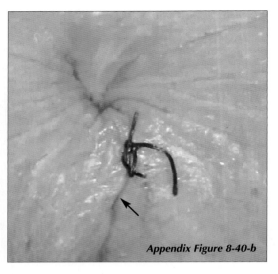

Appendix Figure 8-40-b

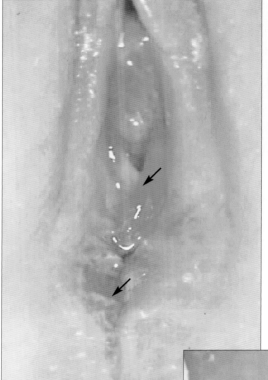

Appendix Figure 8-40-a: *Photo was taken 3 days after surgical repair of a deep laceration of the posterior fourchette that extended across the perineum almost to the anal sphincter. The 2 parts of the transected hymen were overlapped (upper arrow), when the posterior fourchette tear was sutured shown at 6 o'clock. Reprinted with permission from "The Sexual Abuse CD ROM Teaching Set" published by the North American Society for Pediatric and Adolescent Gynecology, NASPAG.org.*

Appendix Figure 8-40-b: *This photograph shows the extent of the laceration and the suture repair at 6 o'clock, extending almost to the anal verge.*

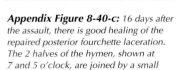

Appendix Figure 8-40-a

Appendix Figure 8-40-c: *16 days after the assault, there is good healing of the repaired posterior fourchette laceration. The 2 halves of the hymen, shown at 7 and 5 o'clock, are joined by a small band of scar tissue at 6 o'clock. Reprinted with permission from "The Sexual Abuse CD ROM Teaching Set" published by the North American Society for Pediatric and Adolescent Gynecology, NASPAG.org.*

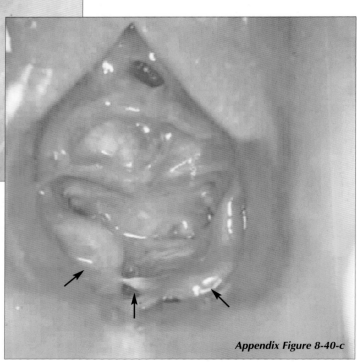

Appendix Figure 8-40-c

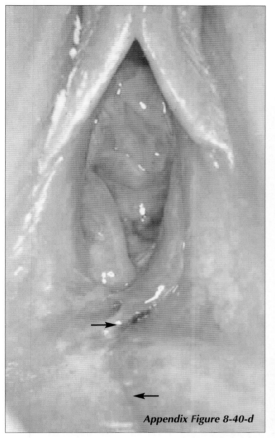

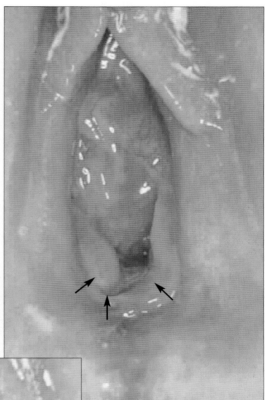

Appendix Figure 8-40-d: *At 16 days, the left half of the torn hymen is bound down to the fossa with scar tissue (top arrow). The thin line across the perineum is the scar from the repaired laceration at 6 o'clock. Reprinted with permission from "The Sexual Abuse CD ROM Teaching Set" published by the North American Society for Pediatric and Adolescent Gynecology, NASPAG.org.*

Appendix Figure 8-40-d

Appendix Figure 8-40-e

Appendix Figure 8-40-e: *One month post assault, there is still a small band of scar tissue shown at 6 o'clock connecting the 2 halves of the hymen.*

Appendix Figure 8-40-f: *Six months post assault, white, flat scar tissue, at 5 to 6 o'clock, has developed in the fossa adjacent to the site of the hymenal laceration.*

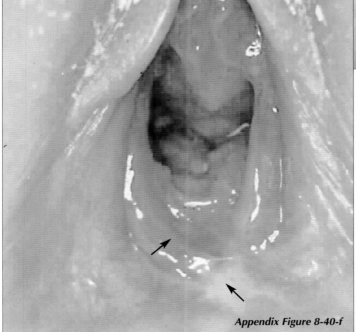

Appendix Figure 8-40-f

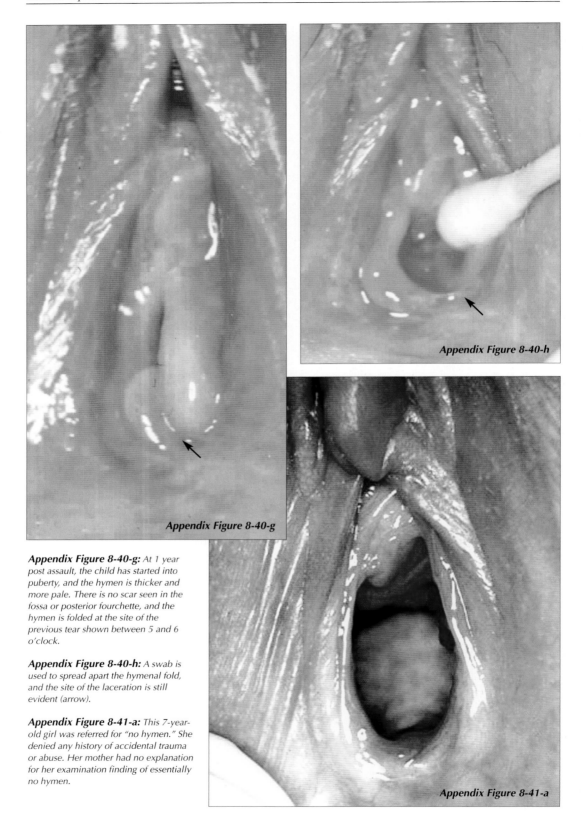

Appendix Figure 8-40-h

Appendix Figure 8-40-g

Appendix Figure 8-40-g: *At 1 year post assault, the child has started into puberty, and the hymen is thicker and more pale. There is no scar seen in the fossa or posterior fourchette, and the hymen is folded at the site of the previous tear shown between 5 and 6 o'clock.*

Appendix Figure 8-40-h: *A swab is used to spread apart the hymenal fold, and the site of the laceration is still evident (arrow).*

Appendix Figure 8-41-a: *This 7-year-old girl was referred for "no hymen." She denied any history of accidental trauma or abuse. Her mother had no explanation for her examination finding of essentially no hymen.*

Appendix Figure 8-41-a

Appendix Figure 8-41-b: *Using labial traction, there are only minute remnants of hymen remaining.*

Appendix Figure 8-41-c: *In the prone knee-chest position, it is still not possible to identify any hymenal tissue between 9 o'clock and 4 o'clock. The cause for this disruption was never determined.*

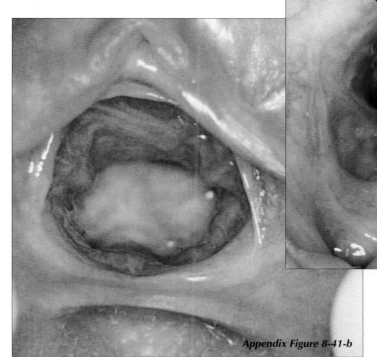

Appendix Figure 8-41-c

Appendix Figure 8-41-b

Appendix Figure 8-42: *16-year-old girl who has been consensually sexually active for 1 year. There is a transection in the hymen at 5 o'clock.*

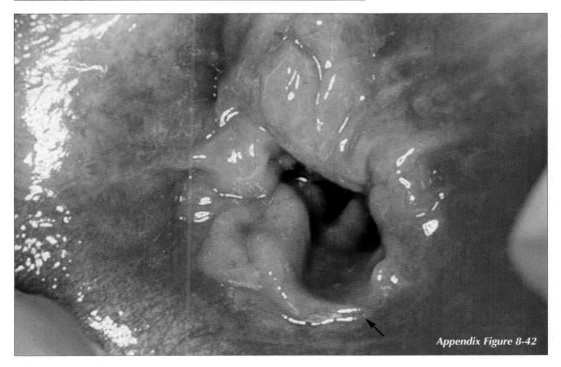

Appendix Figure 8-42

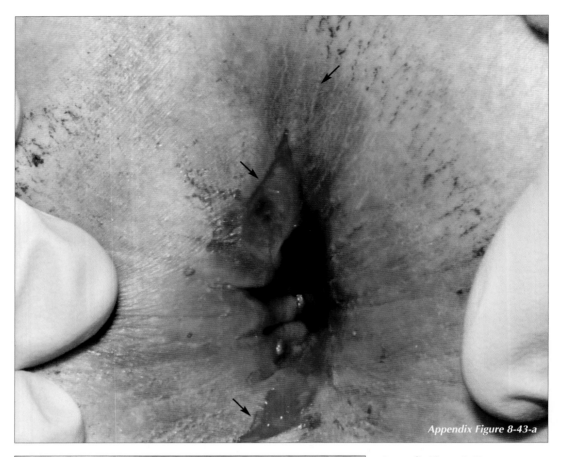

Appendix Figure 8-43-a

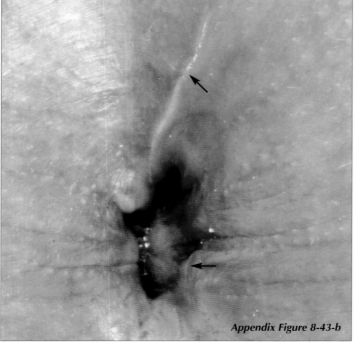

Appendix Figure 8-43-b

Appendix Figure 8-43-a: *This 7-year-old boy asked his mother: "Is my bottom still supposed to be hurting?" When asked for details, he revealed that a 14-year-old male cousin had put his penis in his bottom and told him it would only hurt for a little while. On examination, there is extensive bruising all around the anus and 2 deep anal lacerations at 6 and 11 o'clock.*

Appendix Figure 8-43-b: *10 days after the assault, the bruising has resolved, and there is a white scar at the site of the larger laceration at 12 o'clock.*

REFERENCES

1. Adams J, Harper K, Knudson S. A proposed classification of anogenital findings in children with suspected sexual abuse. *Adolesc Pediatr Gynecol*. 1992;5:73-75.

2. McCann J, Voris J, Simon M, Wells R. Perianal findings in prepubertal children selected for non-abuse: a descriptive study. *Child Abuse & Neglect*. 1989; 13:179-193.

3. McCann J, Wells R, Simon M, Voris J. Genital findings in prepubertal girls selected for non-abuse: a descriptive study. *Pediatrics*. 1990;86:428-439.

4. Berenson A, Heger A, Andrews S. Appearance of the hymen in newborns. *Pediatrics*. 1991;87:458-465.

5. American Academy of Pediatrics, Committee on Child Abuse and Neglect. Guidelines for the evaluation of sexual abuse of children. *Pediatrics*. 1991;87:254-259.

6. Berenson AB, Heger AH, Hayes JM, et al. Appearance of the hymen in prepubertal girls. *Pediatrics*. 1992;89:387-394.

7. Myhre AK, Berntzen K, Bratlid D. Genital anatomy in non-abused preschool girls. *Acta Paediatr*. 2003;92:1453-1462.

8. McCann J, Voris J, Simon M. Genital injuries resulting from sexual abuse: A longitudinal study. *Pediatrics*. 1992;89:307-317.

9. McCann J, Voris J. Perianal injuries resulting from sexual abuse: a longitudinal study. *Pediatrics*. 1993;91:390-397.

10. Heppenstall-Heger A, McConnell G, Ticson L, et al. Healing patterns in anogenital injuries: a longitudinal study of injuries associated with sexual abuse, accidental injuries, or genital surgery in the preadolescent child. *Pediatrics*. 2003;112:829-837.

11. Adams JA. Approach to the interpretation of medical and laboratory findings in suspected child sexual abuse: a 2005 revision. *The APSAC Advisor*. 2005;17:7-13.

12. Berenson AB, Chacko MR, Wiemann CM, et al. A case-control study of anatomic changes resulting from sexual abuse. *Am J Obstet Gynecol*. 2000;182:820-834.

13. Adams JA, Botash AS, Kellogg N. Differences in hymenal morphology between adolescent girls with and without a history of consensual sexual intercourse. *Arch Pediatr Adolesc Med*. 2004;158:280-285.

14. Heger AH, Ticson L, Guerra L, et al. Appearance of the genitalia in girls selected for non-abuse: review of hymenal morphology and non-specific findings. *J Pediatr Adolesc Gynecol*. 2002;15:27-35.

15. Berenson AB, Grady JJ. A longitudinal study of hymenal development from 3 to 9 years of age. *J Pediatr*. 2002;140:600-607.

16. Adams JA, Harper K, Knudson S, et al. Examination findings in legally confirmed child sexual abuse: it's normal to be normal. *Pediatrics*. 1994;94:310-317.

17. Myhre AK, Berntzen K, Bratlid D. Perianal anatomy in non-abused preschool children. *Acta Paediatr*. 2001;1321-1328.

18. Heger A, Emans SJ, Muram D, eds. *Evaluation of the Sexually Abused Child: A Medical Textbook and Photographic Atlas*. 2nd Edition. New York: Oxford University Press;2000.

19. Heger A, Ticson L, Velasquez O, et al. Children referred for possible sexual abuse: medical findings in 2384 children. *Child Abuse Negl.* 2002;26:645-659.

20. Boos SC. Accidental hymenal injury mimicking sexual trauma. *Pediatrics.* 1999;103:1287-1289.

21. Herrmann B, Crawford J. Genital injuries in prepubertal girls from inline skating accidents. *Pediatrics.* 2002;110:e16. http://www.pediatrics.org/cgi/content/full/110/2/e16. Accessed June 16, 2009.

22. Boos SC, Rosas AJ, Boyle C, et al. Anogenital injuries in child pedestrians run over by low-speed motor vehicles: four cases with findings that mimic child sexual abuse. *Pediatrics.* 2003;112:e77. http://www.pediatrics.org/cgi/content/full/112/1/e77. Accessed June 16, 2009.

23. McCann J, Miyamoto S, Boyle C, Rogers K. Healing of hymenal injuries in prepubertal and adolescent girls: a descriptive study. *Pediatrics.* 2007;119:e1094-e1106. http://www.pediatrics.org/cgi/content/full/119/5/e1094. Accessed May 16, 2007.

24. McCann J, Miyamoto S, Boyle C, Rogers K. Healing of nonhymenal genital injuries in prepubertal and adolescent girls: a descriptive study. *Pediatr.* 2007;120:1000-1011.

25. Boyle C, McCann J, Miyamoto S, Rogers K. Comparison of examination methods used in the evaluation of prepubertal and pubertal female genitalia: a descriptive study. *Child Abuse Neglect.* 2008; 32:229-243.

26. Kellogg ND, Menard SW, Santos A. Genital anatomy in pregnant adolescents: "normal" doesn't mean "nothing happened." *Pediatr.* 2004;223:e67-e69. http://www.pediatrics.org/cgi/content/full/113/1/e67. Accessed June 16, 2009.

27. Jones JS, Rossman L, Hartman M, et al. Anogenital injuries in adolescents after consensual sexual intercourse. *Acad Emerg Med.* 2003;10:1378-1383.

28. Huppert JS, Gerber MA, Deitch HR, et al. Vulvar ulcers in young females: a manifestation of apthosis. *J Pediatr Adolesc Gynecol.* 2006;19:195-204.

29. Adams JA, Kaplan RA, Starling SP, et al: Guidelines for medical care for children who may have been sexually abused. *J Pediatr Adolesc Gynecol.* 2007; 20:163-172

30. Adams JA. Guidelines for medical care of children evaluated for suspected sexual abuse: an update for 2008. *Curr Opin Obstet Gynecol.* 2008;20:435-441.

Chapter 9

MEDICAL CONDITIONS THAT MIMIC SEXUAL ABUSE

Lori Frasier, MD

One of the most common reasons for medical referrals in alleged child abuse cases is to evaluate allegations of sexual abuse. As noted in Chapter 7, physical findings resulting from sexual abuse are exceedingly rare. The child abuse specialist often has special expertise and training in evaluation of a broad variety of anogenital conditions and as such may become the point of referral for these conditions. The referral may be initiated because of a possible history of abuse disclosed by the child, behavioral findings, medical signs, or symptoms. Occasionally, a disclosure of abuse accompanies signs or symptoms. The examining clinician must always remain objective in such examinations and not allow the history from the child to overly influence the interpretation of medical findings. The coincidental occurrence of an anogenital condition should not lead the examiner to suggest the condition results from the abuse. Preexamination bias should especially be guarded against when referrals are exclusively for anogenital complaints by the child or when an observation by a parent or referring medical provider indicates that the child has some finding that may be due to sexual abuse. The differential diagnosis of any anogenital symptom must include a variety of conditions unrelated to sexual abuse because there are many symptoms and diseases that may 'mimic' findings of sexual abuse.

In this chapter, many of the "medical mimics" of child sexual abuse (CSA) that have both been described in the literature and clinically observed will be reviewed. Because many patients are referred on the basis of symptoms, the approach of this chapter will be symptom-based rather than systems-based. A differential diagnosis for a variety of symptoms and a diagnostic approach will be presented.

MEDICAL MIMICS OF CSA
GENITAL IRRITATION/ERYTHEMA
A common reason that a clinician may see a child is to address anogenital redness or erythema discovered or reported by a parent or caregiver. Even in the context of recent abuse allegations, it may be difficult to differentiate erythema of nonabusive origins from erythema of sexually abusive origins. The clinician should not be too adamant that such a finding is the direct result of sexual trauma, but this possibility should be included in the analysis of the case. The erythema may involve the keratinized epithelium of the vulvar area, the perineum, the perianal area, the penis, or the mucosa of the vestibule (anatomically, the area between the labia minora and that includes the periurethral and perihymenal areas, the hymen, and the posterior navicular fossa). The most common causes of genital redness are poor hygiene and contact dermatitis. Also, in prepubertal girls, the mucosa of the vestibule may appear erythematous, and what is thought to be an abnormality is a normal appearance due to the highly vascular nature

of these tissues; therefore, what might be thought by the layperson to be an abnormality might in fact be a normal anatomic appearance.

A variety of products can result in a contact irritation of the genital area. These products can be perfume-containing soaps, lotions, bubble baths, toilet paper, and laundry products or any other product that contains irritants. Overzealous cleansing occurring occasionally may also cause such irritation. The diagnosis is usually made after clinical observation of erythema and loss of skin markings. Scaling, crusting, or even blistering can occur. Protected skin folds are usually spared. Edema can be marked if the contact dermatitis involves the penis or the foreskin. The clinical approach to a child with anogenital irritation and redness is first to recommend a regimen of excellent genital hygiene with avoidance of such products. Use of a bland emollient such as zinc oxide or bland occlusive ointment may help to protect the skin as it heals. If skin barrier integrity is lost, overgrowth of bacterial or fungal pathogens may result. These should be treated with appropriate antibiotics or antifungals. A rapid resolution of the condition will assure the parent and clinician the cause of the child's irritation/redness was related to these products or practices.

Other conditions that mimic chronic genital irritation include psoriasis and seborrheic dermatitis. Psoriasis usually occurs as skin lesions that are sharply demarcated and have fine, silvery scales. Inverse psoriasis is a distinct form of the condition that involves the anogenital area, axillae, and ear canals. Erythema is often the predominant clinical feature, and scaling is minimal, leading to confusion with candidiasis, contact dermatitis, or seborrhea. Skin biopsy is diagnostic and usually recommended only after multiple unsuccessful attempts at topical medications. Treatment of psoriasis is aimed at preventing irritation, with high-potency topical steroids given in short bursts.

Seborrheic dermatitis is a common skin condition that mainly affects the scalp and posterior auricular area but can also be present in the diaper area leading to a concern of sexual abuse. The condition is usually characterized by greasy, yellow scales. In severe cases, fissures may develop and become secondarily infected. Infantile seborrheic dermatitis generally spontaneously improves by the end of the first year of life.

Anogenital Bruising
Bruising or apparent bruising of the anogenital area raises a reasonable concern of sexual abuse; however, a careful examination may reveal other conditions. A child may have either what appears to be a significant injury without a history of trauma or an injury history that seems out of context with very minor trauma.

Lichen Sclerosus
Descriptions of childhood lichen sclerosus (LS) et atrophicus first appeared in the literature in the 1950s. However, Jenny et al[1,2] noted that LS was being confused with trauma caused by sexual abuse. Since that time, other authors[3,4] have described this condition as one of the most common mimics of anogenital trauma. Lichen sclerosus is commonly seen in postmenopausal women as a skin condition of unknown origin. Various causative factors have been suggested. These causes range from infections with Borrelia species to immunologic association with certain HLA antigens to familial incidence.[5-7] In children, the classic case is seen in a prepubertal child with a history of waxing and waning genital irritation. There is often a history of frequent treatments for supposed yeast infections because of the prominent symptom of pruritus. Fissuring and stricture in the perianal area have also been reported to cause constipation, a symptom of perianal lichen sclerosus. The skin of the vulva is hypopigmented and atrophic, often in a "figure of 8 pattern" (**Figures 9-1-a, b,** and **c**). This pattern may not be as apparent

in very fair-skinned individuals. Subcutaneous hemorrhage and hemorrhagic bullae are often the hallmark of LS (**Figure 9-2**). Interestingly, the mucosa, including the hymen, is spared, and appears normal.

In severe cases of LS, the act of wiping or sliding off of the toilet may result in denudation of the atrophic epithelium, with pain and bleeding. Upon examination, the child appears to have both bruising and ulcerations, raising concerns of trauma and other infections caused by sexual abuse. Lichen sclerosus is not just a condition of girls. In a study of 140 boys undergoing circumcision, histologic evidence of LS was found in six (4.3%) of the patients.[8] Balanitis xerotica obliterans (BXO) is a subcategory of LS that is limited to the male genitalia and is associated with destructive inflammation, phimosis, urethral stenosis, and squamous cell carcinoma. BXO usually surfaces in adulthood. There are no longitudinal studies in either male or female children with LS that suggest such children are at risk for the development of squamous cell carcinoma.

Treatment of LS is aimed at palliation during symptomatic periods. Most cases are mild and respond to the avoidance of irritants, clothing, and activities that cause trauma. More difficult cases have been treated with a variety of agents such as progesterone, topical estrogens, high-potency corticosteroids, immunosuppressants, and topical nonsteroidal antiinflammatory

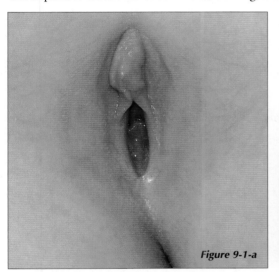

Figure 9-1-a

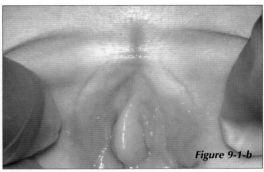

Figure 9-1-b

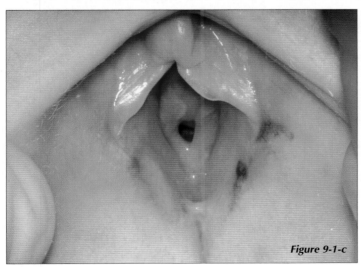

Figure 9-1-c

Figure 9-1-a. *Generalized erythema of the genital mucosa has a variety of causes, but often raises a concern about sexual abuse. Removal of irritants and good genital hygiene result in clearing of the skin.*

Figure 9-1-b. *Pale skin anterior to the clitoris in Lichen Sclerosis et atrophicus. The fissuring is due to friability of the tissue and is a common feature seen in patients with Lichen Sclerosis.*

Figure 9-1-c. *Typical presentation of Lichen Sclerosis et atrophicus, with pale atrophic skin and subcutaneous hemorrhage. The mucosa is not involved.*

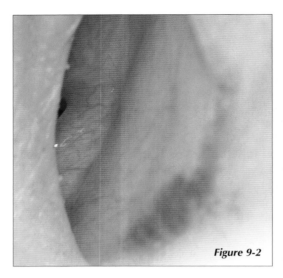

Figure 9-2

Figure 9-2.
Another view of the same patient in Figure 9-1-c. Subcutaneous hemorrhage can resemble traumatic injury.

agents.[9-11] In children who have constipation or anal stricture, a stool softener may be helpful. On average, the condition resolves in adolescence.

HEMANGIOMAS/VASCULAR MALFORMATIONS

A vulvar hemangioma that had undergone ulcerative changes and was thought initially to be an abusive burn was described by Levin et al in 1992.[12] Vascular malformations of the genital area are rare and may not be present at birth. When they become apparent, they could raise concern of abuse. Venous, lymphatic, and capillary-lymphatic-venous malformations are the most common. These can manifest in a variety of ways: as cutaneous marks resembling bruises, genital swelling, deformity, bleeding, fluid leakage, or infection (**Figures 9-3 and 9-4**).[13] Sacral hemangiomas can be associated with imperforate anus. Small vascular malformations or strawberry hemangiomas (**Figure 9-4**) on the genital area may appear as bruises. Unlike bruises, these are relatively stable lesions that do not change or resolve over a short period of times such as weeks; therefore, reevaluation of the area usually leads the clinician to make a diagnosis of a stable vascular lesions, rather than a traumatic bruise or contusion. It is advisable that high-quality photodocumentation be performed in any case that appears to be acute injury. These photos can be compared with ones taken at a later date.

Treatment is difficult in some cases. Because genital cavernous hemangiomas tend to ulcerate, more aggressive treatments such as intralesional steroids or laser ablations may be in order. For large vascular lesions, surgical sclerosis of feeding vessels may result in a reduction of the hemangioma.

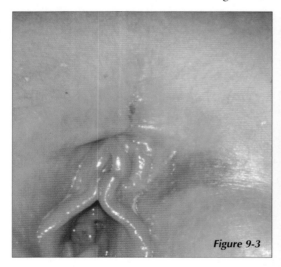

Figure 9-3

Figure 9-3. *Clitoral hood vascular lesion and a small anterior fissure due to poor hygiene. The child was examined one week later; the vascular malformation was stable and the small fissure had resolved.*

Figure 9-4. *Hemangioma.*

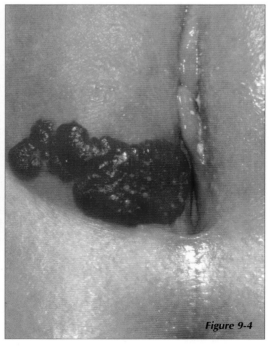

Figure 9-4

PURPURA AS A MIMIC OF BRUISING

Purpura is a common, unspecific symptom indicative of a pathologic condition in which blood leaks into the tissues. Purpuric disorders can be classified according to the pathophysiologic processes outlined in **Table 9-1**.

Purpuric lesions can occur in the genital area only, but their manifestation on the genitalia could simply be the first location of a sequence of symptoms that lead to concerns of sexual abuse. More commonly these conditions have been described as physical abuse mimics. Often, as in Henoch-Schönlein purpura (HSP), if the first symptom appears in the genital area, the extent of the purpura will manifest in a matter of hours to days[14-16] (**Figure 9-5**). Also, the child frequently has classic accompanying symptoms such as abdominal or joint pain, hematuria, and bloody stools.

ACCIDENTAL GENITAL INJURIES

Differentiating an accidental anogenital injury from one (we don't like the term *intentional* in the abuse world; we don't know the "intent" of the abuser) due to abuse is usually straightforward. The child or parent often gives a clear history of some type of impact to the genital area followed by bleeding and pain. On occasion, the child is too young to interview, but the injury is typical of a straddle and the child is ambulatory and has the capability of falling accidentally; however, unusual injuries may be more difficult to evaluate and, therefore, of more concern. Most impact or straddle injuries in girls occur when there is impact between the child and a hard object such as a bicycle or a metal bar of playground equipment. The soft tissues are compressed between the hard object and the ischial tuberosities, causing contusions, lacerations, and even injuries reflecting transmitted trauma to different areas. Most straddle injuries are more anterior, external to the hymen, and unilateral (**Figures 9-6** and **9-7**). If there is a history of impalement, a more internal injury such as tearing of the hymen or perineum may be observed.[17] Unusual injuries have been reported in the literature. In one case, a child who fell while water-skiing had a jet of water injected into her vagina, tearing the vaginal wall without injury to the hymen.[18] Other unusual injuries have occurred when a child's pelvic area was crushed by a car rollover.[18] Another accidental perineal injury is described in which a sudden abduction of the legs during rollerblading caused a perineal "split" injury.[19, 20]

Table 9-1. Classification of Purpuric Disorders
PLATELET DISORDERS
— Primary thrombocytopenic purpura such as idiopathic thrombocytopenic purpura
— Secondary thrombocytopenic purpura caused by conditions such as leukemia or aplastic anemias
VASCULAR DISORDERS
— Vasculitis, as in the case of Henoch-Schönlein purpura (HSP)
COAGULATION DISORDERS
— Disseminated intravascular coagulation resulting from shock or infection; such children are extremely ill
— Hemophilias
— von Willebrand disease

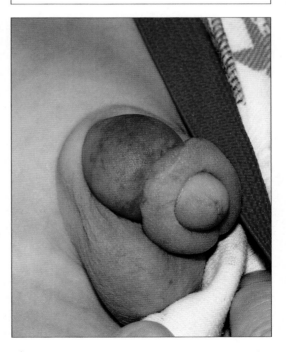

Figure 9-5. *A child who has Henoch Schönlein purpura with involvement of the penis mimicking bruising.*

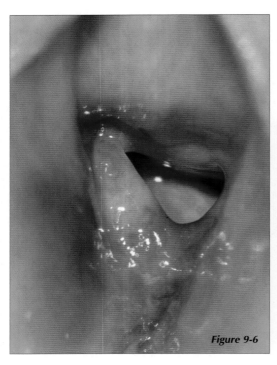

Figure 9-6. *Straddle injuries can involve the hymen if there is external to internal injury, as seen in the child who fell astraddle a diving board and has a posterior fourchette injury, external bruise, and hymenal hematoma.*

Figure 9-7. *This child fell astraddle the handle of a child's toy wagon. The hymen is not well visualized but is normal. There is a hematoma in the fossa from the straddle injury.*

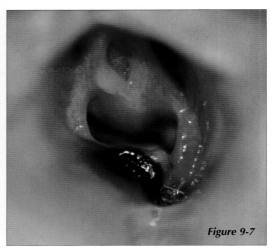

Figure 9-6

Figure 9-7

Merritt's[21] review of genital injuries revealed that the history from the child regarding how the injury occurred remained the most important indicator of whether that injury was accidental or due to sexual abuse. Good photodocumentation with peer review is also helpful in determining the etiologic background of injuries. Occasionally, injuries may be repaired surgically prior to consultation with a child abuse expert. In these cases, it is important to review the provided clinical description and the history. Photography by the repairing surgeon should be encouraged.

SKIN DISCOLORATIONS FROM DYES, SURGICAL ADJUNCTS, AND PLANTS

Although not frequently reported in the literature, marks from dyes (especially those used in colored clothing) can cause discoloration of the skin that resembles a bruise. In addition, this author encountered a patient whose parents had used an aloe vera plant as a diaper rash ointment. This resulted in black streaks on the buttocks that resembled bruises. The clinical test involved wiping the area gently with an alcohol-based wipe, which resulted in removal of the discoloration.

One case of a "Betadine tattoo" has been reported in a child who underwent a surgical procedure. After being cleansed with povidone-iodine (Betadine), the child had circular markings of the buttocks form that resembled fingertip bruises. The grounding for the electrocautery had caused the Betadine to temporarily "tattoo" the skin, resulting in a concern that the child was abused during surgery. The concern regarding sexual abuse was resolved with the explanation for this lesion.

Phytophotodermatitis is a phototoxic dermatitis resulting from contact with psoralen-containing plants such as celery, limes, parsley, figs, eggplant, tomatoes, and carrots. Berloque dermatitis is a variant of phytophotodermatitis and is caused by high concentrations of psoralen-containing fragrances—most commonly, oil of bergamot. The result of exposure to such products and then sunlight may mimic bruises or burns on the skin.

BLEEDING

Blood on the child's underwear is often called "vaginal bleeding" by caregivers and referring clinicians. However, only when blood is observed coming from the vagina is this condition considered truly "vaginal" in origin, which necessitates a far different diagnostic approach than blood originating in structures other than the vagina. The source of the bleeding may be the skin, the urinary tract, or the gastrointestinal tract. All such sources should be considered in an investigation of bleeding.

A careful examination proceeding from external cutaneous structures to more internal genital structures may lead to a determination of the source of the bleeding and subsequently the appropriate diagnosis. A clinician inexperienced in examining children will often try to see the hymen and vagina first without properly assessing other structures. If the origin of blood is not clear, a urinalysis for hematuria as well as a test on the stool for occult blood should be performed to further attempt to locate the source of the bleeding. Brown staining of a child's underwear with stool can sometimes indicate the source of the "blood." Having the parent bring in the child's underwear is often helpful. Frank red blood or slight serosanguineous streaking versus saturation of the underclothing may also guide the clinician in the diagnostic approach.

Skin

Maceration with Irritant Contact

Any of the conditions noted in the earlier contact irritant section can result in extreme maceration with bleeding of the skin. Superficial abrasions either caused by assault or that are self-inflicted can create enough bleeding to raise concerns (**Figure 9-8**).

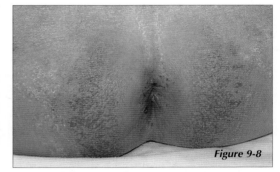

Figure 9-8

Urinary Tract

A urinalysis and careful external examination of the periurethral area may reveal the source of bleeding. Urinary tract infections, hematuria from renal origin, and hemorrhagic cystitis may be diagnosed and appropriately treated.

One frequently reported apparent cause of vaginal bleeding is urethral prolapse. A review of the literature spanning 50 years indicates that urethral prolapse has been reported worldwide.[22-28] Urethral prolapse is most often observed as bleeding, presumably vaginal in origin; furthermore, when examined, the prolapsed, doughnut-shaped urethral tissue is swollen and bleeding and it obscures the anatomy of the hymen (**Figure 9-9**). It is therefore not surprising that genital trauma is immediately considered. Although the incidence is not known, urethral prolapse is rare in all ethnic groups. Anecdotal evidence suggests that the condition may be more common in children of African origin. It is rare in Caucasian children, and the reason for this racial disparity is unknown.

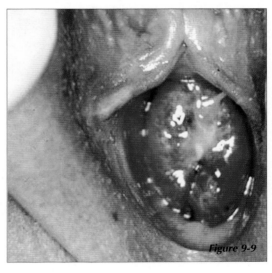

Figure 9-9

Figure 9-8. *This child presented with blood in his underwear and severe maceration of eczematous skin. This was the cause of the bleeding.*

Figure 9-9. *Urethral prolapse.*

Various treatments have been proposed, ranging from excision of the prolapsed tissue to conservative approaches of sitz baths and topical estrogens.[29,30] On some occasions the prolapse does not resolve with such treatment and referral to a pediatric urologist for surgical reduction of the prolapsed tissue may be necessary.

Perivaginal

The perivaginal area may be the source of bleeding. Usually the amount is scant, but it can still be alarming to the caregiver. The clinician should take special care to examine all of the external structures for evidence of bleeding prior to assessing the vaginal area.

Group A, Beta-Hemolytic Streptococci

Group A beta-hemolytic streptococcus causes vulvitis in prepubertal girls. Although such infections may be accompanied by discharge, the mucosa of the perivaginal area is often extremely swollen, beefy in appearance, and bleeding (**Figures 9-10-a** and **b**). Evidence of group A streptococcus dermatitis may be apparent with small satellite lesions consisting of papules, progressing to impetiginous changes. A culture of the perivaginal area is all that is needed to diagnose this condition, which is often quickly responsive to appropriate broad-spectrum oral antibiotics. The child may or may not have evidence of streptococcus pharyngitis.

Shigella Vaginitis

Another bacterial cause of vaginal bleeding is shigella vaginitis. Shigella is a gram-negative bacteria that typically causes enterocolitis (**Figure 9-11**). Vaginal shigellosis

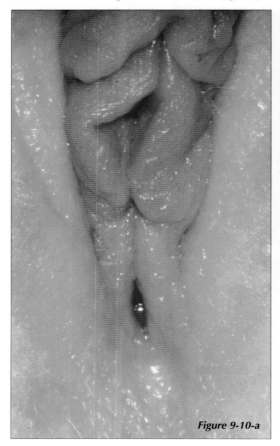

Figure 9-10-a.

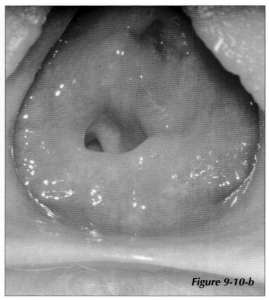

Figure 9-10-b

Figure 9-10-a. *External genital redness in a child with a history of discharge, odor, and slight blood streaking of the underwear.*

Figure 9-10-b. *Extreme erythema of the genital mucosa in the same child as Figure 9-10-a. Both external and mucosal erythema can be a sign of group A strep vulvovaginitis, as seen in this child.*

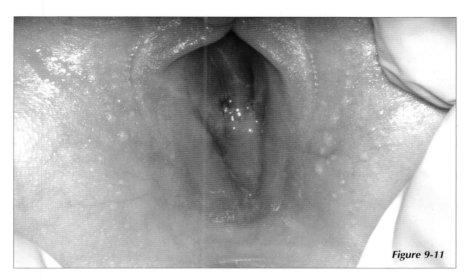

Figure 9-11.
This child's vaginal culture grew Shigella enterocolitica. She presented with vaginal bleeding and a concern of sexual abuse. There is significant redenss and swelling of the mucosa.

Figure 9-11

may not be accompanied by bloody diarrhea or fever.[31] Most shigella infections in the United States are due to shigella sonnei or flexneri.

Topical Irritant or Contact Dermatitis

Any topical irritant or contact dermatitis can result in the perivaginal area being so macerated that bleeding occurs. This is difficult clinically to differentiate from other conditions such as group A streptococcus vulvitis and may respond to similar treatment approaches.

Vaginal Bleeding

Blood observed to originate from beyond the hymenal opening is true vaginal bleeding. The differential diagnosis is very broad. Without evidence of penetrating trauma (ie, injury to the hymen or the external structures), it would be difficult to speculate that the bleeding results from direct vaginal trauma. With signs of sexual development (breast budding, growth acceleration, pubic hair), an endocrine etiology becomes the leading diagnosis; in this case, referral to an endocrinologist is recommended. Vaginal bleeding without sexual development is rare. In a study by Uli et al,[32] only 3 of 33 cases of prepubertal vaginal bleeding in the absence of sexual development were the result of prepubertal menarche. The majority were vaginitis (30%) or vaginal foreign bodies (30%), with the remainder being benign and malignant vaginal or vulvar tumors. A thorough history and physical examination would have revealed the need for a comprehensive endocrinologic examination in only the minority of cases.

Endocrine

Newborn Withdrawal Bleeding

Withdrawal bleeding may occur in the newborn female as the result of the discontinuation of maternal estrogens at birth.[31] Mothers should be instructed about the potential for this bleeding, because they might be alarmed when they notice blood in the diapers.

Prepubertal Menarche

This is an unusual condition resulting in intermittent or cyclic vaginal bleeding in children without the development of secondary sex characteristics. The vagina and uterus are normal, as are the ovaries. In one study of girls with this condition,[32] prepubertal levels of gonadotropins as well as the response to luteinizing hormone-releasing hormone (LHRH) were encountered. This resulted in plasma estradiol levels being elevated, suggesting that the ovaries are prematurely stimulated.[33] Congenital adrenal hypoplasia and severe hypothyroidism have both been reported to cause premenarchal genital bleeding.[32,34]

Precocious Puberty

In general the definition of *precocious puberty* has been the development of breasts or pubic hair before age 8 in girls. This is no longer considered valid in the United States in that significant numbers of girls develop breast budding prior to age 8 years.[35] Vaginal bleeding resulting from precocious puberty (premature menarche) is often accompanied by a growth spurt and breast development. In true isosexual precocious puberty, menarche is either idiopathic or the result of a variety of cerebral disorders or prolonged exposure to sex steroids from any source (**Table 9-2**). Another form of precocious puberty is termed *pseudoprecocious puberty* and is the result of a variety of factors (**Table 9-3**).

Pertinent historical factors for precocious puberty include a family history of early development and idiopathic central puberty or previous central nervous system damage. The physical examination should include a careful evaluation for the presence of accelerated growth and advanced skeletal maturation determined radiologically, a skin examination for odor and sweat, and palpation of the thyroid. Laboratory studies may involve testing of levels of serum LH, follicle-stimulating hormone, estradiol, dehydroepiandrosterone sulfate, and thyrotropin. Imaging modalities include pelvic ultrasound to ascertain whether ovarian cysts are present and to determine uterine size and configuration; computed tomography; and magnetic resonance imaging of the brain.[36]

Table 9-2. Causes of Isosexual Precocious Puberty

Central Precocious Puberty

— Idiopathic

— Cerebral disorders

  — Space-occupying lesions: hypothalamic hamartomas, brain tumors, neurofibromatosis, brain abscess, hydrocephalus, tuberous sclerosis suprasellar infiltrative lesions (eg, sarcoid, chronic granulomatous disease)

  — Sequelae of cellular damage

  — Meningitis

  — Encephalitis

  — Head trauma

  — Cerebral edema

  — Cranial radiation

Secondary Central Precocious Puberty

— Prolonged exposure to sex steroids for any reason

— Undertreated or late-treated congenital adrenocortical hyperplasia

— Androgen-secreting tumors

Table 9-3. Characteristics of Pseudoprecocious Puberty
— Ovarian tumors
— Adrenal disorders (eg, adrenal carcinoma [estrogen-secreting])
— Gonadotropin-independent sexual precocity: recurrent ovarian follicular cysts or McCune-Albright syndrome
— Gonadotropin-producing tumors: tumors that secrete luteinizing hormone (LH) and LH-like substances (eg, human chorionic gonadotropin, estrogen)
— Iatrogenic disorders: prolonged use of estrogen-containing creams or exogenous administration or ingestion of estrogens (replacement oral contraceptive pills)
— Primary hypothyroidism

Vaginal Foreign Body

A common cause of vaginal bleeding can be a foreign body in the vagina. The bleeding is accompanied by a foul-smelling purulent discharge. Staphyloccocus aureus may grow in pure colonies on culture (**Figure 9-12**). The foreign body may be visible with the child in the frog-leg supine position. The prone knee-chest position is ideal for noninvasively evaluating the length of the vagina. An excellent light source and magnification are helpful. Most vaginal foreign bodies are bits of toilet paper that can flushed out with saline irrigation.[37] Different techniques for visualizing the foreign body include ultrasound and radiography. Foreign bodies have been known to be retained for months, even years. A vaginal examination with the patient under anesthesia is indicated if the following sequence of events has been carried out without success in locating a foreign body (**Figure 9-13**): the history and physical examination reveal the presence of intermittent bleeding accompanied by a foul discharge, both suggestive of a foreign body. If no such body is seen during direct visualization of the vagina, flushing the vagina with saline may remove it. A vaginal examination under anesthesia may be indicated if the concern for vaginal foreign body remains high and the child continues to have symptoms.

Neoplasms

Neoplasms of the vagina are rare. Lymphangiomas are congenital lymphovascular neoplasms that tend to bleed spontaneously. They can involve the hymen and the vagina (**Figures 9-14** and **9-15**).

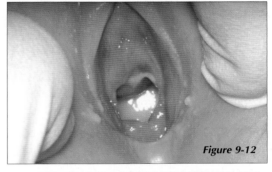

Figure 9-12

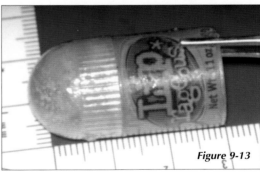

Figure 9-13

Figure 9-12. A foul-smelling sero sanguinous vaginal discharge can be a sign of a vaginal foreign body. In this case, the child had complained for 2 months, and a routine culture grew staphylococcus aureus. An attempt at repeat culture met with a hard resistant green object.

Figure 9-13. The top of a lip gloss tube was removed from this child's vagina while she was under anesthesia.

Hemangiomas can involve the vagina or the cervix. Some hemangiomas will be fed through large vessels that can be treated through sclerosis. Müllerian papillomas, benign papillomata derived from müllerian epithelium, are rare. In one 18-month-old, the primary symptom was vaginal bleeding.[38,39]

Rhabdomyosarcoma, of a subtype embryonal rhabdomyosarcoma, is one of the most common tumors of the pediatric urogenital systems, arising almost exclusively prior to age 5. This tumor is often misdiagnosed in its early stages because the child has vaginal discharge and bleeding. The diagnosis is usually made when the grapelike clusters extrude through the hymenal opening. The diagnosis of this tumor requires referral to a pediatric center with surgical and oncologic services.[40]

Bleeding of Gastrointestinal Origin

Bleeding from the anus, rectum, or higher gastrointestinal (GI) sources can be confused with blood originating from genital structures. Alternatively, anal or rectal bleeding may raise the specter of sexual abuse. Bleeding from the anus also has a wide-ranging differential diagnosis that includes the entire GI tract.

Fissures

Anal fissures may bleed a surprising amount. The blood may be streaked on the outside of the stool or in the underwear. There may or may not be a history of significant constipation or large, hard stools (**Figure 9-16**). Fissures are exceedingly common, and the only way to determine if a fissure is from sexual abuse is to compare the history, timing, and symptoms in relationship to the examination. Anal tears that involve the sphincters are probably not innocent in origin. Conversely, a small fissure may not be evidence of sexual abuse.

Perianal Bleeding

Group A streptococcus dermatitis can cause a beefy, red, sharply demarcated perianal inflammation that can result in bleeding, pain, and fissuring (**Figure 9-17**). A culture of the area will confirm the diagnosis. Treatment is usually a combination of topical (mupirocin) and oral antistreptococcal antibiotics.[41]

Red or maroon blood in the stools is *hematochezia* and indicates distal bleeding or massive higher GI bleed above the distal ileum. Moderate blood from above this site tends to cause tarry-appearing stools, or melena. Diarrhea accompanied by blood suggests an infection or inflammatory bowel disease. Crohn's disease can be accompanied by remarkable anal findings such as fissures, tags, fistulas, pits, scarring, and anal dilatation. Vulvar conditions can also accompany Crohn's disease. There are many case reports of Crohn's disease initially reported as sexual abuse.[42-46] Blood streaked on the stools indicates a distal rectal or anal source such as a fissure or external trauma.

The differential diagnosis of GI bleeding in a child is extensive. **Table 9-4** lists the major causes of GI bleeding by site. It is helpful to keep this differential diagnosis in mind when a child produces blood in the underwear or toilet. Children who may be sexually abused can have coexisting medical conditions.

DISCHARGE

Discharge may be vaginal, anal, or genital in origin. Prepubertal children evaluated for vaginal discharge are often brought to clinicians because of concerns of sexual abuse. In reality, only a very small percentage of children who are sexually abused are diagnosed with a sexually transmitted infection (STI).[47] On rare occasions the evaluation of a scant to moderate discharge reveals sexually transmitted organisms. A variety of organisms cause discharge in prepubertal girls and the evaluation of discharge should include an evaluation for common nonvenereal pathogens, and if indicated, tests for STIs.

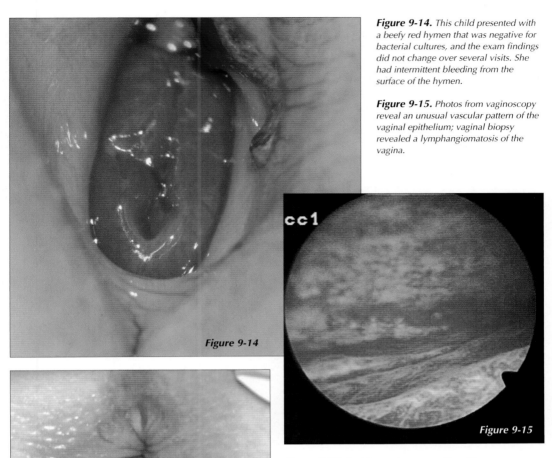

Figure 9-14. *This child presented with a beefy red hymen that was negative for bacterial cultures, and the exam findings did not change over several visits. She had intermittent bleeding from the surface of the hymen.*

Figure 9-15. *Photos from vaginoscopy reveal an unusual vascular pattern of the vaginal epithelium; vaginal biopsy revealed a lymphangiomatosis of the vagina.*

Figure 9-14

Figure 9-15

Figure 9-16. *Anal fissure. Image contributed by Joyce Adams, MD.*

Figure 9-17. *Severe perianal maceration. A culture revealed pure group A beta-hemolytic strep.*

Figure 9-16

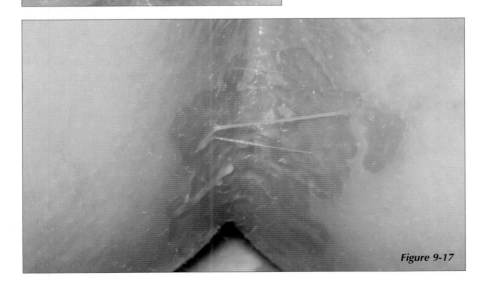

Figure 9-17

157

> ## Table 9-4. Significant Factors in Gastrointestinal Bleeding
>
> FACTORS
>
> **Upper GI Bleeding**
> — Peptic ulcer/gastritis   — Esophageal varices
>
> — Swallowed blood from epistaxis   — Esophagitis
>
> — Mallory-Weiss syndrome
>
> **Midbowel**
> — Intussusception   — Meckel's diverticulum
>
> **Lower GI Bleeding**
> — Bacterial enteritis   — Foreign body
>
> — Anal fissure   — Hemolytic uremic syndrome
>
> — Colonic polyps   — Inflammatory bowel disease
>
> — Lymphonodular hyperplasia   — Hemorrhoids
>
> — Henoch-Schönlein purpura
>
> **All Locations**
> — Hemangioma, arteriovenous   — Coagulopathy
>   malformation
>
> *Data adapted from* Nelson Textbook of Pediatrics, *Behrman et al.*[48]

During a clinical examination, a scant vaginal discharge may be found to be normal (physiologic leukorrhea) or caused by a variety of nonvenereal pathogens. Smegma, the accumulation of exfoliated skin cells and bacteria, is white and cheesy in appearance and is usually found in the folds between the labia. Some children may have what appears on the underwear to be discharge, when they fail to empty their bladder completely and small reflux of urine into the vagina results in some drainage. Any bacteria found normally in the respiratory tract can be found in the genital area. Nonspecific vaginitis is a condition of poor hygiene or exposure to irritants. On culture a nonspecific vaginitis generally grows mixed normal flora. Nonspecific vaginitis generally responds to a program of topical bland emollients, excellent hygiene, and avoidance of irritants (eg, bubble bath, perfumed soaps, detergents).

A heavy growth of a single organism suggests a possible infection with that organism and may require antibiotic treatment. Yeast infections caused by *Candida albicans* are uncommon in toilet-trained prepubertal children. Children who have just completed a course of broad-spectrum antibiotics, who have diabetes mellitus, or who are immunocompromised are exceptions. Clinicians tend to overtreat children with antifungal creams when children appear for diagnosis of nearly any condition resulting in genital redness, irritation, or itching, presuming it to be candida.

NONVENEREAL PATHOGENS
Many commonly occurring, nonvenereal organisms can cause vaginitis. **Table 9-5** lists the common bacterial organisms. In a child with vaginal discharge, STIs are often a

major concern. However, STIs are found rarely in sexually abused children; therefore, in addition to cultures for chlamydia and gonorrhea, routine cultures should be performed to identify these common nonvenereal pathogens.

PAPULES, MACULES, AND NODULES

Papules and Nodules

Lesions that appear to be genital warts, such as papules and macules in the genital area, raise the specter of sexual abuse. Recent evidence suggests that although human papillomavirus can be transmitted via sexual abuse, vertical and fomite transmission also exist.[47-49]

Molluscum Contagiosum

Molluscum contagiosum is a DNA poxvirus for which humans are the only known reservoir. There appears to be bimodal distribution in childhood and then in young adulthood. Mollusca appear as pearly papules on an erythematous base with a central umbilication (**Figure 9-18**). The lesions can appear clustered in the anogenital area, and

---

Table 9-5. Nonvenereal Pathogens Causing Vulvitis/Vulvovaginitis/Vaginitis

BACTERIAL

— Group A *Streptococcus*	— *Neisseria meningitidis*
— Group B *Streptococcus*	— *Staphylococcus aureus*
— *Haemophilus influenzae*	— *Staphylococcus epidermidis*
— *Streptococcus pneumoniae*	— *Gardnerella vaginalis*

Gram-negative Enteric Pathogens

— *Escherichia coli*	— *Pseudomonas* spp.
— *Streptococcus faecalis*	— *Salmonella* spp.
— *Klebsiella* spp.	— *Shigella* spp.
— *Proteus* spp.	

Gram-negative Anaerobes

— *Peptococcus* spp.	— *Bacteroides* spp.
— *Peptostreptococcus* spp.	

VIRAL

— Rubella (measles)	— Kawasaki disease
— Epstein-Barr virus (infectious mononucleosis)	— Nonspecific viral infections

FUNGAL

— *Candida albicans*	— Tinea corporis

PARASITIC

— Pinworms (*Enterobius vermicularis*)

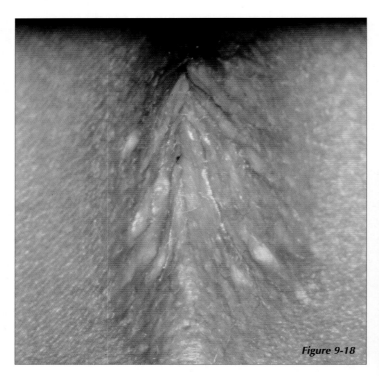

Figure 9-18

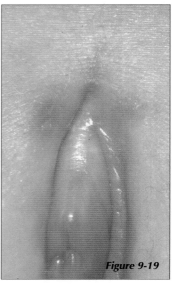

Figure 9-19

Figure 9-18. *Perianal molluscum contagiosum that can mimic genital warts and raise the suspicion of sexual abuse.*

Figure 9-19. *Pseudoverrucous papules and nodules. Small nodules near the clitoris of this child raised a concern of genital herpes. On careful examination the lesions were nodular and not painful. They cleared with removal of the irritant.*

the localization of the outbreak in this is often what raises the red flag of sexual abuse. When the child is carefully examined, as are as siblings or close playmates, extragenital mollusca are often found. There may be some risk that the lesions are transmitted sexually; however, mollusca are so common and so easily transmitted from person to person that innocent transmission is most likely the rule.

Perianal Pseudoverrucous Papules and Nodules

Perianal Pseudoverrucous Papules and Nodules (PPN) is an underreported benign cutaneous condition of flat-topped papules and nodules (**Figure 9-19**). It is a variant of Jacquet's dermatitis (called also erosive dermatitis, diaper dermatitis, or colloquially as diaper rash). Jacquet's dermatitis is a chronic ulcerative condition of the diaper area first described in 1886.[50] It was reported in children who had undergone surgery for Hirschsprung's disease and whose skin was exposed to chronic fecal soiling. Described in peristomal areas, it is also observed in children with urinary or fecal incontinence. The condition clears with removal of the irritant.[51-53]

A variety of rare conditions have been reported to be confused with genital warts, which, in turn raise the concern of sexual abuse. The differential diagnosis of papular and nodular lesions of the anogenital area is broad. **Table 9-6** lists conditions that have been reported or observed in this context.

VESICLES AND ULCERS

Vesicles and ulcerations of the genital area suggest infections such as herpes virus and therefore hoist the specter of sexual abuse. However, acquiring herpes simplex virus (HSV) from sexual abuse is one of the lowest risks among all STIs. It is not screened for, and, therefore, only patients with overt symptoms such as vesicles come to the attention of the medical community. Please see Chapter 10 for a review of HSV as an STI.

Several non-HSV infections can cause vesicles or ulcerations of the genital area. None are known to have any risk for being sexually transmitted. Genital ulcerations caused by Epstein-Barr virus (EBV) have been described infrequently. In studies reviewing 26 cases, the average age is reported as 14.5 years, and sexual contact is rare.[59-61] EBV serologic testing may be helpful, but one must keep in mind that the results are not positive unless testing occurs several days after the development of lesions. Polymerase chain reaction tests of the lesions have yielded positive, confirmatory results of EBV in one study and may be helpful in diagnosis.[61] Another class of herpes viruses, varicella-zoster virus, can cause lesions of the genital area in children. An early occurrence of chicken pox or a later occurrence of shingles in a sacral dermatome may look very much like HSV. Coxsackievirus, first described in 1955 is known to cause oral and cutaneous lesions in children, also can cause genital lesions.[62] Deitch and colleagues[60] described 9 patients who developed vulvar ulcerations and denied sexual abuse or activity. All were negative for HSV. Six of the patients had systemic symptoms suggestive of a nonspecific viral illness. In a child with other symptoms suggestive of a viral illness and without a history of sexual contact, the clinician must consider genital ulcers as an uncommon occurrence of nonspecific, systemic viral illnesses such as influenza.

Table 9-6. Differential Diagnosis of Papules and Nodules
— Benign pigmented apocrine vulvar hamartomas[40]
— Langerhans cell histiocytosis[54]
— Heck disease: focal epithelial hyperplasia[55]
— Epidermal nevus[56]
— Inflammatory linear epidermal nevus Crohn's disease[45]
— Lymphangioma circumscriptum[57]
— Vulvar syringomas[58]
— Bowenoid papulosis
— Xanthogranulomas
— Tuberous sclerosis

Other conditions that have been reported to cause genital ulcerations include localized vulvar pemphigoid in a young girl.[63] Juvenile bullous pemphigoid manifests as localized grouped or single vesicles on the genitals, face, neck, palms, and soles. At least 2 cases that were confused with sexual abuse are reported in the literature.[63,64] The diagnosis of localized genital pemphigoid requires a high index of suspicion, and confirmation depends upon biopsy results.

Behçet's disease is a rare systemic condition associated with oral aphthae, genital ulcers, skin lesions, arthritis, and GI involvement. Neuropsychiatric symptoms and the presence of HLA-B51 are also associated with this rare cause of progressive, destructive, painful genital ulcers.[65]

Stevens-Johnson syndrome, or erythema multiforme major, occurs as a reaction to a variety of drugs, mycoplasmas, viruses, or other triggers. The result is a severe vesiculobullous reaction of the mucous membranes that can include the genitalia. In severe cases, vaginal stenosis can result from scarring after involvement of the distal vaginal mucosa.[66-68] Drug reactions can cause genital ulcers (**Figures 9-20** and **9-21**). Usually, exposure to a sulfa-containing antibiotic results in a stereotypic reaction that can be duplicated upon reexposure to the drug.

In evaluating lesions of the genital area, a careful history of irritants and potential allergic contact irritants should be sought. Nickel, for example, can be extremely sensitizing. One classic case of allergic contact was that of a child using a bed-wetting

Figures 9-20 and **9-21.** *Fixed drug eruption. These severe, shallow, painful genital ulcers in an adolescent were initially thought to be caused herpes simplex virus. However HSV culture and PCR were negative. The patient was on a sulfa-containing antibiotic for a urinary tract infection. The ulcers cleared with discontinuation of the antibiotic and were felt to be a drug reaction.*

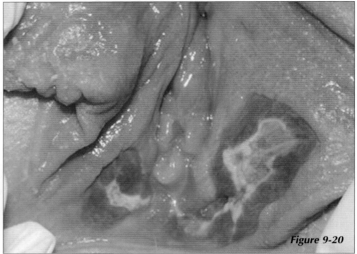

Figure 9-20

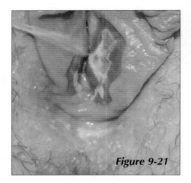

Figure 9-21

alarm, where the contact was nickel. The child was removed from the home and placed in foster care because of the concern that the localized vesicles on the genitals were herpes simplex.[69] This case report demonstrates the potential harm to a child and family when there is a misdiagnosis of sexual abuse.

CONCLUSION

It is challenging to evaluate any child who has injuries or illness suggestive of sexual abuse. When children or adolescents have anogenital signs or symptoms, a differential diagnosis must be developed. This diagnosis should encompass a variety of acquired and congenital conditions. The cooccurence of an unusual anogenital condition in the context of a sexual abuse allegation may be coincidental to the allegations. Such conditions should not be considered as evidence of abuse, as normal examination results should not be thought of as definitive evidence of nonabuse. Children who are referred for genital involvement may have other conditions that can mimic the appearance of sexual abuse or an STI. High-quality photodocumentation and review of cases by experienced clinicians, including dermatologists, gynecologists, urologists, and infectious disease specialists, can be critical in coming to a correct diagnosis.

REFERENCES

1. Jenny C, Kirby P, Fuquay D. Genital lichen sclerosus mistaken for child sexual abuse. *Pediatrics.* 1989;83(4):597-599.

2. Ditkowsky SP, Falk AB, Baker N, Schaffner M. Lichen sclerosis et atrophicus in childhood. *AMA J Dis Child.* 1956;91(1):52-54.

3. Al-Khenaizan S, Almuneef M, Kentab O. Lichen sclerosus mistaken for child sexual abuse. *Int J Dermatol.* 2005;44(4):317-320.

4. Loening-Baucke V. Lichen sclerosus et atrophicus in children. *Am J Dis Child.* 1991;145(9):1058-1061.

5. Hagedorn M. [Genital vulvar lichen sclerosis in 2 siblings]. *Z Hautkr.* 1989;64(9):810, 813-814.

6. Breier F, Khanakah G, Stanek G, et al. Isolation and polymerase chain reaction typing of Borrelia afzelii from a skin lesion in a seronegative patient with

generalized ulcerating bullous lichen sclerosus et atrophicus. *Br J Dermatol.* 2001;144(2):387-392.

7. Buechner SA, Winkelmann RK, Lautenschlager S, Gilli L, Rufli T. Localized scleroderma associated with Borrelia burgdorferi infection. Clinical, histologic, and immunohistochemical observations. *J Am Acad Dermatol.* 1993;29(2 Pt 1):190-196.

8. Flentje D, Benz G, Daum R. [Lichen sclerosis et atrophicus as a cause of acquired phimosis—circumcision as a preventive procedure against penis cancer?]. *Z Kinderchir.* 1987;42(5):308-311.

9. Beattie PE, Dawe RS, Ferguson J, Ibbotson SH. UVA1 phototherapy for genital lichen sclerosus. *Clin Exp Dermatol.* 2006;31(3):343-347.

10. Wright JE. The treatment of childhood phimosis with topical steroid. *Aust N Z J Surg.* 1994;64(5):327-328.

11. Serrano G, Millan F, Fortea JM, Grau M, Aliaga A. Topical progesterone as treatment of choice in genital lichen sclerosis et atrophicus in children. *Pediatr Dermatol.* 1993;10(2):201.

12. Levin AV, Selbst SM. Vulvar hemangioma simulating child abuse. *Clin Pediatr (Phila).* 1988;27(4):213-215.

13. Vogel AM, Alesbury JM, Burrows PE, Fishman SJ. Vascular anomalies of the female external genitalia. *J Pediatr Surg.* 2006;41(5):993-999.

14. Brown J, Melinkovich P. Schonlein-Henoch purpura misdiagnosed as suspected child abuse. A case report and literature review. *JAMA.* 1986;256(5):617-618.

15. Daly KC, Siegel RM. Henoch-Schonlein purpura in a child at risk of abuse. *Arch Pediatr Adolesc Med.* 1998;152(1):96-98.

16. Harley JR. Disorders of coagulation misdiagnosed as nonaccidental bruising. *Pediatr Emerg Care.* 1997;13(5):347-349.

17. Rothamel T, Burger D, Debertin AS, Kleemann WJ. Vaginorectal impalement injury in a 2-year-old child—caused by sexual abuse or an accident? *Forensic Sci Int.* 2001;119(3):330-333.

18. Perlman SE, Hertweck SP, Wolfe WM. Water-ski douche injury in a premenarcheal female. *Pediatrics.* 1995;96(4 Pt 1):782-783.

19. Boos SC, Rosas AJ, Boyle C, McCann J. Anogenital injuries in child pedestrians run over by low-speed motor vehicles: four cases with findings that mimic child sexual abuse. *Pediatrics.* 2003;112(1 Pt 1):e77-84.

20. Herrmann B, Crawford J. Genital injuries in prepubertal girls from inline skating accidents. *Pediatrics.* 2002;110(2 Pt 1):e16.

21. Merritt DF. Evaluation of vaginal bleeding in the preadolescent child. *Semin Pediatr Surg.* 1998;7(1):35-42.

22. Johnson CF. Prolapse of the urethra: confusion of clinical and anatomic characteristics with sexual abuse. *Pediatrics.* 1991;87(5):722-725.

23. Shetty AK, Coffman K, Harmon E. Urethral prolapse. *J Pediatr.* 1998;133(4): 552.

24. Templeman C, Hertweck P, Perlman S, Nakajima S. Urethral prolapse in a 7 year old girl. *Aust N Z J Obstet Gynaecol.* 2000;40(4):480.

25. Valerie E, Gilchrist BF, Frischer J, Scriven R, Klotz DH, Ramenofsky ML. Diagnosis and treatment of urethral prolapse in children. *Urology.* 1999;54(6): 1082-1084.

26. Rudin JE, Geldt VG, Alecseev EB. Prolapse of urethral mucosa in white female children: experience with 58 cases. *J Pediatr Surg.* 1997;32(3):423-425.

27. Esposito JM. Circular prolapse of the urethra in children: a cause of vaginal bleeding. *Obstet Gynecol.* 1968;31(3):363-367.

28. Neuwirth RS. Urethral Prolapse—a Cause of Vaginal Bleeding in Young Girls. Report of 5 Cases. *Obstet Gynecol.* 1963;22:290-292.

29. Falandry L. [Prolapse of the urethra in black girls. Personal experience in 11 cases]. *Med Trop (Mars).* 1994;54(2):152-156.

30. Richardson DA, Hajj SN, Herbst AL. Medical treatment of urethral prolapse in children. *Obstet Gynecol.* 1982;59(1):69-74.

31. Baiulescu M, Hannon PR, Marcinak JF, Janda WM, Schreckenberger PC. Chronic vulvovaginitis caused by antibiotic-resistant Shigella flexneri in a prepubertal child. *Pediatr Infect Dis J.* 2002;21(2):170-172.

32. Uli N, Chin D, David R, et al. Menstrual bleeding in a female infant with congenital adrenal hyperplasia: altered maturation of the hypothalamic-pituitary-ovarian axis. *J Clin Endocrinol Metab.* 1997;82(10):3298-3302.

33. Blanco-Garcia M, Evain-Brion D, Roger M, Job JC. Isolated menses in prepubertal girls. *Pediatrics.* 1985;76(1):43-47.

34. Campaner AB, Scapinelli A, Machado RO, Dos Santos RE, Beznos GW, Aoki T. Primary hypothyroidism presenting as ovarian tumor and precocious puberty in a prepubertal girl. *Gynecol Endocrinol.* 2006;22(7):395-398.

35. Slyper AH. The pubertal timing controversy in the USA, and a review of possible causative factors for the advance in timing of onset of puberty. *Clin Endocrinol (Oxf).* 2006;65(1):1-8.

36. Emans S, Laufer M, Goldstein D, eds. *Pediatric and Adolescent Gynecology.* Fourth ed. Philadelphia, PA: Lippincott, Williams and Wilkins; 1998.

37. Smith YR, Berman DR, Quint EH. Premenarchal vaginal discharge: findings of procedures to rule out foreign bodies. *J Pediatr Adolesc Gynecol.* 2002;15(4):227-230.

38. Lane BR, Ross JH, Hart WR, Kay R. Mullerian papilloma of the cervix in a child with multiple renal cysts. *Urology.* 2005;65(2):388.

39. Luttges JE, Lubke M. Recurrent benign Mullerian papilloma of the vagina. Immunohistological findings and histogenesis. *Arch Gynecol Obstet.* 1994;255(3): 157-160.

40. Stephens-Groff SM, Hansen RC, Bangert J. Benign pigmented apocrine vulvar hamartomas. *Pediatr Dermatol.* 1993;10(2):123-124.

41. Herbst R. Perineal streptococcal dermatitis/disease: recognition and management. *Am J Clin Dermatol.* 2003;4(8):555-560.

42. Bourrat E, Faure C, Vignon-Pennamen MD, Rybojad M, Morel P, Navarro J. [Anitis, vulvar edema and macrocheilitis disclosing Crohn disease in a child: value of metronidazole]. *Ann Dermatol Venereol.* 1997;124(9):626-628.

43. Porzionato A, Alaggio R, Aprile A. Perianal and vulvar Crohn's disease presenting as suspected abuse. *Forensic Sci Int.* 2005;155(1):24-27.

44. Sellman SP, Hupertz VF, Reece RM. Crohn's disease presenting as suspected abuse. *Pediatrics.* 1996;97(2):272-274.

45. Stratakis CA, Graham W, DiPalma J, Leibowitz I. Misdiagnosis of perianal manifestations of Crohn's disease. Two cases and a review of the literature. *Clin Pediatr (Phila).* 1994;33(10):631-633.

46. Wardinsky TD, Vizcarrondo FE, Cruz BK. The mistaken diagnosis of child abuse: a three-year USAF Medical Center analysis and literature review. *Mil Med.* 1995;160(1):15-20.

47. Girardet RG, Lahoti S, Howard LA, et al. Epidemiology of sexually transmitted infections in suspected child victims of sexual assault. *Pediatrics.* 2009;124(1):79-86.

48. Behrman R, Kliegman R, Jenson H, eds. *Nelson Textbook of Pediatrics.* Sixteenth ed. Philadelphia: WB Saunders Company; 2000; No. 1.

49. Hornor G. Ano-genital warts in children: Sexual abuse or not? *J Pediatr Health Care.* 2004;18(4):165-170.

50. Siegfried E, Frasier L. The spectrum of anogenital disease in children. *Current Problems in Dermatology.* 1997;9(9):33-80.

51. Goldberg NS, Esterly NB, Rothman KF, et al. Perianal pseudoverrucous papules and nodules in children. *Arch Dermatol.* 1992;128(2):240-242.

52. Rodriguez Cano L, Garcia-Patos Briones V, Pedragosa Jove R, Castells Rodellas A. Perianal pseudoverrucous papules and nodules after surgery for Hirschsprung disease. *J Pediatr.* 1994;125(6 Pt 1):914-916.

53. Rodriguez-Poblador J, Gonzalez-Castro U, Herranz-Martinez S, Luelmo-Aguilar J. Jacquet erosive diaper dermatitis after surgery for Hirschsprung disease. *Pediatr Dermatol.* 1998;15(1):46-47.

54. Papa CA, Pride HB, Tyler WB, Turkewitz D. Langerhans cell histiocytosis mimicking child abuse. *J Am Acad Dermatol.* 1997;37(6):1002-1004.

55. Cohen PR, Hebert AA, Adler-Storthz K. Focal epithelial hyperplasia: Heck disease. *Pediatr Dermatol.* 1993;10(3):245-251.

56. Mahto M, Ashworth J, Vickers DM. A case of linear epidermal naevus presenting as genital warts—a cautionary tale. *Int J STD AIDS.* 2005;16(3):267-269.

57. Darmstadt GL. Perianal lymphangioma circumscriptum mistaken for genital warts. *Pediatrics.* 1996;98(3 Pt 1):461-463.

58. Tay YK, Tham SN, Teo R. Localized vulvar syringomas—an unusual cause of pruritus vulvae. *Dermatology.* 1996;192(1):62-63.

59. Cheng SX, Chapman MS, Margesson LJ, Birenbaum D. Genital ulcers caused by Epstein-Barr virus. *J Am Acad Dermatol.* 2004;51(5):824-826.

60. Deitch HR, Huppert J, Adams Hillard PJ. Unusual vulvar ulcerations in young adolescent females. *J Pediatr Adolesc Gynecol.* 2004;17(1):13-16.

61. Halvorsen JA, Brevig T, Aas T, Skar AG, Slevolden EM, Moi H. Genital ulcers as initial manifestation of Epstein-Barr virus infection: two new cases and a review of the literature. *Acta Derm Venereol.* 2006;86(5):439-442.

62. Mitchell SC, Dempster G. The finding of genital lesions in a case of Coxsackie virus infection. *Can Med Assoc J.* 1955;72(2):117-119.

63. Levine V, Sanchez M, Nestor M. Localized vulvar pemphigoid in a child misdiagnosed as sexual abuse. *Arch Dermatol.* 1992;128(6):804-806.

64. Hoque SR, Patel M, Farrell AM. Childhood cicatricial pemphigoid confined to the vulva. *Clin Exp Dermatol.* 2006;31(1):63-64.

65. Pivetti-Pezzi P, Accorinti M, Abdulaziz MA, La Cava M, Torella M, Riso D. Behçet's disease in children. *Jpn J Ophthalmol.* 1995;39(3):309-314.

66. Graham-Brown RA, Cochrane GW, Swinhoe JR, Sarkany I, Epsztejn LJ. Vaginal stenosis due to bullous erythema multiforme (Stevens-Johnson syndrome). Case report. *Br J Obstet Gynaecol.* 1981;88(11):1156-1157.

67. Marquette GP, Su B, Woodruff JD. Introital adenosis associated with Stevens-Johnson syndrome. *Obstet Gynecol.* 1985;66(1):143-145.

68. Murphy MI, Brant WE. Hematocolpos caused by genital bullous lesions in a patient with Stevens-Johnson syndrome. *J Clin Ultrasound.* 1998;26(1):52-54.

69. Hanks JW, Venters WJ. Nickel allergy from a bed-wetting alarm confused with herpes genitalis and child abuse. *Pediatrics.* 1992;90(3):458-460.

Chapter 10

SEXUALLY TRANSMITTED INFECTIONS

Michelle I. Amaya, MD, MPH
Nancy D. Kellogg, MD

The identification of sexually transmitted infections (STI) in possible victims of sexual abuse has presented clinical and diagnostic challenges. Each STI may present with varying or no clinical features and the incubation period may extend up to 4 years in the case of human papillomavirus. Once a clinician has decided to test for an STI, there are a number of diagnostic tests available, each with varying sensitivity and specificity rates as well as site-specific restrictions. Even when an STI is identified in a child, the determination that the infection was sexually transmitted can be problematic (**Table 10-1**). Clinicians must be knowledgeable about the indications for STI testing, the appropriate tests to utilize, and the possible modes of transmission in order to accurately interpret and treat an STI in a child or adolescent.

Interpreting the presence of an STI within the context of sexual abuse or assault also presents challenges for the clinician who works with investigative agencies. The clinician must become knowledgeable about sensitivities and specificities for various testing modalities, in addition to the positive predictive values when such tests are utilized in low- and high-prevalence populations. Investigative agencies are most interested in testing that is considered the legally acceptable standard with little or no possibility of false-positive results. The clinician, on the other hand, must consider the low sensitivities of some "gold standards," and may wish to utilize a test that optimizes detection of the STI. In some situations, such as a sexually active adolescent who is also sexually assaulted, the presence of an STI will have no forensic significance, but is significant as a public health issue, so using the most sensitive test in this high-prevalence population is optimal. Confirming the STI in a sexually active adolescent also enables treatment of presumably infected sexual contacts as well. The sexual abuse or assault examination is often the first time a sexually active adolescent has ever been screened for STIs, and the first opportunity for clinicians to impact this problem on a public health level.

A medical evaluation of a child or adolescent for sexual abuse or assault may include testing and treating for STIs. The American Academy of Pediatrics has recommended that testing for STIs in child and adolescent victims of sexual abuse include a serum rapid plasma reagin test (RPR); a vaginal smear for *Trichomonas vaginalis*; throat, rectal, and genital cultures for *Neisseria gonorrhoeae*; and rectal and genital cultures for *Chlamydia trachomatis*.[1] More recently, the US Centers for Disease Control and Prevention[2] (CDC) have recommended cultures for *Neisseria gonorrhoeae* from the anus and pharynx for both male and female children, and from the vagina (females) or urethra (males). Cultures for *Chlamydia trachomatis* are recommended from the anus of both males and females, from the vagina (females), and from the urethra (males) when discharge is present. Additional tests recommended by the CDC are culture and vaginal smear for *Trichomonas vaginalis* infection and bacterial vaginosis, and serum samples for *Treponema pallidum*, human immunodeficiency virus (HIV), and hepatitis B surface antigen (HbsAg) (**Table 10-2**). Even when such recommendations are employed, the prevalence of sexually transmitted infections in prepubertal children evaluated for sexual abuse is low. In one study of over 3000 boys and girls ages 12 and younger who were examined for STIs as part of the medical evaluation for sexual abuse, the most common STI in boys was clinically diagnosed condyloma acuminata (2.2%) and in girls was genital chlamydia (2.0%).[3] Syphilis (0.2% in boys and 0.2% in girls), rectal gonorrhea (0% in boys and 0.8% in girls), rectal chlamydia (0% in boys and 0.25% in girls), oral gonorrhea (0% in boys and 0.04% in girls), and condyloma acuminata in girls (1.5%) were all less common.[3]

CONSIDERATIONS FOR SEXUALLY TRANSMITTED INFECTION TESTING

Testing for STIs in children and adolescents can be uncomfortable, intrusive, and traumatic. Obtaining blood for syphilis, hepatitis, and HIV testing is certainly uncomfortable; repeat testing is often recommended for up to 6 months past the last abusive sexual contact. Vaginal sampling for gonorrhea and chlamydia cultures involves the insertion of a cotton-tipped applicator past the hymenal ring into the vaginal vault; gentle scraping is required to harvest cells because *Chlamydia trachomatis* is an obligate intracellular organism. Smaller Dacron swabs may be less traumatic, as they are easier to

Table 10-1. Implications of Commonly Encountered STIs for the Diagnosis and Reporting of Sexual Abuse of Infants and Prepubertal Children

STI CONFIRMED	SEXUAL ABUSE	SUGGESTED ACTION
Gonorrhea[a]	Diagnostic[b]	Report[c]
Syphilis[a]	Diagnostic	Report
HIV infection[d]	Diagnostic	Report
C *trachomatis* infection[a]	Diagnostic[b]	Report
T *vaginalis* infection	Highly suspicious	Report
C *acuminata* infection[a] (anogenital warts)	Suspicious	Report
Herpes simplex (genital location)	Suspicious	Report[e]
Bacterial vaginosis	Inconclusive	Medical follow-up

[a] *If not perinatally acquired and rare nonsexual vertical transmission is excluded.*
[b] *Although the culture technique is the "gold standard," current studies are investigating the use of nucleic acid–amplification tests as an alternative diagnostic method in children.*
[c] *To the agency mandated in the community to receive reports of suspected sexual abuse.*
[d] *If not acquired perinatally or by transfusion.*
[e] *Unless there is a clear history of autoinoculation.*

Adapted with permission from Kellogg N and Committee on Child Abuse and Neglect. American Academy of Pediatrics Clinical Report. The evaluation of sexual abuse in children. Pediatrics. 2005;116(2):506-512.

STI	Initial[b]	2 Weeks	12 Weeks	6 Months
Gonorrhea	X	X		
Chlamydia	X	X		
Trichomonas	X	X		
Syphilis	X		X	
Hepatitis	X		X	
HIV	X		X	X
Human papillomavirus[c]	X		X	X

Table 10-2. Suggested Testing Schedule for Sexually Transmitted Infections[a]

[a] *Schedule is based on examination conducted within 5 days of sexual assault. If abuse is chronic, or last abusive sexual contact occurred several weeks prior to examination, testing schedule should be established based on timing of last sexual contact.*
[b] *Not all these tests are appropriate for every patient; testing should be tailored based on type of sexual contact, age of child, symptomatology, and patient/parent requests.*
[c] *The diagnosis of human papillomavirus is made clinically, but due to the prolonged incubation period of this disease, follow-up examinations 6 months to 1 year from the last abusive sexual contact are recommended.*

pass into the vagina without touching the more sensitive hymen. In post-pubertal patients, cervical samples should be obtained if the patient is able to tolerate speculum insertion or has had a previous speculum examination; when appropriate, upper vaginal samples may be substituted according to patient comfort and tolerance. Rectal cultures for gonorrhea and chlamydia are obtained with cotton-tipped or Dacron swabs inserted into the rectum up to a few centimeters. Swabs can be moistened with non-bacteriostatic saline, which may improve the comfort level of the child. Oral samples are gathered near the tonsillar pillars and may produce a gagging reflex. Once the testing is complete, chlamydia samples are refrigerated and gonorrhea samples are incubated if there is a delay in transport to the laboratory.

Testing for STIs can also be costly. For example, at one large urban hospital, an RPR costs $44, an HIV test costs $105, serologic screening for hepatitis B surface antigen and hepatitis C antibody costs $175, each chlamydia culture costs $71, and each gonorrhea culture costs $196. If a vaginal smear is examined by pathology personnel for Trichomonas, the cost is $25. In a female child undergoing the standard testing for STIs as recommended by the American Academy of Pediatrics,[4,5] the total cost for vaginal and serologic samples would be from $660 to $1632, depending on whether serologic testing for HIV, syphilis, and hepatitis is repeated 6, 12, and 24 weeks later. If a female child undergoes STI testing recommended by the CDC,[2] the costs would be approximately $1200.

Because testing can be costly and traumatic, numerous publications have provided recommendations and criteria for selective testing.[1,6,7] Rationale for selective testing includes the low prevalence of STIs in prepubertal victims of sexual abuse. Criteria for selective testing are based on the type of sexual contact and the presence of signs and symptoms that predict disease. Criteria proposed for STI testing in prepubertal children include the following: sibling, sexual offender, or patient with an STI; history of genital-genital contact; vaginal discharge noted on examination; or abnormal hymenal exam.[1,6,7] Vaginal discharge noted on examination and genital findings consistent with trauma are 2 factors common to these 3 papers. Criteria for testing postpubertal children are generally broader because of the higher proportion of asymptomatic infected patients and because sexually active adolescents have a higher prevalence of STIs. In two studies,[6,7] all of the children infected with gonorrhea or chlamydia would have been detected if they were tested based on the presence of one of the following major risk markers: genital discharge by history or exam, history of suspected sexual contact with an individual thought to have an STI, suspicious anogenital examination findings, or a history of penile-rectal or penile-vaginal contact. Additional testing criteria included the presence of two minor risk factors: vaginitis and a sibling thought to have been sexually abused.[6] Utilizing these major and minor criteria, testing would have been avoided in 56% of the children in this study. As a result of these and other studies, fewer children than in previous years are tested for STIs during their medical evaluation for sexual abuse.

An alternative approach to the detection of STIs in prepubertal children evaluated for sexual abuse is sequential testing. In one study of prepubertal females referred for sexual abuse evaluations with vaginal discharge, utilizing a non-culture test with high sensitivity followed by a culture with high specificity in testing for gonorrhea provided optimal results with the lowest false-negative and -positive rates.[8] This approach entails gathering samples for both the non-culture and culture techniques initially, processing the non-culture results first and withholding treatment on positive results until confirmation can be made with the culture technique. Advantages to this approach include better detection of gonorrhea; disadvantages are the high cost and potential trauma of obtaining additional tissue samples for testing. Such an approach may be most advantageous in detection of *Chlamydia trachomatis*, which has low culture sensitivity.

Proposed criteria for testing clearly delineate prepubertal and sexually naive children from pubertal and sexually active adolescents. Typically, protocols recommend testing for STIs in the prepubertal group and prophylactic antibiotic treatment for STIs in the sexually active group. The rationale for this approach is that identification of an STI in sexually active adolescents is forensically insignificant, and may, in fact, make the victim appear "promiscuous" to a jury. In addition, the cost of prophylactic antibiotic treatment with Azithromycin, Cefixime, and Metronidazole is approximately $130, which is much less expensive than the costs of STI testing. However, the prevalence of STIs in the adolescent population is high and many infected individuals are asymptomatic, undetected, and untreated. Because of risks of ascending infection and poor compliance with follow-up examinations, prophylaxis is generally recommended in adolescents (in addition to testing). If infected adolescents are treated but not tested, their infected partners will likely be undetected and untreated.

NEISSERIA GONORRHOEAE AND CHLAMYDIA TRACHOMATIS

Because symptomatology, indications for testing, and co-infection are similar or common for *Neisseria gonorrhoeae* and *Chlamydia trachomatis*, these STIs will be discussed jointly. Among sexually abused children, the reported rates of gonorrhea or chlamydia infection range from 3% to 20%, with higher prevalence among adolescents.[7,9] Currently, *Chlamydia trachomatis* is more common than *Neisseria gonorrhoeae* in the adult population, so a similar trend is anticipated among children and adolescents sexually victimized by adults. Pediatric and adult populations infected with these STIs may be asymptomatic, although symptoms such as vaginal discharge and vaginitis are more commonly seen among prepubertal females infected with gonorrhea (**Figures 10-1, 10-2,** and **10-3**).[10] Genital and anal chlamydia infections are often asymptomatic; discharge, dysuria, abdominal pain, and rectal pain are reported symptoms in some infected patients.[11] Genital chlamydia and gonorrhea infections in adolescents may also progress to pelvic inflammatory disease and infertility, while pelvic inflammatory disease is not commonly seen among prepubertal children with chlamydia or gonorrhea.[2,5] The incubation period for chlamydial disease is variable but usually at least a week. Neonatal chlamydia conjunctivitis typically develops 5 to 12 days after birth, but may occur up to 30 days after birth. The incubation period for gonorrhea is usually 2 to 7 days.[2,5]

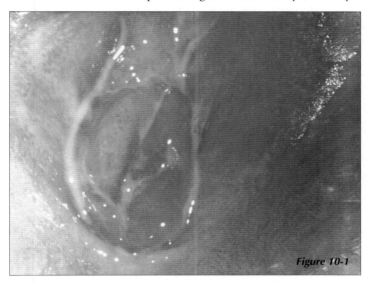

Figure 10-1

Figure 10-1. The yellow vaginal discharge present is consistent with Neisseria gonorrhoea, *which grew in the vaginal culture of a 4-year-old Hispanic child.*

Figure 10-2. Photo of a 3-year-old girl with yellow-green vaginal discharge and history that "Daddy hurt my pee pee." Culture was positive for N. gonorrhoea including confirmatory testing.

Figure 10-3. Photo of same child as seen in Figure 10-2, examined 2 weeks after treatment for gonorrhea. This photo shows a hymen with no signs of injury and an opening that was estimated to be 2 to 3 mm wide. Gonorrhea causes a vulvovaginitis in prepubertal girls; penetration beyond the hymen is not necessary to transmit the infection.

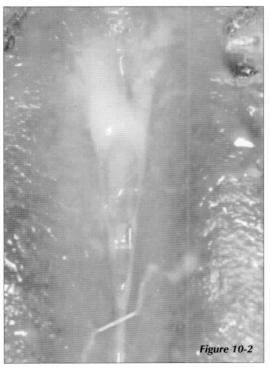

Figure 10-2

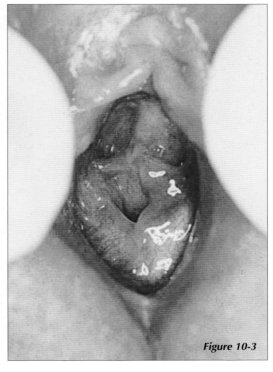

Figure 10-3

The selection of sampling sites depends primarily on the history from the patient in addition to clinical signs. Because oral gonorrhea infections may be asymptomatic, it is recommended that testing of the oropharynx be conducted when history or examination suggests contact between the patient's mouth and another individual's genitals; sometimes through contiguous spread the patient may present with conjunctivitis. Testing for oral or pharyngeal chlamydia infection is not recommended because the yield is low, perinatally acquired infection may persist past age 2 years,[12] and some laboratories do not distinguish between *Chlamydia trachomatis* and *Chlamydia pneumonia.*[2] Similarly, the patient's history should dictate the need for vaginal or cervical, urethral, and anal testing for gonorrhea and chlamydia, as patients may be asymptomatic. The patient's comfort, especially during an assessment for sexual abuse or assault, is of paramount importance, and the clinician may opt to alter sampling sites to reduce trauma. For example, urine nucleic acid amplification tests may be conducted instead of urethral or vaginal swabs in children; if the urine test is positive, those patients could return for urethral or vaginal swabs for culture. This sequential testing may reduce trauma in a significant number of children by reducing the number of required vaginal or urethral swabs. Genital swabs are usually tolerated without much difficulty in older children and adolescents.

Criteria for testing children have been based on studies that utilize culture techniques for the detection of *Neisseria gonorrhoeae* and *Chlamydia trachomatis.* A positive gonorrhea culture must be validated with 2 confirmatory tests such as carbohydrate degradation and enzyme substrate tests, or by alternative independent methods. These tests will differentiate *Neisseria gonorrhoeae* from other *Neisseria* species. The isolation of *Chlamydia trachomatis* can be confirmed by microscopic identification of inclusions by staining with fluorescein-conjugated monoclonal antibody specific for *Chlamydia trachomatis.* While there is little risk of bacterial cross-contamination in chlamydia cultures, oral and rectal bacteria overgrowth may make the test impossible to interpret. In addition, menstrual blood may interfere with interpretation of vaginal swabs submitted for chlamydia cell culture.

Other detection techniques for these organisms have been tested extensively in adult populations, some with promising results. These techniques include enzyme immunoassay, direct fluorescent antibody, nucleic acid hybridization (or probe) tests, and nucleic acid amplification tests (NAAT). Examples of NAATs include polymerase chain reaction, ligase chain reaction, transcription mediated assay (APTIMA), and Becton-Dickinson probe. Of particular note is the distinction between NAATs and DNA hybridization, often confused because both detect DNA sequences. Sensitivity rates are significantly lower with DNA hybridization tests than with NAATs.[3,5,13] Only the culture has been approved for pharyngeal and rectal samples, and antibiotic susceptibility tests can only be done from culture samples.

The CDC has endorsed the use of NAATs in the population of sexually active adults.[2] Among adults, reported prevalence of *Neisseria gonorrhoeae* utilizing NAATs ranges from 5% to 16%, with sensitivities of 89% to 100% and specificities of 99% to 100%.[14-16] NAATs detect both viable and nonviable organisms. While both false-negative and false-positive results are uncommon with these assays, false-negative results are in fact more common than false-positive results; they can occur due to the presence of inhibitors of the amplification process found most often in cervical specimens.[17] A source of false-positive results includes carryover contamination during sample processing. Clinicians must ensure that any object or surfaces that come in contact with patient samples other than culture or NAAT materials are effectively decontaminated since carryover of only a few organisms will produce false-positive results. Laboratory measures to reduce the likelihood of carryover contamination with probe amplification methods, such as ligase chain reaction (LCR), or signal amplification methods, include the use of the Gap Junction LCR and the establishment of a unidirectional workflow that physically separate the reagent and specimen storage area, sample processing area, and amplification/detection area.[18] Instruments should be decontaminated prior to each run of assays in accordance with manufacturer instructions and weekly swipe tests should be performed to ensure effective decontamination.

Reported prevalence in adult populations of *Chlamydia trachomatis* utilizing NAATs ranges from 10% to 16%, with sensitivities of 99% to 100% and specificities of 98% to 100%.[14,15,19] In particular, the sensitivity of NAATs for chlamydia generally exceeds culture techniques; NAATs have been found to detect an additional 25% to 30% of infected adults.[20] In one laboratory, LCR costs $88 and the polymerase chain reaction (PCR) test costs $128 for both *Neisseria gonorrhoeae* and *Chlamydia trachomatis*.

While these techniques have been extensively tested in the adult population, very few comparative studies have been done in the pediatric population. One study compared 95 vaginal cultures to PCR tests performed on the same swab, several months after the swab had been frozen.[21] Of the samples, 12 of the vaginal samples were positive by PCR for *Chlamydia trachomatis*, 3 of which were either negative or indeterminate by culture technique. Another study compared urine-based LCR tests to cultures in 154 children referred for sexual abuse examinations.[22] In this study, 18 children and adolescents had positive urine-based LCR tests for *Chlamydia trachomatis*; 8 of the 18 also had positive culture results from the urethra, anus, vagina, or cervix. Positive urine-based LCR tests were found in 5 subjects for *Neisseria gonorrhoeae*, 2 of 5 also tested positive for gonorrhea by culture of the anus and urethra. No study subject had a positive culture/negative urine LCR combination for either *Chlamydia trachomatis* or *Neisseria gonorrhoeae*. A third study compared cultures to PCR tests performed on vaginal washes in 29 premenarchal girls referred for sexual abuse evaluations.[23] *Neisseria gonorrhoeae* was detected by PCR in 2 children, one of whom was also culture-positive. Polymerase chain reaction tests detected 4 children with *Chlamydia trachomatis*, 2 of whom were also positive by culture. None of these 3 studies compared vaginal cultures to NAATs performed simultaneously on urine and vaginal samples.

Another study has compared culture results to both urine and vaginal LCR samples for *Neisseria gonorrhoeae* and *Chlamydia trachomatis*; confirmatory testing with PCR was done on 85% of the urine samples and 89% of the LCR vaginal swabs.[24] Cultures and at least one LCR test were collected in 251 females, ages 6 to 20 years. By at least one LCR test, 28 girls (11%) were positive for chlamydia; only 2 of these subjects were also positive by culture. Among the 151 subjects in which cultures, urine LCR, and vaginal LCR were collected for *Chlamydia trachomatis*, one subject was positive for all 3 tests, 13 subjects were positive for urine and vaginal LCR, and 4 subjects were positive for vaginal LCR only. Of the subjects in which urine and vaginal swabs were submitted for culture and LCR, 122 of 151 also had their urine and LCR vaginal swabs tested by PCR. Overall, there was excellent agreement between LCR and PCR results but poor agreement between both LCR and PCR with the culture technique. All positive PCR results were also positive by LCR. The following factors predicted chlamydia positivity: patient history of consensual sexual contact, patient history of vaginal discharge, and the presence of suggestive or definite examination findings of genital trauma. While 4 of 28 patients with a positive LCR test for *Chlamydia trachomatis* did not have one of these risk factors, all 4 did have a history of genital-genital contact. By at least one LCR test, 8 subjects (3.2%) were positive for gonorrhea; 6 of these subjects also had positive gonorrhea cultures. Among the subjects in which cultures and both LCR samples were collected for *Neisseria gonorrhoeae*, 2 subjects were positive for all 3 tests, and 2 subjects were positive for vaginal LCR only. An increased number of white blood cells seen on vaginal smear predicted a positive gonorrhea result by culture or LCR; all patients were either co-infected with *Chlamydia trachomatis* (and had one of the risk factors for *Chlamydia trachomatis*) or had leukocytosis on vaginal smear. While LCR and culture techniques were comparable for detecting *Neisseria gonorrhoeae*, LCR techniques detected 26 additional patients with *Chlamydia trachomatis* when compared with the culture technique. In addition, LCR vaginal samples detected more patients with *Chlamydia trachomatis* and *Neisseria gonorrhoeae* than LCR urine samples. These findings are similar to that of adult studies[20]; however, other publications[17,25] caution against comparing results from a high-prevalence adult population to a low-prevalence pediatric population as the positive predictive value for a new test in a low-prevalence (<5%, as determined by the "gold standard" culture) population could be as low as 35% depending on reporting sensitivities and specificities.[17] The reagents for LCR are no longer available, so most laboratories have ceased LCR testing. The study referenced here suggests comparable clinical experience with PCR.

A recent recommendation[25] states that "Data, experience, and court cases are insufficient to assess the applicability of NAATs to detect *Chlamydia trachomatis* or *Neisseria gonorrhoeae* in investigating sexual abuse and assault." The focus of this recommendation is the use of a test as an investigative tool and the defensibility of a positive result in court. However, the medical evaluation of suspected victims of child and adolescent sexual abuse has a dual purpose[25]:

Examination of victims (of sexual abuse and assault) is required for two purposes: (1) to determine if an infection is present so that it can be successfully treated; and (2) to acquire evidence for potential use in a legal investigation. Testing to satisfy the first purpose requires a method that is highly sensitive, whereas satisfying the second purpose requires a method that is highly specific. Because of the health and legal implications of test results, the additional time, labor, and cost of performing tests that are sensitive and highly specific are justified.

The latter statement is true if the forensic implications of the test (which require minimizing false-positive results) are more important than detection and treatment of the disease (which require minimizing false-negative results). The risk of attributing a false-positive NAAT to sexual abuse is small if there is other compelling evidence of abuse. The child's history is the most important "evidence" and is the only evidence in the majority of child sexual abuse cases. Screening a general population of children for gonorrhea or chlamydia with NAATs and interpreting a positive result as conclusive evidence of sexual abuse in the absence of a clear history or other compelling evidence is misleading and inappropriate. In children with consistent and detailed histories of sexual abuse, the greatest risk would occur in a legal setting when the physician is asked to interpret a positive result by NAAT coupled with a negative result by culture; in such settings, the culture remains the "gold standard" and positive NAATs may provide further "suspicious" or "suggestive" evidence of abuse. However, the number of children and adolescents presenting for medical evaluations of suspected sexual abuse far exceeds the number of such cases that result in court testimony. While all medical evaluations of suspected victims of child and adolescent sexual abuse involve diagnosis and treatment of the physical and emotional consequences of abuse, few also involve testimony. For example, in San Antonio, Texas, fewer than 5% of child sexual abuse cases that include a medical evaluation result in a criminal trial. Far more cases do result in a guilty plea and no trial; accurate and appropriate interpretation of positive

NAATs in such cases is also required. The risks of treating a false-positive result by NAAT are small. The cost is less than $100 for outpatient antibiotic therapy. For example, the side effects of antibiotic treatment for *Neisseria gonorrhoeae* with Ceftriaxone include diarrhea (2.7%); pain, induration, and tenderness at injection site (1%); headache or dizziness (<1%); nausea and vomiting (<1%); and rash (1.7%).[26] The side effects of Azithromycin for treatment of *Chlamydia trachomatis* include diarrhea/loose stools (7%), nausea (5%), abdominal pain (5%), vomiting (2%), and dyspepsia (1%).[26] The benefits of treating additional victims infected or possibly infected with chlamydia or gonorrhea (as detected by NAATs) include a reduction in the probability of pelvic inflammatory disease, infertility, and ectopic pregnancy. Treatment can also provide reassurance to the victim that the sequelae of abuse are effectively addressed and treated.

While culture remains the optimum standard and is defensible in court, NAATs may be more sensitive, particularly for detecting *Chlamydia trachomatis*. A more sensitive test is better suited to identifying and treating disease when legal implications are a secondary, rather than primary, concern. Clinicians who evaluate children and adolescents for sexual abuse and assault may opt to use both culture and NAATs to maximize useful outcomes for both the patient and the legal system. An initial positive NAAT test for gonorrhea or chlamydia in a victim of acute assault may reflect perpetrator secretions rather than victim infection. Subsequent testing (repeating the NAAT and collecting cultures if the child will tolerate it) is indicated, particularly for prepubertal children, and may provide information that allows the clinician to appropriately interpret the results.

Once gonorrhea or chlamydia infection is reliably identified with the appropriate test, the probability of sexual transmission is addressed. Infection with these organisms confirms mucosal contact with infected (and infective) genital secretions. Overall, possible modes of transmission include the following (see **Table 10-3**):

— *Vertical transmission from mother to infant during birth.* Congenital chlamydia infections involving genital and non-genital sites have been documented in rare cases up to almost 3 years after birth.

— *Horizontal transmission through sexual contact.*

— *Close non-sexual contact between individuals.* There is limited research available to support the transmission of these diseases through close nonsexual contact between individuals and even less (aside from anecdotal reports) to support transmission between individuals and fomites. Chlamydia is an obligate intracellular organism and does not survive on inanimate surfaces; gonorrhea survives under strict growth requirements, such as a specific carbon dioxide concentration. **Table 10-3** summarizes studies on the transmission of chlamydia and gonorrhea.

The treatment of gonorrhea and chlamydia includes providing prophylaxis and treating identified disease. The most current CDC recommendation for prophylactic treatment[2] (for adolescents >12 years of age) is azithromycin one gram orally in a single dose or doxycycline 100 mg orally twice a day for 7 days (*Chlamydia trachomatis*), and Ceftriaxone 125 mg IM in a single dose (*Neisseria gonorrhoeae*).

Recommended treatment of *Chlamydia trachomatis* for children between ages 6 months to 12 years is erythromycin or azythromycin.[2,5] The recommendation for infants younger than 6 months of age is erythromycin base or ethylsuccinate 50 mg/kg/day orally divided into 4 doses daily for 14 days. Treatment with erythromycin is approximately 80%

effective so follow-up assessment is recommended to determine whether retreatment is necessary. Infants treated with erythromycin who are under age 6 weeks have an increased risk of infantile hypertrophic pyloric stenosis. Azithromycin 20 mg/kg/day orally given as a single dose daily for 3 days may be effective, however data are limited and reassessment post-treatment is recommended. This test of cure may be best done at least 3 weeks after treatment is completed, as NAATs (if used) will detect viable and nonviable organisms for up to 3 weeks. Children heavier than 45 kg or older than 12 years of age may receive a single 1-gram oral dose of Azithromycin. Doxycycline 100 mg orally twice a day for 7 days is a recommended alternative, however should not be given to pregnant adolescents or children under age 8 years.[2,5]

In adults, a minority of untreated chlamydia infections (up to 30%) may resolve on their own without treatment or when the patient is treated for syphilis with benzathine penicillin. In a study that assessed 74 evaluable patients, 24 patients (32%) had negative follow-up cultures. Culture transport media for these 24 culture-negative patients were tested with direct immunofluorescence (DFA) or PCR assays for chlamydial infection, and 3 (13%) were positive (for a net negative rate of 28%). Culture positivity rates declined significantly with increasing age and duration of follow-up. Neither a history of symptomatic chlamydia infection nor treatment with cefixime, metronidazole, or antifungal agents was associated with clearance of infection.[27] While notification, testing, and treatment of partners/perpetrators is a recommended public health initiative, negative test results of a named perpetrator does not exclude that person from perpetration.

Recommended treatment of gonococcal infections is intramuscular ceftriaxone or oral cefixime in adolescents with uncomplicated infection.[2,5] Safety and effectiveness of using oral cefixime to treat gonorrhea in children has not been studied. Prevalence of Quinolone-resistant *Neisseria gonorrhoeae* (QRNG) is high in Europe, Asia, the Middle East, and the Pacific (including California and Hawaii) and is increasing in the United States. It is also more common among men having sex with men (MSM). In April, 2007, the CDC recommended removal of quinolones as an option for treatment of *Neisseria gonorrhoeae* in the United States.[28] Gonococcal infections of the pharynx are more difficult to eradicate than anogenital infections with an approximately 90% cure rate; therefore, a single intramuscular dose of ceftriaxone is the treatment of choice.

Because NAATs have high sensitivity for chlamydia infections, adolescents with a negative chlamydia NAAT result at the time of *Neisseria gonorrhoeae* treatment do not need chlamydia treatment. If NAAT results are not available or Chlamydia testing is negative with a test other than NAAT, patients treated for gonorrhea should also be treated for chlamydia. Recommendations apply for pharyngeal gonorrhea infection because of risk of coinfection of a genital site (see **Table 10-4**).

The differential diagnosis for gonorrhea and chlamydia infections includes numerous infectious agents that may produce vaginitis; urethritis; and secretions from oral, ocular, and rectal tissues. If the appropriate confirmatory tests for gonorrhea are not done, then a positive culture may indicate the presence of other species such as *Neisseria meningitidis, Neisseria lactimica, Neisseria cinerea, Neisseria sicca, Neisseria subflava biovar perflava, Neisseria mucosa, Neisseria flavescens, Neisseria polysaccharea, Branhamella catarrhalis,* and *Kingella dentrificans.*[29] If the diagnostic tests and interpretation are appropriately conducted to minimize false-positive results, then a positive test for gonorrhea or chlamydia is reliable and other infectious causes can be excluded from the differential diagnosis.

Table 10-3. Summary of Studies on the Transmission of Chlamydia and Gonorrhea

Neisseria gonorrhoeae

1. Argent AC, Lachman PI, Hanslo D, Bass D. Sexually transmitted diseases in children and evidence of sexual abuse. *Child Abuse Negl.* 1995;19:1303-1310.

   — A retrospective study of STDs diagnosed in 107 children up to age 14 years; diagnosed sexual abuse by history or physical in 36 of 61 children with gonnorhea (GC); in 17 with GC transmission was unknown; it is unclear in this study how the remaining 8 of the 61 were infected with GC.

2. Bump RC, Sachs LA, Buesching WJ. Sexually transmissible infectious agents in sexually active and virginal asymptomatic adolescent girls. *Pediatrics.* 1986;77:488-494.

   — Compares 68 sexually active girls with 52 virginal girls, all of whom underwent STI testing. None of the virgins had GC.

3. Paradise JE, Campos JM, Friedman HM, Frishmuth G. Vulvovaginitis in premenarchal girls: clinical features and diagnostic evaluation. *Pediatrics.* 1982;70:193-198.

   — Looks at 54 premenarcheal girls presenting with vulvovaginitis; not all cultures for all STDs were done in all patients. Compared with 52 age-matched controls. GC found in 4 of 36 in the test group, none of the controls. Authors assume the transmission is sexual; not clear if sexual abuse was identified by history or other means.

4. Alexander JW, Griffith H, Housch JG, Holmes JR. Infections in sexual contacts and associates of children with gonorrhea. *Sex Transm Dis.* 1984;11:156-158.

   — Investigated 244 individuals who were identified as either sexual contacts, household associates, or nonhousehold associates of 36 children infected with GC. Ten of the 21 sexual contacts of the children had GC; 21 of the household associates (out of 41 children under 15 that were tested, 4 had GC) and 14 of the nonhousehold associates (out of 51 children under 15 that were tested, 5 had GC) out of the remaining 223 had GC. A history of sexual contact was elicited from 18 of the 36 index/infected children. The mode of transmission for the other 18 children is not addressed.

5. Nair P, Glazer-Semmel E, Gould C, Ruff E. Neisseria gonorrhoeae in asymptomatic prepubertal household contacts of children with gonococcal infection. *Clin Pediatr.* 1986;25:160-163.

   — Looks at prepubertal contacts of 12 females and 2 males presenting with vaginitis (11), sexual behavior (1), and "peculiar gait and unusual tonsillitis" (2); all were diagnosed with GC. GC was recovered from the vagina/urethra (10), the rectum (6), and the throat (9). The authors state "We were unable to determine the source of *N. gonorrhoeae* in this survey."

6. Hammerschlag MR, Alpert S, Rosner I, Thurston P, Semine D, McComb D, McCormack WM. Microbiology of the vagina in children: normal and potentially pathogenic organisms. *Pediatrics.* 1978;62:57-62.

   — Vaginal cultures in 100 girls, ages 2 months to 15 years. GC found in one 4-year-old girl; while source was not determined, cultures from the other family members were negative.

7. Gardner JJ. Comparison of the vaginal flora in sexually abused and nonabused girls. *J Pediatrics.* 1992;120:872-877.

   — Prospective study of 209 sexually abused girls and 108 controls. No GC found among the nonabused group.

(continued)

Table 10-3. Summary of Studies on the Transmission of Chlamydia and Gonorrhea *(continued)*

Neisseria gonorrhoeae

8. Sgroi, SM. Pediatric gonorrhea beyond infancy. *Pediatr Ann.* 1979;8:326-336.

   — Prospective study of 15 children with genitourinary GC denominator, 8 of whom eventually disclosed sexual abuse, 3 of whom had "strong contributing evidence" of sexual abuse but no history, and 4 of whom had no history or other evidence of sexual contact. Three of the 4 in the latter group were siblings from a "large and disorganized family… with extensive neglect."

9. Branch GB and Paxton R. A study of gonococcal infections among infants and children. *Public Health Rep.* 1965;80:347-352.

   — Identified 180 children ages birth to 14 with GC. Based on public health nurse interview, all 19 children with GC one year and under were infected via "birth canal" or "contamination" via mother's hands and all mothers of these 19 children were infected with GC. Sexual contact was confirmed in 126 of the remaining 161 children; 32 of these 161 were said to be infected via "casual acquaintances" but this is not further clarified. Of interesting note, one child with GC between 5 and 9 years of age was determined to have been infected through "boyfriend-girlfriend relationship"; this also was not further elucidated.

10. Shore WB and Winkelstein JA. Nonvenereal transmission of gonococcal infections to children. *J Pediatr.* 1971;79:661-663.

    — Chart review of 15 children with GC; method of transmission was presumed as "indirect contact," "sexual contact," and "unknown." Three of 15 were determined as sexual transmission due to their history of rape. Five cases were unknown transmission. The remaining 7 all co-slept with their parents and either one or both parents were noted to have GC. The gender of the infected parent was not given, but in the 5 of 7 cases where the child and one parent had GC, the other parent who was in the same bed did not have GC.

11. Shapiro, RA, Schubert CJ, Siegel RM. Neisseria gonorrhea infections in girls younger than 12 years of age evaluated for vaginitis. *Pediatrics.* 1999;104:e72.

    — Prospective study of 93 girls without a history of sexual abuse presenting for evaluation of genital symptoms. Four of 43 with signs of vaginal discharge had GC.

12. Farrel MK, Billmire ME, Shamroy JA, Hammond JG. Prepubertal gonorrhea: A multidisciplinary approach. *Pediatrics.* 1981;67:151-153.

    — Followed 46 children under 12 years with GC for 4.5 years. Twenty-nine of 46 were victims of sexual assault, and the authors were able to establish a "history of exposure" in some of the remaining patients. Modes of transmission are not well described.

13. Ingram DL, White ST, Durfee MF, Pearson AW. Sexual contact in children with gonorrhea. *Am J Dis Children.* 1982;136:994-996.

    — Study of 31 children with GC; all children older than 4 "had a sexual contact" and 6 of 17 children from 1 to 4 years old "named a sexual contact" while 6 of the 1 to 4 year olds did not name sexual contacts they "lived with older males who had gonorrhea." "Four of the six also lived with older females who also had gonorrhea."

(continued)

Table 10-3. *(continued)*

Chlamydia trachomatis

1. Argent AC, Lachman PI, Hanslo D, Bass D. Sexually transmitted diseases in children and evidence of sexual abuse. *Child Abuse Negl.* 1995;19:1303-1310.

   — A retrospective study looking at STDs diagnosed in 107 children up to 14 years; found sexual abuse by history or physical in 5 of 12 children with CT; in the remaining 7 with CT the transmission was unknown. A limitation of this study is that the CT infections were diagnosed using direct immunofluorescence.

2. Bump RC, Sachs LA, Buesching WJ. Sexually transmissible infectious agents in sexually active and virginal asymptomatic adolescent girls. *Pediatrics.* 1986;77:488-494.

   — Compares 68 sexually active girls with 52 virginal girls, all of whom underwent STD testing. One of the virgins had CT while 13 of the sexually active group were infected with CT. Tissue culture was used.

3. Rettig PJ, Nelson JD. Genital tract infection with *Chlamydia trachomatis* in prepubertal children. *J Pediatr.* 1981;99:206-210.

   — Examined 23 prepubertal children with nongonococcal urethritis and vaginitis for CT; none had CT. In another group with gonococcal anogenital infection (N= 31) found 9 of 33 "episodes" of GC complicated by CT. Tissue culture techniques used. Only 1 of 9 patients had a history of sexual contact. The study does not address the mode of transmission for the other 8 children but does state that a sibling of 1 child, and a father, 2 siblings, and a cousin of another child were all positive for CT and/or GC.

4. Schachter J, Grossman M, Sweet RL, Holt J, Jordan C, Bishop E. Prospective study of perinatal transmission of *Chlamydia trachomatis. JAMA.* 1986;255:3374-3377.

   — Followed 131 infants of 262 pregnant women infected with CT for 5 years. Conjunctivitis was found in 23 of the infants, pneumonia in 21 infants, and subclinical rectal and vaginal CT infections in 18 of the infants (only 126 had rectal cultures and 36 had vaginal cultures with 17 and 5 positive results, respectively). Rectal infections were detected in the second or third month and vaginal infections were detected between 70 and 154 days.

5. Ingram DL, Runyan DK, Collins AD, White ST, Durfee MF, Pearson AW, Occhiuti AR. Vaginal *Chlamydia trachomatis* infection in children with sexual contact. *Pediatr Infect Dis.* 1984;3:97-99.

   — Compared vaginal, throat, and rectal cultures for CT in 50 children ages 1 to 12 with a history of sexual contact and 34 children without such history. Three of the 50 study children and none of the control group had CT. One of the 3 with CT had a history of vaginal intercourse and all were asymptomatic.

6. Bell TA, Stamm WE, Wang SP, Kuo CC, Holmes KK, Grayston JT. Chronic *Chlamydia trachomatis* infections in infants. *JAMA.* 1992;267:2188.

   — Found evidence of persistent or recurring CT infections in 22 infants, one of whom had oropharynx CT 28.5 months after birth; 35% were still infected at one year of age. Serologic tests supported acquisition of infection at birth. Vaginal and/or rectal cultures were positive in the third/fourth month of life.

Table 10-4. Treatment Recommendations for Gonorrheal and Chlamydial Infections			
INFECTIONS	INFANTS	CHILDREN (6 MONTHS TO 12 YEARS OR < 45 KG)	CHILDREN/ADOLESCENTS ≥ AGE 8 AND ≥ 45 KG
C. trachomatis	Erythromycin base orally 50 mg/kg/day divided into 4 doses x 14 days (retest)	Erythromycin; OR Azithromycin orally 20 mg/kg/day daily x 3 days (retest)	Azithromycin 1 gm orally as a single dose; OR Doxycycline 100 mg orally twice daily x 7 days
N. gonorrhoeae (uncomplicated anogenital)	25-50 mg/kg IV or IM single dose; not to exceed 125 mg	Ceftriaxone 125 mg IM single dose; OR Spectinomycin 40 mg/kg IM single dose	Ceftriaxone 125 mg IM single dose; OR cefixime 400 mg orally single dose
N. gonorrhoeae (pharyngeal)	25-50 mg/kg IV or IM, single dose, not to exceed 125 mg	Ceftriaxone 125 mg IM single dose	Ceftriaxone 125 mg IM single dose

HUMAN PAPILLOMAVIRUS

Condyloma acuminata (venereal warts) is one of the most frequently diagnosed infections in sexually abused children (**Figures 10-4, 10-5, 10-6,** and **10-7**). In adults, transmission of this disease is considered sexual, and human papillomavirus (HPV) is considered the most common STI worldwide. Twenty million Americans are currently infected, with 6 million new cases reported annually. Half of those infected are between ages 15 to 24 years. Some are infected with multiple HPV types.[30] A recent National Health and Nutrition Examination Survey (NHANES) study estimates point prevalence of genital HPV in women ages 14 to 49 years to be 27%, with 45% of women ages 20 to 24 years infected.[31] Though varying widely, estimates of genital HPV prevalence in adult men are greater than 20%.[32] How HPV is transmitted to children is controversial and has remained so despite ongoing active research in this area for the last 20 years. Because of the strong association of this disease with sexually abused children, dilemmas particularly arise when confronted with a young child with visible condyloma who lacks a disclosure of abuse. What does the presence of condyloma mean? Was the infection sexually transmitted?

More than 100 types of human papillomaviruses have been identified and are grouped into mucosal and cutaneous subtypes based on their predilection to infect particular types of epithelium.[2,5] Most often, nongenital warts are cutaneous types and anal, genital, oral, and respiratory papillomas/dysplasias are mucosal types. There are 40 identified mucosal types of HPV that infect the genital tract. Because of detection of some types in genital cancers, mucosal HPVs are further grouped into high-risk and low-risk types. Most HPV infections (up to 90% of infections within 2 years)[31,33,34] are thought to be cleared by the immune system before they cause any harm, though it is unclear whether infected persons completely clear infection or HPV infection simply becomes dormant and undetectable. While there are more than 18 high-risk types, the most common are HPV-16 (found in 50% of cancers), and HPV-18, which together

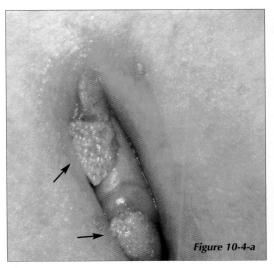

Figure 10-4-a

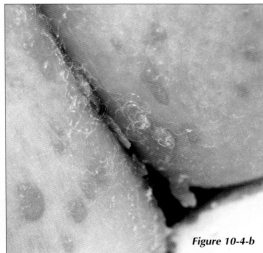

Figure 10-4-b

Figure 10-4-a. *3-year-old child is supine. There are 2 cauliflower-like, warty clusters of* Condyloma acuminata (HPV). *One is on the periurethral area and the other on the posterior hymen. There are several isolated warts on the labia majora.*

Figure 10-4-b. *Flat and sessile warts visible on the buttocks of the child.* Gardnerella vaginalis *and group B streptococcus were cultured from the vagina (35mm).*

Figure 10-5. Condyloma acuminata *is evident in the perianal area (35mm).*

Figure 10-6. *Condyloma at the base of the penis in a 3-year-old boy. Child did not give a disclosure of abuse.*

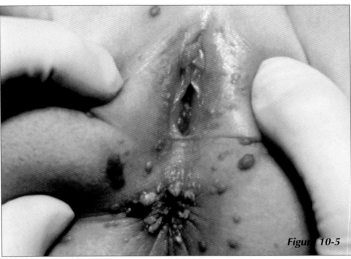

Figure 10-5

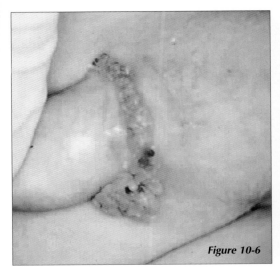

Figure 10-6

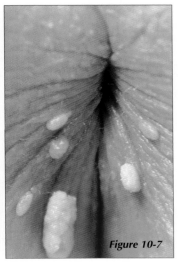

Figure 10-7

Figure 10-7. *Condyloma in the anal area of a 4-year-old girl who gave no disclosure of sexual abuse. Mother had a history of an abnormal PAP smear several years previously.*

181

cause 70% of cervical cancers worldwide.[5,30,35] Other common high-risk genital types are 31, 33, 35, 39, 45, 51, 52, 56, 58, 59, 68, and 82. Low-risk types include HPV-6 and HPV-11, which together cause more than 90% of genital warts.[30]

Though transmission of genital HPV in adults is believed to be almost always sexual, mechanisms of transmission in children remain controversial and are theorized to occur by multiple mechanisms (**Figures 10-7, 10-8, 10-9,** and **10-11**). Sufficient data to clearly define mechanisms of HPV transmission in children are still lacking. Transplacental transmission has been postulated due to rare reports of infants developing laryngeal papillomatosis as early as 1 day of age,[36] presence of non-genital condyloma acuminata in a newborn delivered by Cesarean section (C-section) with intact membranes,[37] identification of HPV in amniotic fluid and umbilical cord blood from infants delivered to mothers with HPV infection,[38,39] and identification of HPV-16 in peripheral blood mononuclear cells.[40] These reports involve very few numbers of cases, despite the high prevalence of adult HPV.

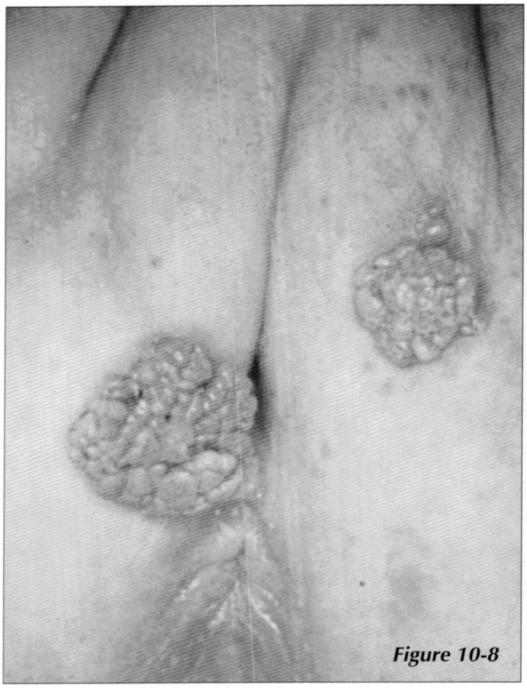

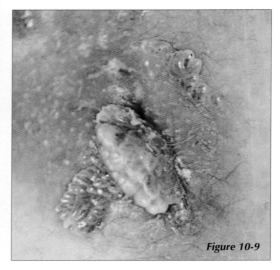

Figure 10-8

Figure 10-9

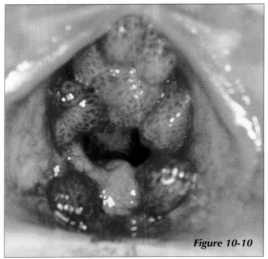

Figure 10-10

Figure 10-8. *Giant, pedunculated condyloma in an 8-month-old female. Both parents had genital warts at the time of the baby's birth. The source of the baby's HPV could have been from either parent. No other STIs were found in the infant.*

Figure 10-9. *Anal condyloma in a 2-month-old breastfed infant. This child was removed from the parents because the physician who examined the baby said that the warts could only have been spread by sexual contact. Further history revealed that mother had a past history of genital warts but currently had no lesions. The mode of transmission in this infant was most likely not sexual.*

Figure 10-10. *This 6-year-old girl gave a history of penile-genital contact by her stepfather. She had been brought for an examination because of genital bleeding, determined to have been caused by the condyloma. In this case, the transmission was likely sexual.*

Vertical and postnatal transmission has been studied by assessing frequency of positive HPV DNA in oral or genital swabs in infants and children.[41-45] Chatterjee et al found 16% (5 of 31) newborn buccal smears to be positive for HPV DNA (types 6,11,16,18).[44] Summersgill et al collected oral squamous cells from swabs or oral saline solution from 268 healthy infants, children, and adolescents who were 20 years old or younger.[43] HPV DNA was detected in 6% of subjects; 5% of the adolescents (over 12 years old) were positive, none of the children aged 7 to 12 years old were positive, and 9% of the children under age 7 years were positive. In Japan, 45% of healthy 3-year-olds and 50% of healthy 5-year-olds attending the same nursery school had HPV DNA detected on oral buccal swabs, especially HPV-16, HPV-1, HPV-2, and HPV-75.[42] These studies raise the unanswered question: is this colonization, infection, or contamination?

Finnish researchers addressed this question with a prospective study of 324 infants and their parents over 36 months, assessing oral and genital swabs for 12 high-risk HPV DNA types.[41] While these researchers did not report concordance of mother/baby HPV DNA or whether subjects had any visible warts or condyloma, they described acquisition, clearance, and persistence of high-risk HPV DNA detected in infant oral and genital specimens (**Figure 10-12**). Patterns were very similar for oral and genital mucosa. At delivery, HPV DNA was detected in 14% of infant oral swabs. Of these infants, 10% (1.4% of total) had persistent HPV carriage at 36 months of age and 11% cleared the

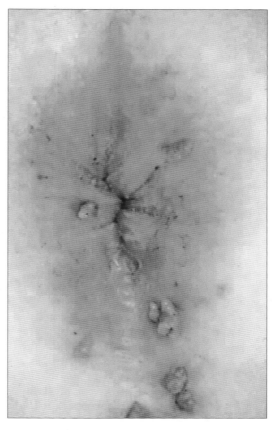

Figure 10-11. This 3-year-old child has anal warts, noticed first at 12 months. Mother had noted one small wart for several years, then the warts appeared to spread and she brought him for an examination. The child denied any abuse. Several others in the family had warts on their hands. These warts were not biopsied, but were treated with topical medication and resolved.

HPV. No HPV DNA was ever detected in oral specimens from 37% of all infants. New (or acquisition of) HPV DNA in oral mucosa was demonstrated in 42% of the infants. Persistent oral carriage of high-risk HPV types in infants was significantly associated with high-risk oral HPV types in the mother at month 36 and in the father at month 24, young age of mother at initiation of sexual activity and use of oral contraception, and presence of maternal hand warts. With regard to infant genital specimens, 15% were HPV DNA–positive at birth. Only 1.5% (5) of these infants had persistent positive genital HPV DNA testing at age 36 months, and 14% of infants with initial positive genital testing cleared the HPV. No genital HPV was detected at any point in the study for 47% of infants, and 36% of infants acquired genital HPV DNA during the follow-up period (see **Figure 10-12**). Persistent infant genital HPV carriage was significantly predicted by mother's history of recent genital warts at age over 20 years, and maternal history of smoking initiation at age 18 to 21 years. The authors did not comment on the relationship of acquired infant oral and genital HPV types to each other or to mother's or father's HPV types. Importantly, persistent HPV carriage occurred infrequently, though persistent carriage of HPV was more common in oral than genital mucosa of infants. Persistent oral carriage of HPV in infants appears related to oral HPV carriage in the parents and to presence of hand warts in the mother. Infant genital HPV carriage was uncommon and appeared related to mother's recent history of genital warts.

Another study of buccal samples from 267 children ages 3 to 11 years showed much higher prevalence of HPV DNA in children when using type-specific PCR testing (HPV-16, a high-risk mucosal type).[45] Prevalence of HPV-16 was 52% compared to 17% by generic PCR. All controls and 20 tested fomite surfaces in the school environment all tested HPV negative. This author also summarized serologic studies demonstrating presence of antibodies by EIA to HPV-16 in 4% to 14% of children aged 1 to 13 years, as well as detection of IgM antibody to HPV-16 among 50% of children aged 1 to 10 years presented as evidence for recent or persistent HPV-16 infection in children. This study did not differentiate vertical transmission from early childhood acquisition. A follow-up study by the same group tested for persistence of oral HPV-16 in 20 children ages 4 to 9 years, comparing them to a negative control group.[46] Time interval tested was 30 months. Of the HPV-16 positive group, 40% were subsequently negative and 63% of the negative control group had become HPV-16 positive. The authors concluded that (asymptomatic) oral HPV-16 DNA in children is likely transient. It is possible that the high rates may reflect false-positive PCR results.[47]

The high rates of infant HPV DNA detection in some of the above studies and lack of comparison to parent HPV DNA rates are in contrast to two large prospective longitudinal studies of infant and parent HPV DNA.[48,49] Both studies describe women with relatively high rates of genital/cervical HPV DNA (Smith et al 29%; Watts et al 41% cervical but 74% with cervical, vulvovaginal, and history of condyloma or abnormal Pap smear). Infants had very low rates of oral or genital HPV (Smith et al 1.6%; Watts et al 1.5% genital, 1.2% anal, none oral or nasopharyngeal). Further, the infants with HPV DNA were not concordant with their mother HPV DNA types. Results from both of these studies support the conclusion that vertical transmission of HPV infection is rare.

An unanswered question is whether presence of HPV DNA represents true infection. Respiratory papillomatosis (RP) is interesting to study because it clearly represents infection, not colonization or carriage. Frequently, RP is presumed to occur through vertical transmission, as most of the affected children with this disorder have HPV-6 or HPV-11 and obstetric delivery of women with genital HPV by C-section may be

Figure 10-12.
High-risk HPV DNA detected in infant oral and genital specimens, describing acquisition, clearance, and persistance.

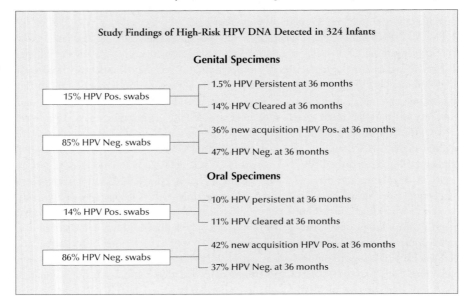

Study Findings of High-Risk HPV DNA Detected in 324 Infants

Genital Specimens

15% HPV Pos. swabs
— 1.5% HPV Persistent at 36 months
— 14% HPV Cleared at 36 months

85% HPV Neg. swabs
— 36% new acquisition HPV Pos. at 36 months
— 47% HPV Neg. at 36 months

Oral Specimens

14% HPV Pos. swabs
— 10% HPV persistent at 36 months
— 11% HPV cleared at 36 months

86% HPV Neg. swabs
— 42% new acquisition HPV Pos. at 36 months
— 37% HPV Neg. at 36 months

associated with lower rates of infant laryngeal infection,[50] though C-section to prevent transmission of HPV to the newborn is currently not indicated.[2] Vertical transmission as explanation for all or even most cases of respiratory papillomas has been challenged, as the disease also develops in older children and adults. There are no reported cases of respiratory or laryngeal papillomas in siblings, marital partners, or family members.[38] Sinclair et al highlight the bimodal age distribution for peak diagnosis of RP (between ages 2 and 5 years in children, and between ages 20 and 30 years in adults). They also point out the paucity of studies that consider acquisition of RP from child sexual abuse, despite adult RP being attributed to oral-genital contact.[51] Wiatrak et al have published a 10-year longitudinal prospective study of 74 children with recurrent respiratory papillomatosis followed from time of diagnosis.[38] In this series, the mean age of diagnosis was 4 years old, with the youngest child diagnosed at age 4 months and the oldest at age 12 years. No type of screening for sexual abuse was described.

Horizontal transmission and autoinoculation are additional proposed modes of transmitting HPV to children's genitals. It is unknown how commonly this occurs; however, HPV types 2, 3, 27, and 57 have been shown to be present in pediatric anogenital warts.[47,52] Because these 4 types are commonly seen in cutaneous warts, it is speculated that children may transfer HPV to their genitals when scratching, toileting, et cetera. Additionally, horizontal transmission is theorized to occur from an adult caregiver when assisting with diaper changes or toileting, or during sexual abuse of the child, as many disclosures of sexual abuse involve fondling and digital penetrative acts. HPV DNA has been found in finger brush samples of adults with genital HPV disease. It is unknown whether this transient hand carriage is adequate to allow transmission without abraded skin.[52]

Attempts to demonstrate fomite transmission of HPV from floors, toys, humid surfaces of bathhouses, and so on have not yielded any positive HPV DNA samples.[45,47] Fomite transmission is speculated to be a cause of plantar warts; however, demonstration of fomite transmission has not been reported.

Evaluation of a child, especially an older child (>3 years of age) who presents with genital or oral warts should include consideration of sexual abuse, as sexual transmission of HPV is known to occur commonly. A complete medical evaluation is recommended, including a child forensic interview, caretaker interview to assess maternal history of condyloma or abnormal Pap smears, and history of cutaneous warts affecting the child or family members. Although vertical transmission does not appear to be common, absence of a clear maternal history does not preclude it. Physical exam of the entire child including the oral cavity should be performed and testing for other STIs should be done. Consensus is currently lacking on when to report these cases to child protective services (CPS). Routine reporting to CPS has been suggested for children over age 4 years presenting with anogenital warts, with referral to CPS for younger children guided by overall history, forensic interview, and clinical findings.[51]

Other methods of transmission including nonsexual horizontal transmission and autoinoculation are possible. Fomite transmission is unlikely though described.[51] Blood transfusion is a theoretical risk with limited, inconclusive data.[40] Host factors also influence viral transmission, persistent carriage of HPV, and rate of HPV disease. Patients with immunosuppression—either from immunodeficiency, HIV infection, or iatrogenic immunosuppression—have higher rates of HPV disease. Patients with mucosal breaks (ie, ulcerative diseases including herpes simplex virus [HSV]) may also be at increased risk of HPV disease; however, data are lacking to support skin disorders such as eczema as a factor increasing infection rate with HPV.

The diagnosis of condyloma acuminata (venereal warts) is primarily clinical. During clinical examination, application of acetic acid (ie, TCA or BCA used for treatment) to a suspicious skin lesion may elicit a characteristic "white frosting" of HPV-infected tissue, which is not expected to occur in HPV-uninfected lesions, though not a specific test for HPV. Application of acetic acid can be quite painful.[53] Other diagnostic tests include histologic examination and detection of HPV DNA in biopsied material. HPV DNA can be detected with dot blot hybridization, DNA blotting, and modifications of PCR.[54] While costly and labor intensive, the DNA blot is considered the "gold standard."[55] Although genital HPV subtypes have been detected in oral mucosal scrapings of asymptomatic prepubertal children,[56] subtyping of HPV appears to have no diagnostic or therapeutic value when performed on asymptomatic patients. HPV colonization can occur via sexual and nonsexual transmission. Subtyping of HPV in patients with clinically apparent lesions does not assist physicians in determining whether such lesions are sexually transmitted. A biopsy should be considered if the diagnosis is uncertain, lesions do not respond or appear to worsen during standard treatment, the patient is immunocompromised, or if the warts appear atypical.[2] Histopathologic detection of HPV in cervical scrapings or biopsies of suspicious lesions depends on the identification of koilocytosis; false negatives are problematic with inexperienced personnel.[55] Serology for HPV is being developed and is currently used in research. The antibody response to HPV is generally type-specific and is being used to study epidemiologic spread of type-specific infections (especially those 15 genital types established as oncogenic in humans), and for monitoring HPV vaccine–induced antibody responses.[57] High-throughput, multiplexed antibody analysis (allowing standardized scale-up of up to 100 antigens) is being studied.[58] Currently, HPV researchers have found the presence of cutaneous HPV DNA and antibodies to the same HPV type are not significantly correlated, thus concluding "the biologic meaning of seropositivity as a marker of cutaneous HPV infection" is as yet uninterpretable.[59] HPV serologic tests are not available commercially, and the usefulness of this test for clinical or forensic purposes in child abuse pediatrics is unknown and unstudied, and should not be used at this time.

The quadrivalent HPV vaccine (Gardasil®, Merck) was FDA approved June 2006 to prevent cervical cancer and lesions caused by HPV-6, HPV-11, HPV-16, and HPV-18. International studies confirm the vaccine is nearly 100% effective at preventing HPV-16 and HPV-18 infection. The CDC recommends routine vaccination of girls 11 to 12 years old, with catch-up vaccination for young women who missed routine vaccination between ages 13 to 26 years. Girls as young as 9 years old may be vaccinated at the discretion of health care providers.[30] Prophylactic use of this vaccine in sexually abused or assaulted children and adolescents has not been explored.

A number of treatments for condyloma accuminata are available, however no definitive evidence exists to support best efficacy of any single treatment. Treatment efficacy varies among patients. The effect of treatment on limiting HPV transmission is unknown, so treatment should be considered only for patients with visible lesions. Regardless of treatment, lesions may spontaneously resolve, and are likely to recur. Because most lesions are small in number and asymptomatic, it is likely best to observe without therapy for spontaneous resolution. Decision to treat may be influenced by development of symptoms including pruritis, pain, or bleeding, or by increasing number or size of warts. Ablative surgery should be reserved for extensive lesions, particularly those interfering with function (eg, obstructive, painful). Most warts respond to a course of treatment (or spontaneously involute) within 3 months. Complications are rare but include post-treatment pigmentation change, depressed or hypertrophic scars, and chronic pain syndromes (vulvodynia, analdynia, hyperesthesias, painful defecation, or fistulas), and limited reports of severe systemic side effects from interferon and podophyllin treatments exist.[2] Patient-applied therapies are likely to have optimal response with supervision/follow-up to assist compliance and efficacy, and to monitor for side effects (see **Table 10-5**). Podofilox 0.5% solution or gel is a safe, easy-to-use antimitotic drug. Most patients experience mild to moderate local pain or irritation with treatment. Imiquimod is a topical immune enhancer that stimulates interferon and other cytokines. Treatment is usually associated with mild to moderate redness and irritation. Referral may be made to dermatologists or gynecologists for provider-administered treatments. Side effects may be minimized by limiting treatment cycles to 3 months and allowing sufficient time to heal between therapy regimens. Trichloroacetic acid (TCA) or Bichloroacetic acid (BCA) 80% to 90% may be applied weekly if necessary in the office setting. A small amount is applied only to the warts and allowed to dry (lesions will whiten). Excess acid should be removed by powdering the treated area with talc, baking soda, or liquid soap preparations. Podophyllin resin 10% to 25% may be applied in the office weekly as needed. Toxicity may be associated with systemic absorption; therefore, only a small amount should be used (maximum 0.5 ml) and application should be limited to a small area less than 10 cm^2 per session. Other modalities are cryotherapy, surgical removal (eg, excision, curettage, electrosurgery), carbon dioxide laser surgery, or injection of intralesional interferon.[2] (**Table 10-5**) Differential diagnosis of external warts includes molluscum contagiosum, linear epidermal nevus, syphilis (condyloma lata), skin tags, and penile pearly papules (benign).

Table 10-5. Treatment Modalities for Anogenital Warts

TREATMENT MODALITIES

Anal Warts	Cryotherapy (liquid nitrogen) OR TCA/BCA 80-90% applied to warts OR Surgical removal (if on rectal mucosa)
Vaginal Warts	Cryotherapy (liquid nitrogen—do not use cryoprobe) OR TCA/BCA 80-90% applied to warts
Urethral Meatus Warts	Cryotherapy (liquid nitrogen) OR Podophyllin 10-25% in compound tincture of benzoin OR Podofilox* 0.5% solution or gel OR Imiquimod* 5% cream
External Genital Warts (Patient-Applied)	Podofilox 0.5% solution or gel: twice a day x 3 days (then 4 days no treatment); may repeat up to 4 cycles. Max 0.5 ml/day to max area 10 cm^2 OR Imiquimod 5% cream: 3 times a week once daily at bedtime, up to 16 weeks. Wash treated area 6-10 hours after application
External Genital Warts (Provider-Applied)	Cryotherapy (liquid nitrogen or cryoprobe) every 1-2 weeks OR Podophyllin resin 10-25% in compound tincture of benzoin OR TCA/BCA 80-90% applied to warts OR Surgery (excision, curettage, electrocautery, carbon dioxide laser) OR Intralesional interferon (injection)

Limited data.

TRICHOMONAS VAGINALIS

Infection with *Trichomonas vaginalis* is another STI that can occur in sexually abused children and adolescents (**Figure 10-13**). In the United States, it is considered the second most common STI, and the most common curable STI.[60] Epidemiologically, trichomonas is considered a marker for high-risk sexual behavior in adults and is commonly associated with other STIs, especially gonorrhea. Bacterial vaginosis commonly occurs concurrently with trichomonas in women, and trichomonas infection has been found to be an important cofactor that amplifies HIV transmission.[5,60,61] Incubation period ranges from 4 to 28 days (averaging 1 week).[5,60]

Trichomoniasis is asymptomatic in most men (90%) and half of women infected. The organism is a flagellated protozoan, slightly larger than a white blood cell. Typical symptoms in women, when present, are frothy pale yellow to gray-green vaginal discharge, odor, pruritis, and irritation (vaginal redness and edema, "strawberry" cervix). Dysuria and lower abdominal pain are also common. The urethra is infected in most cases. Males may develop urethritis, epididymitis, or prostatitis, though uncommonly. Reinfection by infected partners is common.[5,60,62]

The diagnosis is typically made by microscopic examination of vaginal secretions or a spun urine sample. Male urine, prostatic secretions, or semen may be tested. Vaginal smear (wet prep) examination has a low sensitivity rate (13% to 80%),[2,5,60,63-66] in part because non-motile trichomonads closely resemble white blood cells and can be overlooked. Hence, detection relies heavily on the microscopic expertise of the examiner as well as appropriate preparation of the vaginal smear to preserve motility of the trichomonads, including inspection of the vaginal smear slide within 10 to 20 minutes of sample collection. Alternative detection techniques for trichomonas include culture, latex agglutination, direct fluorescent antibody, and PCR. Culture is considered the gold standard,[60] as it is the most sensitive and specific commercially available test method,[2] though it has a much lower sensitivity in males.[60] Culture also has a low cost of approximately $2.50 per test (excluding laboratory and pathologist fees). There are 3 culture media available: Diamond's media, Kupferberg's Trichosel media, and InPouch™ TV. In a study that compared the sensitivity of these 3 media, the InPouch™ TV test was significantly more sensitive than either the Diamond's or Trichosel media and detected approximately twice as many infected patients at 48 hours.[67] While the manufacturer's evaluation of latex agglutination indicated good sensitivity and specificity rates, some kits have been discontinued and studies are more limited than with other techniques. Two tests with better clinical utility than vaginal smear, latex agglutination, and DFA are immunochromatographic capillary flow dipstick (OSOM Trichomonas Rapid Test/ Genzyme Diagnostics, Cambridge, Massachusetts) and nucleic acid probe test (Affirm™ VP III/ Becton Dickenson, San Jose, California). They are Federal Drug Administration (FDA) approved tests performed on vaginal secretions with sensitivity greater than 83% and specificity greater than 97%. Unlike with culture, false-positives may occur with these tests, especially in low-prevalence populations.[2] Direct fluorescent antibody (DFA) has been demonstrated to be more sensitive than vaginal smear, but less sensitive than culture or PCR.[66] In the same study, cultures utilizing Trichosel media detected 46 positive results whereas PCR detected 61 positive results. However, PCR is extremely expensive and laborious compared to all other detection techniques for *Trichomonas vaginalis* and no FDA-cleared PCR test for *Trichomonas vaginalis* is available in the United States, though may be available through some research and commercial labs.[2,5]

Figure 10-13.
Appearance of Trichomonas vaginalis on wet preparation examination.

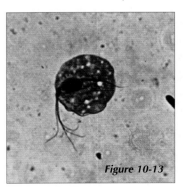

Figure 10-13

Metronidazole is the treatment of choice. Adolescent dose is 2 grams orally in a single dose, or alternatively tinidazole 2 grams orally in a single dose. Patients unable to tolerate the single dose (eg, because of nausea) or with treatment failure are recommended to take metronidazole 500 mg orally twice a day for 7 days.[2] Recommended treatment for children weighing less than 45 kg is oral metronidazole 15 mg/kg per day divided (maximum 2 grams/day) into 3 doses per day for a total of 7 days.[5] Low-grade resistance to metronidazole has been described in vitro but has not yet become clinically important.[2,68]

Differential diagnosis of *Trichomonas vaginalis* includes other infectious and non-infectious causes of vaginitis. Additionally, *Trichomonas vaginalis* must be reliably distinguished from other human trichomonas species, *Trichomonas tenax* and *Pentatrichomonas hominis* (ie, *Trichomonas hominis*), which are nonpathogenic and occur infrequently. *Trichomonas tenax* is found in oral gingival and tracheobronchial secretions. *Pentatrichomonas hominis* is found in the gastrointestinal tract, therefore stool contamination of vaginal/urethral specimens makes identification of *Trichomonas vaginalis* more difficult. Trichomonas species have strict habitat restriction, meaning *Trichomonas tenax* and *Pentatrichomonas hominis* are not viable in the vagina/urethra (and cannot be sexually transmitted). Consequently, the diagnosis of infection with *Trichomonas vaginalis* is best made from vaginal or urethral samples. In young patients, bagged urine samples may be contaminated with Pentatrichomonas. The decision to test for *Trichomonas vaginalis* cannot be based on the presence of patient symptoms or signs as most males and many females are asymptomatic.[2,5,60] Testing criteria for *Trichomonas vaginalis* should complement testing criteria for *Neisseria gonorrhoeoa* and *Chlamydia trachomatis*, and include a patient history for vaginal-penile contact. Published studies support the use of culture, with or without vaginal smear microscopy, as the diagnostic test of choice for *Trichomonas vaginalis*.

Duration of trichomonas infection is not well described, however one study using mathematical models to study epidemiology of trichomonas estimated average duration of trichomonas infection in women to be 3 to 5 years, and in men to be 4 months.[69] Data are lacking on duration of infection in neonates, however newborn infection is considered to be self-limited and treatment unnecessary.[5] Few papers are found describing neonatal or prepubertal infection and duration of infection in these ages. One paper from 1974 with 984 newborn subjects describes 0.6% to 5% of infants of trichomonas positive mothers to have evidence of infection, with infection persisting until treatment (oldest infant 8 weeks of age).[70] The authors postulate that the hyperestrogenic acidic environment of the neonatal vagina allows trichomonas infection to develop (nonetheless rarely described in this population). Once the estrogenic environment subsides and vaginal pH neutralizes (around 6 to 8 weeks of life), conditions are less favorable for trichomonas. Other papers describe case reports of neonatal nasal or respiratory infection.[71,72,61] Vertical transmission is thus possible, though uncommon. Persistence of neonatal infection is not well documented but is thought to be rare outside of the neonatal period. Although fomite transmission is also theoretically possible as trichomonas has been shown to be viable for several hours in urine and washcloths, transmission has not been reported and is likely to be infrequent given the strong association of trichomonas infections with other sexually transmitted infections.[60,70,73,74] Presence of trichomonas infection in an adolescent or child outside of the neonatal period is therefore most likely to be sexually transmitted. Report to social services, investigation, and evaluation of the child for other sexually transmitted infections is indicated.

HERPES SIMPLEX VIRUSES

There are 2 types of herpes simplex viruses and both cause genital herpes infections in children and adults. Herpes simplex type 2 (HSV-2) is considered one of the most prevalent STIs worldwide as it affects both males and females. It accounts for the majority of genital herpes infections.[75,76] Described as "virtually nonexistent in persons younger than age 12 years," HSV-2 seroprevalence infections are almost always acquired between ages 15 to 40 years, "as expected for an STD."[75,77,78] The most recent estimate of HSV-2 seroprevalence using glycoprotein G-based (gG-based) type specific screening, is 17.2%, reported for people ages 14 to 49 years during the time period 1999-2004, according to NHANES data. This figure has decreased from the rate of 22% reported for 1988-1994. Currently lowest for those 14 to 19 years old (0.9%), HSV-2 seroprevalence has also decreased more than for any other included age group compared to 1988-2004 levels (5.8%).[76] Orolabial HSV-2 occurs much less frequently than genital infections, measured by studies of HSV shedding using daily swabs for PCR testing. In these adult studies, oral HSV-2 shedding was not associated with any visible oral lesions, though was usually associated with HSV-2 genital lesions or genital shedding.[75,79,80] The vast majority of people (>85%) with HSV-2 specific antibodies do not report symptoms of genital herpes,[75,76] yet persons infected with HSV-2 have been shown to have asymptomatic HSV-2 shedding by PCR on 20% to 25% of all days. Furthermore, people who are HSV-2 seropositive without symptomatic genital herpes have been shown to be equally likely to shed HSV as those with symptomatic genital herpes.[81] Therefore, most HSV-2 transmission occurs from asymptomatic infected persons. This fact is important to consider when evaluating a child who presents with genital herpes caused by HSV-2, as the infected perpetrator would be expected to lack a history of symptomatic genital or oral HSV-2 most of the time, though would be HSV-2 seropositive (**Figure 10-14**).

Herpes simplex type 1 (HSV-1) is frequently transmitted in childhood by nonsexual contacts, most often via infectious saliva. Seroprevalence is approximately 20% in children younger than age 5 years and then increases linearly to age of 70 years.[75,77] Importantly, HSV-1 seroprevalence has been decreasing as improvements in hygiene and living conditions occur. Seroprevalence in the United Kingdom among 10- to 14-year-olds dropped to 24% in 1994-1995.[82] United States seroprevalence among 14- to 19-year-olds decreased to 39% (1999-2004).[76] Genital HSV-1 infections have been reported

Figure 10-14.
This 3-year-old has extensive herpes simplex type 2 (HSV-2) around her anus and on her perineum and labia majora (35mm).

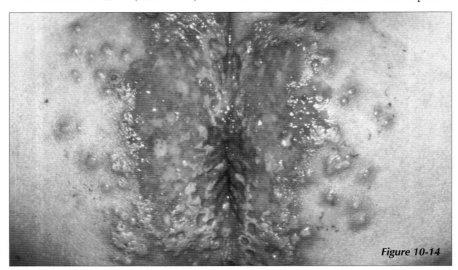

Figure 10-14

more frequently in the United States and Europe during the last 10 years. Nearly half of all first episodes of genital herpes in Canada and the United Kingdom are HSV-1 infections.[81] Genital herpes infections with HSV-1 are associated with receptive oral sex[83] and are less infectious compared to HSV-2, as recurrences are much less frequent and rates of asymptomatic genital shedding are much lower for both men and women.[81,84]

Examples of nonsexual transmission of HSV-1 include herpes gladiatorum (transmission during sports activities with close skin-to-skin contact like wrestling), and more commonly from patients with herpes labialis to health care personnel, especially dentists.[85,86] The risk of transmission from health care personnel with HSV infection is theoretically possible but highly unlikely,[5] with the exception of personnel with herpetic whitlow. There are a very limited number of studies or case reports describing nosocomial (nonsexual) transmission. Most of these papers describe possible but unproven cases involving very few patients. There are no data on whether HSV transmission can occur by an uninfected person via hand contamination with infected secretions. Data are also lacking on nonsexual transmission by persons with genital lesions (eg, while changing diapers). In 1982, Turner et al studied 9 adults with herpes labialis and demonstrated with viral culture that 7 of them (78%) demonstrated HSV-1 viral shedding from the mouth, and 6 of them (67%) had HSV-1 virus isolated from their hands.[87] The study also demonstrated that HSV-1 survives poorly outside of the body (2 to 4 hours on skin, cloth, or plastic).

Autoinoculation is defined as self-infection of another body site and thus another dorsal root ganglion. Transmission by autoinoculation of HSV-1 is known to occur, as exemplified by cases of herpetic whitlow (ie, HSV-1 infection of the hand and one or more fingers) transmitted by patients with herpes labialis to themselves.[88,89] Most people with ocular HSV have herpes labialis. While ocular infection may occur by direct infection of the conjunctivae with infected saliva (via autoinoculation or from someone else), mouse studies have shown that the virus can spread through the nerve system (among branches of the trigeminal ganglion).[81,84] Cases are rarely reported however. A few cases of HSV-2 autoinoculation have been reported. Gill et al describe 79 patients with HSV hand infections, including HSV-2.[90] All the included children under age 10 years had HSV-1 lesions associated with gingivostomatitis. Of the adult cases, 7 of 49 occurred in health professionals (15%). All of the 20 hand infections with HSV-2 occurred in adults over age 20 years with genital herpes.

Herpes infections may present clinically in children in several ways. Most primary infections are asymptomatic except in neonates where asymptomatic infection is not known to occur.[5] When symptomatic, the virus produces a painful vesiculopustular lesion in most cases; however HSV may also cause subtle and even painless ulcers.[82] Lesions may occur on the face and orolabially. Genital herpes infection in children may present with dramatic dysuria and urinary retention, as well as genital discharge (urethral, vaginal), or skin inflammation and irritation (vulvar irritation, perianal, scrotal, or vulvar fissures). Adenopathy is commonly associated. Systemic symptoms are more common with primary infections and include fever, headache, nausea, vomiting, and myalgia. After primary infection, HSV becomes latent, persisting most frequently in the trigeminal (herpes labialis) or sacral ganglia (genital herpes). Reactivation is most often asymptomatic. Symptomatic herpes labialis usually recurs on the vermillion border of the lips, but may also recur on face, nares, or conjunctiva. Genital herpes vesicular lesions recur on the penis, scrotum, vulva, cervix, thighs, buttocks, perianal regions, or lower back.[5] HSV infections may be complicated by meningitis, encephalitis, ascending myelitis, Bell's palsy, neuralgias, and postinfectious encephalomyelitis. The incubation period for newborn disease is usually up to 4 weeks. Beyond the neonatal period, incubation is 2 to 14 days. See **Figures 10-15** through **10-20** for examples of HSV-1 and HSV-2.

Differential diagnosis of herpes ulcers in children depends somewhat on oral versus genital location however includes a) infectious causes: coxsackie-virus, Ebstein-Barr virus, cytomegaloviruses, *varicella*, syphilis (though ulcers are typically non-painful), tuberculosis ulcers (especially oral), chancroid (ie, *Haemophilus ducreyi*), fungal (ie, *mucormycosis*), and *granuloma inguinale* (outside the United States); b) malignancy; c) trauma; or d) autoimmune/other (eg, Behçet's disease, *aphthous stomatitis*, drug-related eruption, and Jacquet's diaper dermatitis). Chancroid is an uncommon infection that is only known to be transmitted sexually. It has an incubation period of typically 3 to 10 days, which presents with painful genital ulcer(s) and tender suppurative inguinal adenopathy. Culture, about 80% sensitive, requires special media, not currently widely available, and PCR, which is available in some clinical laboratories, though there is no FDA-approved test yet available in the United States.[2] It is treated with azithromycin or ceftriaxone.

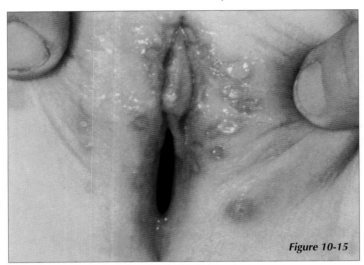

Figure 10-15

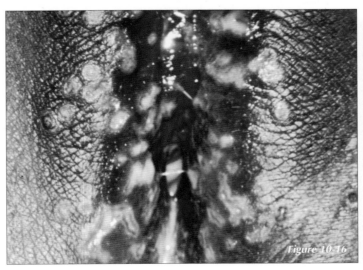

Figure 10-16

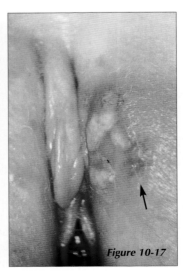

Figure 10-17

Figure 10-15. This photo shows vesicles on the medial aspect of the labia majora and around the introitus (35mm) of a 6-year-old female.

Figure 10-16. Painful sores in genital area in a 4-year-old girl with severe eczema. Child denied sexual contact. Lesions were positive for herpes simplex type 1 (HSV-1). Antibodies were negative for HSV-2 but positive for HSV-1. No one in the family had a history of "cold sores." Mode of transmission was indeterminate.

Figure 10-17. 6-year-old girl with sores on labia. She gave a history of oral-genital contact by mother's boyfriend, who did have a history of cold sores. These lesions cultured positive for HSV-1.

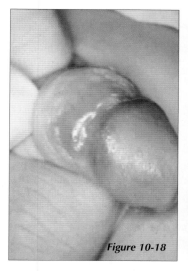

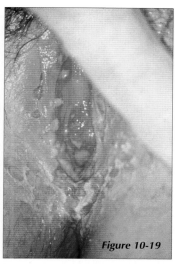

Figure 10-18. *This 3-year-old boy complained of pain in his genital area. He gave no disclosure of abuse. The culture of the penile lesion was positive for HSV-1. The mode of transmission was indeterminate.*

Figure 10-19. *In this 14-year-old patient, the sores appeared one week after being sexually assaulted by a stranger. The lesions were positive for HSV-2.*

Figure 10-20. *This 16-year-old adolescent girl had a history of genital herpes, first appearing at age 15 following consensual sexual activity. She was seen for possible sexual abuse due to the presence of these lesions, which were positive for HSV-2. This likely represents a recurrence of her original infection.*

Figure 10-18

Figure 10-19

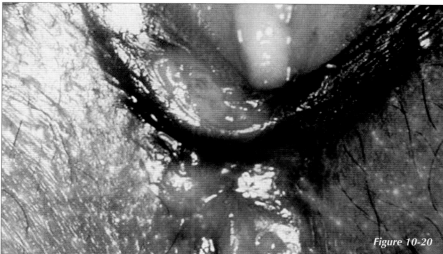

Figure 10-20

Any vesicular, excoriated, or ulcerative lesions should be cultured for HSV. PCR may be performed from the same swab specimen, placed in appropriate liquid viral media. The HSV cell culture becomes less sensitive as viral shedding decreases, typically when lesions are no longer vesicular. Because PCR is highly sensitive and specific, it may be used when suspicious lesions are ulcerative or excoriated. Rapid diagnostic tests such as direct fluorescent antibody staining or enzyme immunoassay detection techniques and histologic identification of multinucleated giant cells and eosinophilic intranuclear inclusions are less sensitive and not recommended.[5]

Obtaining serologic HSV titers for diagnosis of acute disease or for subtyping of HSV-1 and HSV-2 is problematic. Because many victims of sexual abuse or assault do not present clinically during the acute phase of the disease, an acute elevation in titers may be missed. If titers are elevated, and clinical presentation is delayed, then acute primary disease or recurrent disease are both possible explanations.[5] Type-specific assays for HSV-1 and HSV-2 that are not based on detection of glycoprotein G2 (diagnostic for HSV-2) and glycoprotein G1 (diagnostic for HSV-1) do not accurately distinguish HSV-1 from HSV-2, despite the claims of manufacturers and laboratories.[2] FDA-approved, gG-based type-specific assays include the following: POCkit™HSV-2 (Diagnology), HerpeSelect™-1 ELISA IgG or HerpeSelect™-2 ELISA IgG (Focus Technology, Inc.), and HerpeSelect™ 1 and 2 Immunoblot IgG (Focus Technology). One study of 61 patients 1 to 14 years of age reports specificity rates of 97% for HSV-1 and 100% for HSV-2 with the HerpeSelect ELISA (Focus Technologies).[91] The study by Ramos et al of 150 children shows better specificity (less false positives) of the Biokit HSV-2 Rapid Test compared to the HerpeSelect ELISA (Focus Technologies).[92]

As with any antibody test, the statistical odds of a false positive are higher in low-prevalence populations, such as sexually naïve children. While data regarding the use of anti-HSV gG testing in children is limited but promising, certain laboratory measures may reduce the likelihood of false-positive results. Laboratories should be able to reproduce a positive result in at least 2 separate runs, determine that the absorbance reading was at least 3 times higher than the positive cutoff value, and conduct confirmatory testing with enzyme-linked immunosorbent assay (ELISA) or immunoblot (Western blot) for samples detecting the presence of anti-HSV gG.

The distinction between HSV-1 and HSV-2 in children and adolescents evaluated for sexual abuse is important for diagnosis and management. HSV-2 is a sexually transmitted disease; HSV-1 may be sexually or non-sexually transmitted. HSV-2 is more likely to recur in genital regions than HSV-1. It is common for children and adults, especially from lower socioeconomic groups, to have HSV-1 antibodies and no history of clinical disease.[2,5] Fomite transmission has not been documented. Data are lacking regarding sexual transmission of herpes in children[93]; however, sexual abuse includes oral, genital, and digital touching, which are all mechanisms of transmitting herpes viruses. Diagnosis of genital herpes infection in children should be investigated for possible sexual abuse and children with genital herpes should be tested for other STIs including syphilis and HIV. History of neonatal herpes infection should be obtained and is unlikely to be missed as asymptomatic cases are not reported.

Treatment of primary or first clinical episodes of herpes is most effective if initiated within 3 to 6 days of onset of lesions. Treatment of recurrent disease is effective if initiated within 24 hours of appearance of lesions. Valacyclovir and famciclovir have not been FDA approved for children under age 12 years (see **Table 10-6** for dosing recommendations).[2,5]

Table 10-6. Treatment Regimens for Primary and Recurrent Herpes Simplex Outbreaks		
FIRST CLINICAL EPISODE		
Oral Dosing	**Adolescent**	**Child <45 kg (Not Neonate)**
Acyclovir	400 mg 3 times daily for 10 days; OR 200 mg 5 times daily for 10 days	80 mg/kg/day in 3-4 divided doses for 10 days
Valacyclovir	1 g twice a day for 10 days	
Famciclovir	250 mg 3 times a day for 10 days	

(continued)

Table 10-6. *(continued)*

RECURRENT EPISODE

Oral Dosing	Adolescent	Child <45 kg
Acyclovir	400 mg 3 times a day for 5 days; OR 800 mg twice a day for 5 days; OR 800 mg 3 times a day for 2 days	40-80 mg/kg/day in 3 divided doses for 5 days
Valacyclovir	500 mg twice a day for 3 days; OR 1 g daily for 5 days	
Famciclovir	125 mg twice daily for 5 days; OR 1 g twice daily for 1 day	

SYPHILIS (TREPONEMA PALLIDUM)

Syphilis has been described in infants since 1497 and the causative organism, *Treponema pallidum*, was discovered in 1905. Humans are the only natural host of this thin, mobile spirochete, which has very limited survival outside an infected host.[94] In 2000, rates of primary, secondary, and congenital syphilis were the lowest they have ever been since onset of surveillance in 1941 (approximately 2 per 100 000), a rate dramatically lower than the peak rate in 1990. Since 2000, rates of congenital syphilis have remained fairly low (8 cases per 100 000 live births in 2005). Lack of prenatal care is the most important contributor to increased rates of vertical transmission. Vertical transmission rates remain very high (70% to 100%) for 4 years after maternal infection.[95,94] Rates of congenital syphilis increased 26 fold in Russia between 1991-1999 as a result of a lack of available prenatal health services.[94]

Rates of primary and secondary syphilis have been gradually increasing since 2000, with rates highest among African-American men (15.7 cases/100 000 population) and Hispanic men (5.5/100 000), compared to the rate in women (0.8/100 000 population).[96] Disease occurs much more commonly in Sub-Saharan Africa, South and Southeast Asia, and South America. In the United States, syphilis remains an uncommon complication of child sexual abuse, found in fewer than 1% of children screened.[3,95,97,98] There is some thought that this may be due to limited testing, limited recognition of physical manifestations of even classic disease in children, and availability of antibiotics for routine childhood illnesses that may partially treat congenital syphilis and alter appearance of late clinical manifestations.[95,94]

Congenital syphilis may present early (first 2 years of life) or late. Congenital syphilis results from transplacental infection of the developing fetus. Perinatal transmission through infant contact with maternal primary or secondary genital lesions during delivery is possible, but is reported to be extremely uncommon.[99] Symptoms most commonly include mucocutaneous symptoms within the first month of life (as many as 70%), hepatomegaly with or without splenomegaly (70%), leukocytosis, and, most importantly, bone involvement seen on radiographs (60% to 80%). Bony findings appear early, typically with multiple symmetric lesions especially of the femur and humerus, are often painful, and consist of periostitis, cortical demineralization, and osteochondritis. Other symptoms that may be present are intrauterine growth retardation and failure to thrive; generalized lymphadenopathy; syphilitic profuse and sometimes bloody rhinitis ("snuffles"), which may occur as late as age 3 months; anemia and thrombocytopenia; pneumonia alba (ie, fibrosing pneumonitis); nephrotic syndrome; neurosyphilis; and ocular involvement (eg, chorioretinitis, glaucoma, uveitis).[94,100] Late findings of congenital syphilis occur in approximately 40% of untreated survivors and include perforation of the hard palate, Hutchinson teeth (ie, peg-shaped, notched central incisors), sensorineural hearing loss, blindness (eg, interstitial keratitis, secondary glaucoma, or corneal scarring), and bony deformities (eg, saddle nose deformity, frontal bossing, anterior "saber" bowing of shins, thickening of the clavicle, and Clutton joints, which are symmetric, painless sterile joint effusions usually of the knees).[94,100] Description of clinical presentation is provided here to assist in differentiation from acquired syphilis, as acquired syphilis in children is considered to be sexually transmitted except in rare circumstances. Even though the rash of secondary syphilis has been shown to contain viable treponemes, close physical contact with mucosal surfaces is necessary for transmission and transmission from secondary syphilis is rarely described.[74,94,99,101] Children presenting with symptoms of primary syphilis after age 6 months or secondary syphilis after age 15 months should be presumed to be victims of sexual abuse (even if there is no disclosure) and should be evaluated comprehensively for other STIs and abnormal physical findings, be reported to protective services, and undergo forensic interviewing. All infants and children diagnosed with syphilis should be tested for HIV.[2] Medical providers evaluating children older than 1 month of age should conduct a cerebrospinal fluid (CSF) examination for neurosyphilis; obtain long bone films; and review infant birth and maternal prenatal and delivery medical records to assess for evidence of congenital syphilis.[2]

Acquired syphilis in children may be detected when asymptomatic children (latent phase) undergo serologic screening. Primary syphilis may present as marked non-tender adenopathy (especially inguinal). A chancre (not always seen by the patient or on exam) appears at the primary inoculation site 10 to 90 days (average 21 days) after contact and may be vaginal, labial, cervical, penile, scrotal, anal, rectal, oral, or any extragenital site where there has been a break in the epidermal barrier. The chancre is typically a solitary, erythematous papule that rapidly erodes leaving a painless, smooth, yellowish-red ulcer with regular margins (**Figures 10-21** and **10-22**). It contains viable treponemes and may be crusted or there may be a serous and highly infectious discharge, but purulent discharge is uncommon.[101] Lesions heal in 3 to 12 weeks when untreated. Secondary syphilis presents with generalized involvement of skin and mucous membranes and constitutional symptoms. Constitutional symptoms are variable and sometimes vague, but most commonly include malaise, anorexia, headache, and a low-grade fever with generalized lymphadenopathy. The rash (or secondary eruption) usually appears 6 to 8 weeks after the chancre, and in most cases the chancre has resolved. The rash is a polymorphous maculopapular rash typically extending to the palms and soles. Scaling may be prominent especially on hands and feet. Moist areas may develop coalescing small fleshy plaques (ie, condyloma lata) that can be confused with condyloma acuminata (ie, HPV). Mucous patches may occur on any mucous membrane, most often oropharynx and rectum, and appear as painless, grayish-white erosions.[5,101] Neurosyphilis is present in approximately 30% of patients with secondary syphilis. Skin and mucous membrane lesions contain treponemes and are contagious with significant direct contact. Iritis, uveitis, arthritis, and nephrotic syndrome may all occur as part of secondary syphilis, likely secondary to immune complex formation.[94] Primary and secondary syphilis lesions will resolve without treatment, though the infection persists in a latent form. Secondary syphilis signs can recur during the first year after infection (ie, early latency) but not later.[94]

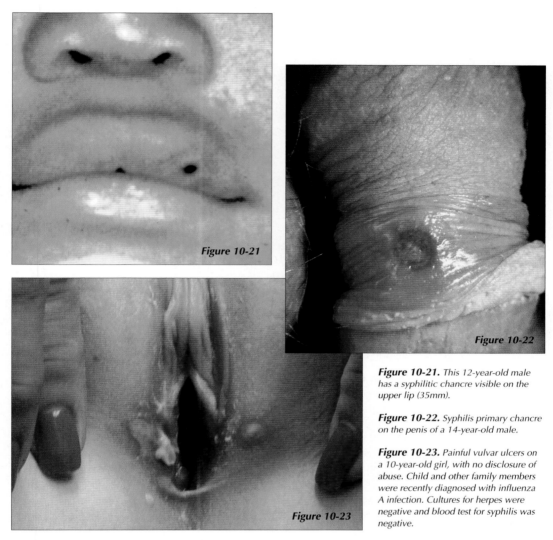

Figure 10-21. *This 12-year-old male has a syphilitic chancre visible on the upper lip (35mm).*

Figure 10-22. *Syphilis primary chancre on the penis of a 14-year-old male.*

Figure 10-23. *Painful vulvar ulcers on a 10-year-old girl, with no disclosure of abuse. Child and other family members were recently diagnosed with influenza A infection. Cultures for herpes were negative and blood test for syphilis was negative.*

Differential diagnosis of primary syphilis includes herpes simplex, trauma, Behçet's disease, Jacquet's diaper dermatitis, furuncle or impetigo, and other ulcerative lesions (**Figure 10-23**). Syphilitic chancres are painless however. Differential diagnosis of secondary syphilis includes pitiriasis rosea, psoriasis, tinea versicolor, drug reactions, nummular eczema, and nonspecific viral exanthems.[94,101]

Definitive diagnosis of acute syphilis infection is made with darkfield microscopy or direct fluorescent antibody (DFA) testing exudate or tissue obtained from a primary or secondary mucocutaneous lesion.[2] This is especially important when skin lesions are present, as serologic tests are usually negative during the first 7 to 10 days of infection.[101] In the absence of a lesion, serologic testing is recommended. Like HIV screening, syphilis screening is a two-step protocol consisting of a highly sensitive but less specific test, then confirmed with a highly specific test. Non-treponemal tests, such as RPR (the more sensitive of the non-treponemal tests)[94] or Venereal Disease Research Laboratory (VDRL) detects nonspecific anti-cardiolipin antibodies and must be confirmed with a test that detects specific anti-treponemal antibodies. Specific treponemal tests include *Treponema pallidum* particle agglutination (TP-PA), fluorescent treponemal antibody absorbed (FTA-ABS), *Treponema pallidum* hemagglutination test (MHA-TP), which has been replaced by the TP-PA test, and ELISA. The FTA-ABS is the most sensitive of these tests (detecting 85% of patients with primary syphilis and 100% of patients with secondary syphilis) but is more difficult to perform.[94] Non-treponemal tests such as RPR and VDRL usually become negative (months to years) after successful treatment, but may remain positive life-long at a persistently low titer, a condition termed serofast. Non-treponemal tests should be reported quantitatively (as a titer). Serial testing using the same test type can give information about disease activity, but importantly, RPR and VDRL titers are not comparable. In contrast, the specific treponemal tests (ie, TP-PA, FTA-ABS) do not give an index of disease activity. Most patients who have a reactive treponemal test will have reactive tests life-long, regardless of disease activity[2]; therefore, a reactive test indicates the patient has had syphilis sometime in life, but is not helpful in determining the time during which infectious contact occurred.

New approaches to screening and diagnosing syphilis involve an initial screen with a treponemal-specific test such as an enzyme immunoassay (EIA), which is more specific and as sensitive as an RPR test.[102] Rapid tests on finger-stick specimens (Abbott Determine TP) are available and have shown sensitivity of 88% and specificity comparable to TP-PA.[103] Other significant advantages relate to laboratory processing; ELISAs are less labor intensive and less dependent on technician interpretation. If an initial screen for anti-treponemal antibodies is positive, an RPR is done to differentiate active from past treated disease.

Syphilis treatment recommendations are based on the child's stage of syphilis infection. Congenital syphilis and neurosyphilis require the most aggressive and prolonged treatment; therefore, the workup of any child with suspected syphilis or positive serologies must exclude congenital or central nervous systems (CNS) involvement. Neurosyphilis in children should be treated with aqueous crystalline penicillin G (200 000 to 300 000 U/kg per day, given every 4 to 6 hours intra-venously for 10 to 14 days) not to exceed the adolescent/adult dose of 18 to 24 million U per day, administered as 3 to 4 million U IV every 4 hours for 10 to 14 days. Some infectious disease experts recommend 3 additional weekly intramuscular injections of benzathine penicillin G (children 50 000 U/kg per dose; adolescents/adults 2.4 million U per dose). Early congenital syphilis is treated with aqueous penicillin G 100 000 to 15 000 U/kg per day given as 50 000 U/kg per dose IV every 12 hours during the first 7 days of life and then every 8 hours to complete a total of 10 days of treatment. Daily IM procaine penicillin G (50 000 U/kg/dose) may be given as an alternate treatment for 10 days. Late congenital syphilis treatment is aqueous penicillin G 200 000 to 300 000 U/kg per day IV for 10 days.[2]

HUMAN IMMUNODEFICIENCY VIRUS

While the majority of children infected with HIV (>90%) acquired infection from their mothers in the perinatal period, transmission to children also occurs sexually.[104] In 1998, Lindegren et al analyzed national HIV/AIDS surveillance data retrospectively and found 26 of 9136 children with HIV/AIDS had acquired HIV through sexual abuse.[104] Of these sexually abused children, 18 (69%) were reported in the 3-year period 1993-1996 after the CDC revised the pediatric HIV/AIDS case report form to collect standardized information about sexual contact with a male or female. The authors concluded that these cases likely represented a minimum estimate because sexual abuse was (and is) under-recognized and under-reported to cps as well as HIV/AIDS surveillance systems. There are few other studies of HIV incidence in sexually abused children. Diagnosis of sexually transmitted HIV in young children requires exclusion of perinatal transmission through review of maternal records of HIV testing and infant birth records.

HIV is transmitted through body secretions and unfixed tissues, especially blood and secretions containing blood. Body secretions that are highly unlikely to transmit HIV (unless mixed with blood) are saliva, urine, feces/diarrhea, and vomit.[105] Receptive anal intercourse is the most successful route of sexual transmission—consensual risk 0.5% to 3% per episode (followed by vaginal intercourse) and consensual risk 0.1% to 0.2%. Oral sex is estimated to convey a lower risk per episode (though increasingly recognized as the sole reported risk factor in a subset of cases).[2] Sexual intercourse combined with trauma (and, therefore, contact with bloody secretions) increases transmissibility, thus forced insertive anal or vaginal intercourse carries a higher risk than consensual or oral contact. Risk is also related to the stage of the infected person. Periods of highest level *viremia* are at the 2 extremes of disease: during the weeks following acute infection (when risk may be 1000 times higher) and at the end stages of untreated AIDS.[106,107] Efficacy of transmission is increased with concurrent genital infections (especially ulcerative STDs), syphilis, and bacterial vaginosis. The local prevalence of HIV is important in estimating the risk of transmitting HIV to a sexually abused child or adolescent. Risk is highest for perpetrators with known HIV infection. For those with unknown HIV status, risk is higher when the alleged perpetrator has a history of intravenous (IV) drug use, crack cocaine drug use, promiscuity, incarceration, infection with other STIs, or is a man who has sex with other men (**Table 10-7**).[2]

Testing for HIV should be voluntary and conducted with the patient's knowledge (or his or her legally authorized representative). Testing should be offered to every patient with an STI or seeking evaluation for an STI.[2] In most states, public health statutes allow for evaluation and treatment of minors for STIs without parental knowledge, allowing adolescents aged 13 and older to give consent for STI (including HIV) testing;

Table 10-7. Transmission Risk by Type of Exposure to HIV-Infected Source	
TYPE OF HIV EXPOSURE	TRANSMISSION RISK, PER HUNDRED EVENTS (%)
Blood Transfusion	95
Perinatal Exposure (untreated)	13-45
Receptive Anal Intercourse (unprotected)	0.5-3.2
Needle Sharing (injection drug use)	0.67
Needlestick (health care)	0.32
Receptive Vaginal Intercourse (unprotected)	0.01-0.3
Insertive Vaginal Intercourse (unprotected)	0.03-0.09
Ingestion of Human Milk (single exposure)	0.001-0.004

Reprinted with permissions from Havens P and Committee on Pediatric AIDS. American Academy of Pediatrics Clinical Report. Postexposure prophylaxis in children and adolescents for nonoccupational exposure to human immunodeficiency virus. Pediatrics. June 2003;111(6):1475-1489.

however, not every state has explicitly included HIV testing as not requiring parental consent.[108] Standard testing is a two-step process consisting of an ELISA for HIV antibodies in the blood (or rapid finger-stick or oral swab test), with positive tests confirmed with a repeated ELISA followed by the highly specific Western blot assay or an immunofluorescence assay (IFA). Western blot results require specialized interpretation and may take 1 to 2 weeks to be reported. In some countries with limited resources, 2 positive tests on 2 different brands of ELISA-based rapid tests are considered definitive for HIV infection in children older than 18 months.[5] The ELISA test detects HIV antibodies in 95% of patients 3 months after infection.[2] Rapid test results are available as soon as 20 minutes (eg, Oraquick) or within 1 hour.[109] Negative antibody tests cannot exclude recent infection and should be repeated in 3 months if clinical suspicion warrants further testing. Sexual abuse victims may present with a history of symptoms that may suggest acute retroviral syndrome. These influenza-like symptoms (eg, fever, malaise, lymphadenopathy, rash) frequently occur in the first 4 to 6 weeks following HIV infection, before the ELISA antibody test becomes positive.[110] Therefore, standard serologic testing will fail to detect these very early cases and direct testing for virus, rather than antibody, is required, typically using PCR-based testing for HIV RNA (ie, "viral load") or testing for the HIV marker, p24 antigen. Infants with perinatal exposure to HIV may have positive ELISA testing in the absence of HIV infection due to presence of maternal antibodies in the infant for up to 18 months. Infant infection may be determined using HIV DNA PCR serial testing consisting of 3 total determinations; once after age 1 month, and one other testing between ages 2 and 4 months in conjunction with evaluation by a pediatric HIV expert. PCR testing is most accurate with HIV DNA PCR assays (a negative RNA PCR may occur in HIV-infected patients), especially in children under age 18 months.[2] Testing of the alleged perpetrator is recommended when obtainable (voluntary or by court order).

Questions are frequently raised about the HIV exposure risk following child sexual abuse and sexual assault, and the utility of HIV post-exposure prophylaxis (PEP). Medical providers may seek to offer treatment with any hope of benefit to sexually traumatized children, particularly for this eventually fatal disease. Current recommendations for HIV prophylaxis are based on very limited data. To date, there are no randomized controlled trials of PEP for nonoccupational exposure (sexual) or occupational exposure. The 1997 case-control study published in the *New England Journal of Medicine* assessing outcomes of occupational exposure in health care settings after percutaneous needle stick with HIV infected blood is the most compelling existing report of PEP effectiveness.[106,111] In this retrospective analysis, zidovudine alone appeared to reduce the risk of transmission by greater than 60%. Despite study limitations, these results are believable because risk reduction is in the same range as perinatal transmission prevention with zidovudine alone. Although uncontrolled and far from definitive, there is also a growing experience with offering PEP following non-occupational sexual exposures in adults.[112] Based on these studies, animal models, the demonstrated effectiveness of perinatal prophylaxis, and the great strides in making antiretroviral regimens more potent, tolerable, and convenient, PEP in acute child and adolescent sexual abuse cases might be effective in preventing HIV transmission.[2,113] Medical providers making the decision to recommend PEP must, therefore, take into consideration risk of infection, likelihood of efficacy of prophylaxis, medication side effects, and likelihood of adherence to medications and medical follow-up.

The most recent guidelines from the CDC and the World Health Organization (WHO) recommend a 28-day course of PEP using highly active anti-retroviral therapy (HAART) only for those persons seeking care within 72 hours of a substantial exposure to blood, genital secretions, or other potentially infectious bodily secretions of a known HIV-infected person.[2,106,113,114] Patients initiating PEP should have baseline HIV and lab testing (ie, CBC, serum chemistry), be able to receive the first dose of PEP as soon as possible after the decision is made to treat, and agree to close medical follow-up in 3 to 5 days. Baseline HIV and lab testing assesses for HIV infection prior to the current exposure and gives a baseline for monitoring antiretroviral toxicities. The sooner PEP is administered after HIV exposure, the more likely it is to interrupt transmission. Use of an FDA-approved rapid HIV test is preferred if available (results within an hour), as patients who test HIV-positive should be excluded from PEP. It is generally not recommended to provide HIV PEP in cases when therapy will not be initiated until more than 72 hours after the exposure. In sexual assault cases where the alleged perpetrator has unknown HIV status, the CDC recommends that clinicians evaluate the risks and benefits of PEP and individualize recommendations on a case-by-case basis. In these cases, it is important to gather as much information about the potential HIV risk factors of the alleged perpetrator(s). When the alleged perpetrator is known to be HIV-infected, exploring his or her detailed treatment history in collaboration with an experienced HIV clinician is critically important for planning an appropriately individualized PEP regimen based on prior drug exposures and documented antiretroviral resistance.

Prior to initiation of PEP, clinicians should explain to patients that the agents used for PEP have unproven benefit and documented toxicities in these circumstances. Patients should also understand the importance of adherence to recommended dosing in order to receive maximum potential benefit and to reduce the risk of selecting for drug-resistant HIV strains. If PEP is given, clinicians should consult with a specialist in HIV treatment, provide a 3- to 5-day starter pack of the recommended antiretroviral regimen, and have patients return to assess tolerance of medication and to make a better assessment of HIV risk.[2,106] If it is possible to test the alleged perpetrator, PCR testing is preferred because of the possibility the perpetrator has acute infection and had not yet seroconverted. If the perpetrator's HIV PCR test is negative, the patient's antiretroviral treatment should be stopped.

Treatment regimens may consist of 2 or 3 antiretrovirals (2 nucleoside analogue reverse transcriptase inhibitors plus either a protease inhibitor or a non-nucleoside reverse transcriptase inhibitor). Two-drug therapy is used most commonly in developing countries, while three-drug therapy is used in areas with available HAART treatment and increased risk for primary transmission of a resistant HIV strain.[5,113,114] Commonly used regimens in children and adolescents include lamivudine and zidovudine (available as liquid formulations or as a single tablet, Combivir, taken twice daily), or zidovudine, lamivudine, and nelfinavir (also taken twice daily).[105,113,115]

Several studies have demonstrated poor adherence of sexual assault survivers to PEP protocols.[113,116] Olshen et al reported 13 of 110 adolescents who had been sexually assaulted and offered HIV PEP completed their 28-day PEP course (12%).[115] Only 37 of these adolescents returned for a follow-up examination, and half of them (46%) developed an adverse reaction to the PEP medicines. Medication adherence may be improved with fewer doses and fewer pills per dose, counseling about importance of adherence and potential side effects, use of supportive medicines like anti-emetics to treat side effects, and access to help/encouragement by phone or office visit.[113]

HEPATITIS A, B, AND C
Serologic testing in children and adolescents evaluated for sexual abuse or assault may include HIV, RPR, and tests for hepatitis A, B, and C. Although hepatitis A is usually transmitted by fecal-oral contact, it can be transmitted during sexual activity.[2] The

diagnosis of acute hepatitis A is based on the presence of serum IgM antibody to Hepatitis A Virus (HAV); total anti-HAV does not differentiate individuals with acute disease, past disease, or hepatitis A immunization.

Among adolescents and adults, sexual activity is the most common mode of transmission for hepatitis B infections[2]; other modes of transmission include mucous membrane contact and intravenous contact with infected needles or syringes. The presence of IgM antibody to hepatitis B core antigen confirms the diagnosis of acute infection. The presence of hepatitis B surface antigen can indicate acute or chronic infection; in uninfected, immunized individuals, only the antibody to hepatitis B surface antigen will be positive.

Hepatitis C is primarily transmitted by percutaneous exposure to blood products and by sexual activity. Screening victims of sexual abuse or assault should include serum antibody to hepatitis C virus (HCV); antibody assays include an initial enzyme immunoassay (EIA), and positive results are confirmed by a recombinant immunoblot assay (RIBA).[5] An alternative diagnostic test for hepatitis C is serum HCV RNA.

The clinician may opt to screen for hepatitis A, B, and C whenever risk factors for HIV are detected, or when the assailant is known to have hepatitis or liver disease. Risk factors in the assailant include, but are not limited to the following: stranger to victim, multiple sexual partners, drug use, history of incarceration, and other health risk markers, such as membership in a gang. In cases where children or adolescents are victims of acute sexual assault, it is prudent to ascertain whether they have been immunized fully against Hepatitis B (3 doses). If the patient is unimmunized, an initial dose of Hepatitis B vaccine should be given, preferably within 24 hours of exposure, with the remainder of the vaccine doses given at appropriate intervals. For patients whose hepatitis B status is unknown and cannot be ascertained within 24 hours of the exposure, practitioners may opt to send a blood specimen for hepatitis B immune status and give the first vaccine dose. Additional doses at follow-up visits would be given only if the test showed the patient to be non-immune. Hepatitis B immune globulin (HBIG) should be given in those cases where the perpetrator is known to be hepatitis B surface antigen positive.[5]

BACTERIAL VAGINOSIS

Bacterial vaginosis (BV) is a clinical syndrome characterized by malodorous vaginal discharge caused by replacement of normal *Lactobacillus* species in the vagina with overgrowth of anaerobic bacteria, *Gardnerella vaginalis*, and *Mycoplasma hominis*. It is described as the most prevalent adult and adolescent vaginal infection worldwide,[5,117] but there are limited studies of prevalence in prepubertal children, especially during the last decade. The incubation period is unknown. The disease state of BV is associated with multiple sexual partners, a new sex partner, lack of vaginal lactobacilli, and douching. Douching itself is also associated with sexual activity.[117] As many as 50% of women with clinical BV are asymptomatic. Diagnosis of BV requires presence of 3 of the following clinical findings[2,5]:

— Homogeneous thin white discharge that smoothly coats the vaginal walls

— "Clue cells" on microscopic examination (vaginal smear) making up at least 20% of vaginal epithelial cells (clue cells are vaginal epithelial cells covered with bacteria so that they appear granular and ragged) (**Figure 10-24**)

— Vaginal fluid pH >4.5

— Positive amine test or whiff test (fishy odor of vaginal discharge before or after addition of 10% potassium hydroxide)

Culture is not recommended because it is not specific.

The mechanism of transmission of BV remains unclear. While women who have never been sexually active are rarely affected, it is still unclear whether BV results from a sexually transmitted pathogen.[2] Part of the confusion stems from the fact that diagnosis of BV cannot be based on isolation of *Gardnerella vaginalis*, as this organism is present in as many as 50% of women without BV, and may also be present in asymptomatic females who are sexually inexperienced.[5,118-120] In a 2005 study by Schwebke and Desmond, the authors followed 94 sexually active women without BV aged 18 years or older for development of BV.[117] Their male partners were also studied. Their data support sexual transmission of BV. Multivariate analysis showed that incident BV was most significantly associated with exposure to a new sexual partner. Use of condoms with occasional partners was also found to be protective. The authors reviewed studies citing evidence for and against sexual transmission of BV and concluded that "while the etiology of BV remains unproven, evidence continues to accumulate in favor of sexual transmission." Evidence for sexual transmission was cited from several studies. Gardner and Dukes induced bacterial vaginosis in a woman by introducing vaginal secretions from an infected woman into the subject's vagina.[121] Schwebke and Desmond also cite studies reporting increased rates of BV and trichomonas associated with increased number of sexual partners, not frequency of intercourse[122]; up to 90% of male partners of women with BV having *Gardnerella vaginalis* and other BV bacteria[121]; balanoposthitis in sexually active males caused by BV organisms[123,124]; and isolating BV organisms (especially *Gardnerella vaginalis*) from semen of asymptomatic males.[125] Evidence cited against sexual transmission includes 2 types of studies. The Bump and Buesching study reports similar rates of *Gardnerella vaginalis* and BV in sexually active versus self-reported sexually inexperienced adolescents.[119] The "virginal" group of 14- to 17-year-old girls was defined by self-report and included one girl with chlamydia cervicitis. Additionally virginal designation excluded only sexual intercourse, with no mention of excluded external rubbing, oral, rectal, or digital touching. There are also a group of studies of male partners that fail to show reduction in BV recurrence rates among women whose male sexual partners were treated with a single 2-gram dose of metronidazole.[126,127] Schwebke and Desmond point out that those studies are now two decades old, do not include a measure of compliance with treatment, and that single-dose therapy has been shown to be marginally effective in infected females and is likely to be poorly effective in infected males. Wahl et al demonstrated *Gardnerella vaginalis* could not be found in urethra, glans, or rectal cultures of asymptomatic non-abused prepubertal boys, while reporting a case of a 3-year-old male with symptomatic balanitis with culture positive for *Gardnerella vaginalis*.[128] These authors concluded that while significance of *Gardnerella vaginalis* as an STI in prepubertal boys is currently unknown, isolation in a symptomatic boy raises questions of sexual abuse, as would isolation in a prepubertal

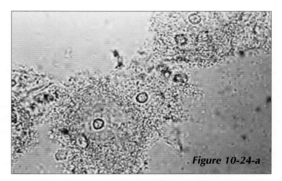

Figure 10-24-a

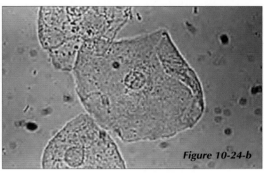

Figure 10-24-b

Figure 10-24-a. *Microscopic appearance of "clue cells," vaginal epithelial cells, using saline wet mount preparation. Provided with permission from Seattle STD/HIV Prevention Training Center.*

Figure 10-24-b. *Microscopic appearance of normal vaginal epithelial cells, using saline wet mount preparation. Provided with permission from Seattle STD/HIV Prevention Training Center.*

girl with symptoms of BV. While studies to date do not conclusively support sexual transmission of BV or a diagnosis of sexual abuse in a prepubertal child with bacterial vaginosis, the child with BV should be tested for other sexually transmitted pathogens (*Neisseria gonorrhea, Chlamydia trachomatis, Trichomonas vaginalis*). Forensic interview and medical examination are recommended.

Treatment for children (<45 kg) with BV is metronidazole, 15 mg/kg per day orally, in 2 divided doses for 7 days (maximum 1 gram/day). Single-dose therapy has the lowest cure rate and is not recommended. Adolescents should be treated with metronidazole 500 mg orally twice a day for 7 days. Alternate regimens are metronidazole gel, 0.75% intravaginally daily for 5 days, or clindamycin cream, 2% intravaginally at bedtime for 7 days. The Clindamycin cream is oil based and may weaken condoms and diaphragms, and may be less efficacious than metronidazole.[2,5]

Differential diagnosis of bacterial vaginosis includes other causes of vaginal discharge. Other infectious causes include *Neisseria gonorrhoeae, Chlamydia trachomatis, Trichomonas vaginalis*, and Shigella species (or other enteric bacteria). Candidiasis, pin worms, and group A streptococcus would be less likely causes, as pain or pruritis are much more prevalent with these infections than in BV. Non-infectious causes include foreign body and nonspecific vaginitis (due to constipation, bubble baths, poor hygiene, et cetera).

TESTING THE SUSPECT

When an STI is identified in a child or adolescent victim of sexual abuse or assault, investigators frequently ask whether testing the suspect for disease would provide important information for criminal investigation. Most of the time testing a suspect for STIs is uninformative, confusing, or even damaging to the prosecution of the suspect. In general, most sexual offenders are males, and males are more difficult to test for STIs than females. Many diseases can resolve without treatment, so a negative test does not preclude prior disease; for example, most venereal HPV lesions resolve within 3 to 5 years without treatment.[129] If the suspect is treated for an STI or for another infection that eradicates an existing STI, then the suspect will be disease-free at the time of testing. Serologic tests for syphilis, hepatitis A, hepatitis B, hepatitis C, and gG-based type-specific assays for HSV-1 and HSV-2 can confirm the presence of past disease in the suspect. Treponemal-specific tests should be performed because non-treponemal tests may become non-reactive with treatment. The presence of total anti-HAV titers, in the absence of HAV immunization, confirms past infection with hepatitis A. The presence of antibody to hepatitis B surface antigen indicates resolved infection or immunity following immunization; the presence of hepatitis B surface antigen would confirm active or chronic disease[5] in a suspect. The presence of antibody to hepatitis C virus confirms disease, and is positive in 80% of infected patients 15 weeks after exposure; in the acute phase, up to 15 weeks after exposure, anti-HCV is sometimes negative.[5] Both ELISA serum antibody testing and HIV PCR testing should be performed, as recently HIV-infected perpetrators may not have yet developed a detectable antibody response. With this dilemma, the bottom line for medical providers remains what is best medical care for the patient.

REFERENCES

1. American Academy of Pediatrics Committee on Child Abuse and Neglect: Guidelines for the evaluation of sexual abuse of children. *Pediatrics*. 1991;87(2): 254-260.

2. Workowski KA, Berman SM. Sexually transmitted diseases treatment guidelines, 2006. *MMWR Recomm Rep*. 2006;55(RR-11):1-94.

3. Everett V, Ingram D, Flick L, Russell T, Tropez-Sims S, McFadden A. A Comparison of Sexually Transmitted Diseases (STDs) Found In A Total Of 696 Boys And 2973 Girls Evaluated For Sexual Abuse (Abstract). *Pediatr Res.* 1998;43(4, Supp 2):91.

4. Kellogg N. The evaluation of sexual abuse in children. *Pediatrics.* 2005;116(2):506-512.

5. Pickering L, Baker C, Long S, McMillan J, eds. *Red Book: 2006 Report of the Committee on Infectious Diseases.* 27th ed. Elk Grove Village, IL: American Academy of Pediatrics; 2006.

6. Ingram DM, Miller WC, Schoenbach VJ, Everett VD, Ingram DL. Risk assessment for gonococcal and chlamydial infections in young children undergoing evaluation for sexual abuse. *Pediatrics.* 2001;107(5):E73.

7. Siegel RM, Schubert CJ, Myers PA, Shapiro RA. The prevalence of sexually transmitted diseases in children and adolescents evaluated for sexual abuse in Cincinnati: rationale for limited STD testing in prepubertal girls. *Pediatrics.* 1995;96(6):1090-1094.

8. Palusci VJ, Reeves MJ. Testing for genital gonorrhea infections in prepubertal girls with suspected sexual abuse. *Pediatr Infect Dis J.* 2003;22(7):618-623.

9. Ingram DL. Neisseria gonorrhoeae in children. *Pediatr Ann.* 1994;23(7):341-345.

10. American Academy of Pediatrics. Committee on Child Abuse and Neglect. Gonorrhea in prepubertal children. *Pediatrics.* 1998;101(1 Pt 1):134-135.

11. Fuster CD, Neinstein LS. Vaginal Chlamydia trachomatis prevalence in sexually abused prepurbertal girls. *Pediatrics.* 1987;79(2):235-238.

12. Bell TA, Stamm WE, Wang SP, Kuo CC, Holmes KK, Grayston JT. Chronic Chlamydia trachomatis infections in infants [published erratum appears in *JAMA* 1992;267(16):2188]. *JAMA.* 1992;267(3):400-402.

13. Pickering L, ed. *2000 Red Book: Report of the Committee on Infectious Diseases.* 25th ed. Elk Grove Village, IL: American Academy of Pediatrics; 2000.

14. Van Dyck E, Ieven M, Pattyn S, Van Damme L, Laga M. Detection of Chlamydia trachomatis and Neisseria gonorrhoeae by enzyme immunoassay, culture, and three nucleic acid amplification tests. *J Clin Microbiol.* 2001;39(5):1751-1756.

15. Carroll KC, Aldeen WE, Morrison M, Anderson R, Lee D, Mottice S. Evaluation of the Abbott LCx ligase chain reaction assay for detection of Chlamydia trachomatis and Neisseria gonorrhoeae in urine and genital swab specimens from a sexually transmitted disease clinic population. *J Clin Microbiol.* 1998;36(6):1630-1633.

16. Buimer M, van Doornum GJ, Ching S, et al. Detection of Chlamydia trachomatis and Neisseria gonorrhoeae by ligase chain reaction-based assays with clinical specimens from various sites: implications for diagnostic testing and screening. *J Clin Microbiol.* 1996;34(10):2395-2400.

17. Hammerschlag MR. Use of nucleic acid amplification tests in investigating child sexual abuse. *Sex Transm Infect.* 2001;77(3):153-154.

18. Laboratories A. Chlamydia trachomatis assay: Abbott LCx Probe System. (*Package insert*). Vol: Abbott Park, IL; 1996.

19. Hook EW, 3rd, Smith K, Mullen C, et al. Diagnosis of genitourinary Chlamydia trachomatis infections by using the ligase chain reaction on patient-obtained vaginal swabs. *J Clin Microbiol.* 1997;35(8):2133-2135.

20. Black CM. Current methods of laboratory diagnosis of Chlamydia trachomatis infections. *Clin Microbiol Rev.* 1997;10(1):160-184.

21. Matthews-Greer J, Sloop G, Springer A, McRae K, LaHaye E, Jamison R. Comparison of detection methods for Chlamydia trachomatis in specimens obtained from pediatric victims of suspected sexual abuse. *Pediatr Infect Dis J.* 1999;18(2):165-167.

22. Girardet RG, McClain N, Lahoti S, Cheung K, Hartwell B, McNeese M. Comparison of the urine-based ligase chain reaction test to culture for detection of Chlamydia trachomatis and Neisseria gonorrhoeae in pediatric sexual abuse victims. *Pediatr Infect Dis J.* 2001;20(2):144-147.

23. Embree JE, Lindsay D, Williams T, Peeling RW, Wood S, Morris M. Acceptability and usefulness of vaginal washes in premenarcheal girls as a diagnostic procedure for sexually transmitted diseases. The Child Protection Centre at the Winnipeg Children's Hospital. *Pediatr Infect Dis J.* 1996;15(8):662-667.

24. Kellogg ND, Baillargeon J, Lukefahr JL, Lawless K, Menard SW. Comparison of nucleic acid amplification tests and culture techniques in the detection of Neisseria gonorrhoeae and Chlamydia trachomatis in victims of suspected child sexual abuse. *J Pediatr Adolesc Gynecol.* 2004;17(5):331-339.

25. Johnson RE, Newhall WJ, Papp JR, et al. Screening tests to detect Chlamydia trachomatis and Neisseria gonorrhoeae infections—2002. *MMWR Recomm Rep.* 2002;51(RR-15):1-38; quiz CE31-34.

26. *Physicians' Desk Reference.* 60th ed. Montvale, NJ: Medical Economics Company, Inc.; 2006.

27. Parks KS, Dixon PB, Richey CM, Hook EW, 3rd. Spontaneous clearance of Chlamydia trachomatis infection in untreated patients. *Sex Transm Dis.* 1997;24(4):229-235.

28. Update to CDC's sexually transmitted diseases treatment guidelines, 2006: fluoroquinolones no longer recommended for treatment of gonococcal infections. *MMWR.* 2007;56(14):332-336.

29. Whittington WL, Rice RJ, Biddle JW, Knapp JS. Incorrect identification of Neisseria gonorrhoeae from infants and children. *Pediatr Infect Dis J.* 1988;7(1):3-10.

30. CDC. *Human Papillomavirus: HPV Information for Clinicians.* Atlanta, GA: US Department of Health and Human Services, Centers for Disease Control and Prevention; November 2006.

31. Dunne EF, Unger ER, Sternberg M, et al. Prevalence of HPV infection among females in the United States. *JAMA.* 2007;297(8):813-819.

32. Dunne EF, Nielson CM, Stone KM, Markowitz LE, Giuliano AR. Prevalence of HPV infection among men: A systematic review of the literature. *J Infect Dis.* 2006;194(8):1044-1057.

33. Moscicki AB, Shiboski S, Broering J, et al. The natural history of human papillomavirus infection as measured by repeated DNA testing in adolescent and young women. *J Pediatr*. 1998;132(2):277-284.

34. Franco EL, Villa LL, Sobrinho JP, et al. Epidemiology of acquisition and clearance of cervical human papillomavirus infection in women from a high-risk area for cervical cancer. *J Infect Dis*. 1999;180(5):1415-1423.

35. Cohen J. Public health. High hopes and dilemmas for a cervical cancer vaccine. *Science*. 2005;308(5722):618-621.

36. Derkay CS. Task force on recurrent respiratory papillomas. A preliminary report. *Arch Otolaryngol Head Neck Surg*. 1995;121(12):1386-1391.

37. Rogo KO, Nyansera PN. Congenital condylomata acuminata with meconium staining of amniotic fluid and fetal hydrocephalus: case report. *East Afr Med J*. 1989;66(6):411-413.

38. Wiatrak BJ, Wiatrak DW, Broker TR, Lewis L. Recurrent respiratory papillomatosis: a longitudinal study comparing severity associated with human papilloma viral types 6 and 11 and other risk factors in a large pediatric population. *Laryngoscope*. 2004;114(11 Pt 2 Suppl 104):1-23.

39. Tang CK, Shermeta DW, Wood C. Congenital condylomata acuminata. *Am J Obstet Gynecol*. 1978;131(8):912-913.

40. Bodaghi S, Wood LV, Roby G, Ryder C, Steinberg SM, Zheng ZM. Could human papillomaviruses be spread through blood? *J Clin Microbiol*. 2005;43(11):5428-5434.

41. Rintala MA, Grenman SE, Jarvenkyla ME, Syrjanen KJ, Syrjanen SM. High-risk types of human papillomavirus (HPV) DNA in oral and genital mucosa of infants during their first 3 years of life: experience from the Finnish HPV Family Study. *Clin Infect Dis*. 2005;41(12):1728-1733.

42. Kojima A, Maeda H, Kurahashi N, et al. Human papillomaviruses in the normal oral cavity of children in Japan. *Oral Oncol*. 2003;39(8):821-828.

43. Summersgill KF, Smith EM, Levy BT, Allen JM, Haugen TH, Turek LP. Human papillomavirus in the oral cavities of children and adolescents. *Oral Surg Oral Med Oral Pathol Oral Radiol Endod*. 2001;91(1):62-69.

44. Chatterjee R, Mukhopadhyay D, Murmu N, Mitra PK. Correlation between human papillomavirus DNA detection in maternal cervical smears and buccal swabs of infants. *Indian J Exp Biol*. 1998;36(2):199-202.

45. Rice PS, Mant C, Cason J, et al. High prevalence of human papillomavirus type 16 infection among children. *J Med Virol*. 2000;61(1):70-75.

46. Mant C, Kell B, Rice P, Best JM, Bible JM, Cason J. Buccal exposure to human papillomavirus type 16 is a common yet transitory event of childhood. *J Med Virol*. 2003;71(4):593-598.

47. Syrjanen S, Puranen M. Human papillomavirus infections in children: the potential role of maternal transmission. *Crit Rev Oral Biol Med*. 2000;11(2):259-274.

48. Smith EM, Ritchie JM, Yankowitz J, et al. Human papillomavirus prevalence and types in newborns and parents: concordance and modes of transmission. *Sex Transm Dis*. 2004;31(1):57-62.

49. Watts DH, Koutsky LA, Holmes KK, et al. Low risk of perinatal transmission of human papillomavirus: results from a prospective cohort study [see comments]. *Am Obstet Gynecol*. 1998;178(2):365-373.

50. Shah K, Kashima H, Polk BF, Shah F, Abbey H, Abramson A. Rarity of cesarean delivery in cases of juvenile-onset respiratory papillomatosis. *Obstet Gynecol*. 1986;68(6):795-799.

51. Sinclair KA, Woods CR, Kirse DJ, Sinal SH. Anogenital and respiratory tract human papillomavirus infections among children: age, gender, and potential transmission through sexual abuse. *Pediatrics*. 2005;116(4):815-825.

52. Jayasinghe Y, Garland SM. Genital warts in children: what do they mean? *Arch Dis Child*. 2006;91(8):696-700.

53. Sinal SH, Woods CR. Human papillomavirus infections of the genital and respiratory tracts in young children. *Semin Pediatr Infect Dis*. 2005;16(4):306-316.

54. Hammerschlag MR. Sexually transmitted diseases in sexually abused children: medical and legal implications. *Sex Transm Infect*. 1998;74(3):167-174.

55. Muram D, Stewart D. Sexually transmitted diseases. In: A Heger SE, D Muram, ed. *Evaluation of the Sexually Abused Child*. 2nd ed. New York: Oxford University Press; 2000.

56. Jenison SA, Yu XP, Valentine JM, et al. Evidence of prevalent genital-type human papillomavirus infections in adults and children. *J Infect Dis*. 1990;162(1):60-69.

57. Dillner J. Toward "serolomics": papillomavirus serology is taking a technologic lead in high-throughput multiplexed antibody analysis. *Clin Chem*. 2005;51(10):1768-1769.

58. Waterboer T, Sehr P, Michael KM, et al. Multiplex human papillomavirus serology based on in situ-purified glutathione s-transferase fusion proteins. *Clin Chem*. 2005;51(10):1845-1853.

59. Andersson K, Waterboer T, Kirnbauer R, et al. Seroreactivity to cutaneous human papillomaviruses among patients with nonmelanoma skin cancer or benign skin lesions. *Cancer Epidemiol Biomarkers Prev*. 2008;17(1):189-195.

60. Schwebke JR, Burgess D. Trichomoniasis. *Clin Microbiol Rev*. 2004;17(4):794-803, table of contents.

61. Rughooputh S, Greenwell P. Trichomonas vaginalis: paradigm of a successful sexually transmitted organism. *Br J Biomed Sci*. 2005;62(4):193-200.

62. Sena AC, Miller WC, Hobbs MM, et al. Trichomonas vaginalis infection in male sexual partners: implications for diagnosis, treatment, and prevention. *Clin Infect Dis*. 2007;44(1):13-22.

63. Blake DR, Duggan A, Joffe A. Use of spun urine to enhance detection of Trichomonas vaginalis in adolescent women. *Arch Pediatr Adolesc Med*. 1999;153(12):1222-1225.

64. Borchardt KA, al-Haraci S, Maida N. Prevalence of Trichomonas vaginalis in a male sexually transmitted disease clinic population by interview, wet mount microscopy, and the InPouch™ TV test. *Genitourin Med*. 1995;71(6):405-406.

65. Ohlemeyer CL, Hornberger LL, Lynch DA, Swierkosz EM. Diagnosis of Trichomonas vaginalis in adolescent females: InPouch™ TV culture versus wet-mount microscopy. *J Adolesc Health*. 1998;22(3):205-208.

66. van Der Schee C, van Belkum A, Zwijgers L, et al. Improved diagnosis of Trichomonas vaginalis infection by PCR using vaginal swabs and urine specimens compared to diagnosis by wet mount microscopy, culture, and fluorescent staining. *J Clin Microbiol.* 1999;37(12):4127-4130.

67. Borchardt KA, Zhang MZ, Shing H, Flink K. A comparison of the sensitivity of the InPouch™ TV, Diamond's and Trichosel media for detection of Trichomonas vaginalis. *Genitourin Med.* 1997;73(4):297-298.

68. Schwebke JR, Barrientes FJ. Prevalence of Trichomonas vaginalis isolates with resistance to metronidazole and tinidazole. *Antimicrob Agents Chemother.* 2006; 50(12):4209-4210.

69. Bowden FJ, Garnett GP. Trichomonas vaginalis epidemiology: parameterising and analysing a model of treatment interventions. *Sex Transm Infect.* 2000;76(4):248-256.

70. al-Salihi FL, Curran JP, Wang J. Neonatal Trichomonas vaginalis: report of three cases and review of the literature. *Pediatrics.* 1974;53(2):196-200.

71. Temesvari P, Kerekes A. Newborn with suppurative nasal discharge and respiratory distress. *Pediatr Infect Dis J.* 2004;23(3):282-283.

72. Szarka K, Temesvari P, Kerekes A, Tege A, Repkeny A. Neonatal pneumonia caused by Trichomonas vaginalis. *Acta Microbiol Immunol Hung.* 2002;49(1):15-19.

73. Emans S, Laufer M, Goldstein D. *Pediatric and Adolescent Gynecology.* 5th ed. Philadelphia: Lippincott Williams and Wilkins; 2005.

74. Neinstein LS, Goldenring J, Carpenter S. Nonsexual transmission of sexually transmitted diseases: an infrequent occurrence. *Pediatrics.* 1984;74(1):67-76.

75. Corey L, Handsfield HH. Genital herpes and public health: addressing a global problem. *JAMA.* 2000;283(6):791-794.

76. Xu F, Sternberg MR, Kottiri BJ, et al. Trends in herpes simplex virus type 1 and type 2 seroprevalence in the United States. *JAMA.* 2006;296(8):964-973.

77. Johnson RE, Nahmias AJ, Magder LS, Lee FK, Brooks CA, Snowden CB. A seroepidemiologic survey of the prevalence of herpes simplex virus type 2 infection in the United States. *N Engl J Med.* 1989;321(1):7-12.

78. Fleming DT, McQuillan GM, Johnson RE, et al. Herpes simplex virus type 2 in the United States, 1976 to 1994. *N Engl J Med.* 1997;337(16):1105-1111.

79. Kim HN, Meier A, Huang ML, et al. Oral herpes simplex virus type 2 reactivation in HIV-positive and -negative men. *J Infect Dis.* 2006;194(4):420-427.

80. Wald A, Ericsson M, Krantz E, Selke S, Corey L. Oral shedding of herpes simplex virus type 2. *Sex Transm Infect.* 2004;80(4):272-276.

81. Sacks SL, Griffiths PD, Corey L, et al. HSV shedding. *Antiviral Res.* 2004;63 Suppl 1:S19-26.

82. Cowan FM, Copas A, Johnson AM, Ashley R, Corey L, Mindel A. Herpes simplex virus type 1 infection: a sexually transmitted infection of adolescence? *Sex Transm Infect.* 2002;78(5):346-348.

83. Lafferty WE, Downey L, Celum C, Wald A. Herpes simplex virus type 1 as a cause of genital herpes: impact on surveillance and prevention. *Infect Dis.* 2000;181(4): 1454-1457.

84. Wald A, Zeh J, Selke S, Ashley RL, Corey L. Virologic characteristics of subclinical and symptomatic genital herpes infections. *N Engl J Med*. 1995;333(12):770-775.

85. Adams G, Stover BH, Keenlyside RA, et al. Nosocomial herpetic infections in a pediatric intensive care unit. *Am J Epidemiol*. 1981;113(2):126-132.

86. Rowe NH, Heine CS, Kowalski CJ. Herpetic whitlow: an occupational disease of practicing dentists. *J Am Dent Assoc*. 1982;105(3):471-473.

87. Turner R, Shehab Z, Osborne K, Hendley JO. Shedding and survival of herpes simplex virus from "fever blisters." *Pediatrics*. 1982;70(4):547-549.

88. Cengizlier R, Uysal G, Guven A, Tulek N. Herpetic finger infection. *Cutis*. 2002; 69(4):291-292.

89. Novick NL. Autoinoculation herpes of the hand in a child with recurrent herpes labialis. *Am J Med*. 1985;79(1):139-142.

90. Gill MJ, Arlette J, Buchan K. Herpes simplex virus infection of the hand. A profile of 79 cases. *Am J Med*. 1988;84(1):89-93.

91. Leach CT, Ashley RL, Baillargeon J, Jenson HB. Performance of two commercial glycoprotein G-based enzyme immunoassays for detecting antibodies to herpes simplex viruses 1 and 2 in children and young adolescents. *Clin Diagn Lab Immunol*. 2002;9(5):1124-1125.

92. Ramos S, Lukefahr JL, Morrow RA, Stanberry LR, Rosenthal SL. Prevalence of herpes simplex virus types 1 and 2 among children and adolescents attending a sexual abuse clinic. *Pediatr Infect Dis J*. 2006;25(10):902-905.

93. Reading R, Rannan-Eliya Y. Evidence for sexual transmission of genital herpes in children. *Arch Dis Child*. 2007;92:608-613.

94. Woods CR. Syphilis in children: congenital and acquired. *Semin Pediatr Infect Dis*. 2005;16(4):245-257.

95. Christian CW, Lavelle J, Bell LM. Preschoolers with syphilis. *Pediatrics*. 1999; 103(1):E4.

96. CDC. *Sexually Transmitted Disease Surveillance 2005 Supplement, Syphilis Surveillance Report*. Atlanta, GA: US Department of Health and Human Services, Centers for Disease Control and Prevention; 2006.

97. Ingram DL, Everett VD, Lyna PR, White ST, Rockwell LA. Epidemiology of adult sexually transmitted disease agents in children being evaluated for sexual abuse. *Pediatr Infect Dis J*. 1992;11(11):945-950.

98. Hammerschlag MR. The transmissibility of sexually transmitted diseases in sexually abused children. *Child Abuse Negl*. 1998;22(6):623-635; discussion 637-643.

99. Rawstron SA, Bromberg K, Hammerschlag MR. STD in children: syphilis and gonorrhoea. *Genitourin Med*. 1993;69(1):66-75.

100. Starling SP. Syphilis in infants and young children. *Pediat Ann*. 1994;23(7):334-340.

101. Ginsburg CM. Acquired syphilis in prepubertal children. *Pediatr Infect Dis*. 1983;2(3):232-234.

102. Egglestone SI, Turner AJ. Serological diagnosis of syphilis. PHLS Syphilis Serology Working Group. *Commun Dis Public Health.* 2000;3(3):158-162.

103. Siedner M, Zapitz V, Ishida M, De La Roca R, Klausner JD. Performance of rapid syphilis tests in venous and fingerstick whole blood specimens. *Sex Transm Dis.* 2004;31(9):557-560.

104. Lindegren ML, Hanson IC, Hammett TA, Beil J, Fleming PL, Ward JW. Sexual abuse of children: intersection with the HIV epidemic. *Pediatrics.* 1998;102(4):E46.

105. Havens P. American Academy of Pediatrics/Committee on Pediatric AIDS Clinical Report. Postexposure prophylaxis in children and adolescents for nonoccupational exposure to human immunodeficiency virus. *Pediatrics.* 2003;111(6):1475-1489.

106. Ellen JM. Human immunodeficiency virus prophylaxis for sexual assault survivors: what we need to know. *Arch Pediatr Adolesc Med.* 2006;160(7):754-755.

107. Pilcher CD, Tien HC, Eron JJ Jr., et al. Brief but efficient: acute HIV infection and the sexual transmission of HIV. *J Infect Dis.* 2004;189(10):1785-1792.

108. Branson BM, Handsfield HH, Lampe MA, et al. Revised recommendations for HIV testing of adults, adolescents, and pregnant women in health-care settings. *MMWR Recomm Rep.* 2006;55(RR-14):1-17; quiz CE11-14.

109. Greenwald JL, Burstein GR, Pincus J, Branson B. A rapid review of rapid HIV antibody tests. *Curr Infect Dis Rep.* 2006;8(2):125-131.

110. Kahn JO, Walker BD. Acute human immunodeficiency virus type 1 infection. N *Engl J Med.* 1998;339(1):33-39.

111. Cardo DM, Culver DH, Ciesielski CA, et al. A case-control study of HIV seroconversion in health care workers after percutaneous exposure. Centers for Disease Control and Prevention Needlestick Surveillance Group. *N Engl J Med.* 1997;337(21):1485-1490.

112. Pinkerton SD, Martin JN, Roland ME, Katz MH, Coates TJ, Kahn JO. Cost-effectiveness of HIV postexposure prophylaxis following sexual or injection drug exposure in 96 metropolitan areas in the United States. *Aids.* 2004;18(15):2065-2073.

113. Smith DK, Grohskopf LA, Black RJ, et al. Antiretroviral postexposure prophylaxis after sexual, injection-drug use, or other nonoccupational exposure to HIV in the United States: recommendations from the US Department of Health and Human Services. *MMWR Recomm Rep.* 2005;54(RR-2):1-20.

114. W.H.O. Occupational and non-occupational post-exposure prophylaxis for HIV infection (HIV-PEP). *Joint ILO/WHO Technical Meeting for the Development of Policy and Guideline; Summary Report.* Geneva: World Health Organization/ International Labour Organization; September 5-7, 2005.

115. Olshen E, Hsu K, Woods ER, Harper M, Harnisch B, Samples CL. Use of human immunodeficiency virus postexposure prophylaxis in adolescent sexual assault victims. *Arch Pediatr Adolesc Med.* 2006;160(7):674-680.

116. Schremmer RD, Swanson D, Kraly K. Human immunodeficiency virus postexposure prophylaxis in child and adolescent victims of sexual assault. *Pediatr Emerg Care.* 2005;21(8):502-506.

117. Schwebke JR, Desmond R. Risk factors for bacterial vaginosis in women at high risk for sexually transmitted diseases. *Sex Transm Dis*. 2005;32(11):654-658.

118. Morris MC, Rogers PA, Kinghorn GR. Is bacterial vaginosis a sexually transmitted infection? *Sex Transm Infect*. 2001;77(1):63-68.

119. Bump RC, Buesching WJ, 3rd. Bacterial vaginosis in virginal and sexually active adolescent females: evidence against exclusive sexual transmission. *Am J Obstet Gynecol*. 1988;158(4):935-939.

120. Bump RC, Sachs LA, Buesching WJ, 3rd. Sexually transmissible infectious agents in sexually active and virginal asymptomatic adolescent girls. *Pediatrics*. 1986;77(4):488-494.

121. Gardner HL, Dukes CD. Haemophilus vaginalis vaginitis: a newly defined specific infection previously classified non-specific vaginitis. *Am J Obstet Gynecol*. 1955;69(5):962-976.

122. Barbone F, Austin H, Louv WC, Alexander WJ. A follow-up study of methods of contraception, sexual activity, and rates of trichomoniasis, candidiasis, and bacterial vaginosis. *Am J Obstet Gynecol*. 1990;163(2):510-514.

123. Kinghorn GR, Jones BM, Chowdhury FH, Geary I. Balanoposthitis associated with Gardnerella vaginalis infection in men. *Br J Vener Dis*. 1982;58(2):127-129.

124. Masfari AN, Kinghorn GR, Duerden BI. Anaerobes in genitourinary infections in men. *Br J Vener Dis*. 1983;59(4):255-259.

125. Hillier SL, Rabe LK, Muller CH, Zarutskie P, Kuzan FB, Stenchever MA. Relationship of bacteriologic characteristics to semen indices in men attending an infertility clinic. *Obstet Gynecol*. 1990;75(5):800-804.

126. Moi H, Erkkola R, Jerve F, et al. Should male consorts of women with bacterial vaginosis be treated? *Genitourin Med*. 1989;65(4):263-268.

127. Swedberg J, Steiner JF, Deiss F, Steiner S, Driggers DA. Comparison of single-dose vs one-week course of metronidazole for symptomatic bacterial vaginosis. *JAMA*. 1985;254(8):1046-1049.

128. Wahl NG, Castilla MA, Lewis-Abney K. Prevalence of Gardnerella vaginalis in prepubertal males. *Arch Pediatr Adolesc Med*. 1998;152(11):1095-1099.

129. Powell LC Jr. Condyloma acuminatum: recent advances in development, carcinogenesis, and treatment. *Clin Obstet Gynecol*. 1978;21(4):1061-1079.

Chapter 11

THE MEDICAL EVALUATION OF ACUTE SEXUAL ABUSE OR ASSAULT IN CHILDREN AND ADOLESCENTS

Allan R. De Jong, MD

The medical evaluation of children and adolescents who are believed to have experienced acute sexual assault or abuse has 2 major components that often are concurrent: (1) providing appropriate medical care and (2) collecting and documenting evidence of a crime. The primary objective should be to provide a sensitive yet thorough evaluation of the physical and emotional needs of the victim. The examiner must be able to obtain a complete history and perform a physical examination on a child or adolescent who has recently experienced a confusing, frightening, violent, or painful event in order to decide upon additional testing, treatment, and prophylaxis for injuries, infections, and pregnancy. The secondary objective of collecting forensic evidence must be accomplished parallel to the primary objective.

This chapter discusses the medical and forensic components of the evaluation process; the collection and interpretation of historical, physical, and forensic evidence; and the medical management of children and adolescents who are victims of acute sexual assault or abuse.

MEDICAL EVALUATION PROCESS

MEDICAL HISTORY

The medical history of the child or adolescent who has been sexually abused or assaulted includes answers to questions of medical and forensic importance; it provides information to help direct appropriate medical care of the victim while obtaining information about the abusive events to help support forensic evidence collection, direct further criminal investigation, and aid in the interpretation of examination findings. The medical history or interview of the victim can provide a unique opportunity to get details of the abuse episode.[1-16] For children who have been victimized, the examiner must decide how much medical information should be obtained directly from the child and how much should be obtained from the child's caregivers. Before obtaining direct history from the child, information should be gathered from all other possible sources. For the adolescent who has been victimized, most of the important medical information is obtained directly from the victim, including the date and time of the assault, pertinent medical history about the anogenital area, any history of prior or subsequent sexual activity, activities since the assault, symptoms occurring at the time of the assault and since the assault, the nature of the assault itself, and information about the suspect. How much information should be collected during the medical evaluation is debatable, and protocols that expand or restrict the questioning done by medical examiners vary among jurisdictions. From the medical perspective, it is always appropriate to collect enough history to allow medical personnel to provide an appropriate medical evaluation, assessment, and treatment of children and adolescents who have been victimized.

Pertinent medical history includes prior injuries, infections, or surgery of the anogenital area; menstrual history; and any recent or current medical treatment. The history of sexual activity before or subsequent to the sexual assault is important to the interpretation of physical findings, sexually transmitted infections, and forensic evidence. Knowledge of activities since the assault will help medical personnel determine the likelihood of finding evidence, because bathing, wiping the anogenital area, urinating, defecating, douching, removing tampons or sanitary pads, rinsing the mouth or gargling, brushing teeth, and eating or drinking can remove forensic materials. Information on whether the victim changed or did not change clothing since the assault is very important because it will direct medical personnel to appropriate clothing to collect for evidence. Symptoms occurring at the time of the assault and since the assault, including anogenital pain or bleeding and nongenital pain or bleeding, are important factors that dictate medical care and evidence collection. The use of drugs or alcohol prior to the assault should prompt drug screening, and memory loss or loss of consciousness should also raise suspicion of drug use. Drug or alcohol use since the assault will alter the results and interpretation of urine or blood drug testing. The description of the nature of the assault itself is helpful for the detection, collection, and interpretation of forensic evidence, as well as for medical treatment. The history of specific types of sexual contact; types of nongenital contact (eg, kissing, licking, biting, or sucking); the use of condoms, lubricants, or other contraception; ejaculation; and the location of the assault should be obtained. The history of the use of weapons, threats, and descriptions of types of force used (eg, hitting, choking, or restraint) can aid in assessing nongenital injuries. Asking the victim whether the suspect may have been injured in the assault through scratching, biting, or other means may help in evidence collection. Some information about the suspect or suspects involved in the assault will help in interpretation of the forensic materials collected.[2-4,9,12,13,16]

The examiner who decides to obtain a medical history or interview about the assault directly from a young child should use appropriate interviewing techniques. Whenever possible, the child should be interviewed alone, because even the presence of a supportive parent may limit or otherwise influence the details disclosed by the child. Sometimes even the presence of another medical or nonmedical support person may interfere with the child's disclosure. The best interview situation is a quiet, non-threatening environment, where the best interviewers are able to assess the child's level of cognitive and language development and use developmentally appropriate questions. It is desirable to avoid leading and suggestive questions and to avoid showing strong emotions.[3] Nonsuggestive, open-ended questions are the best initial questions because they are designed to obtain a narrative response. Examples of such questions include (1) "Why did you come to see the doctor today?"; (2) "Why did your mother bring you to the hospital?"; (3) "Has something happened to you?"; or (4) "Has something happened to you that hurt or scared you?" Initial answers then can often be expanded by using facilitative questions, which include (1) "How did that happen?"; (2) "What happened next?"; or (3) "Can you tell me more about that?" Questions that involve the use of "why" should generally be avoided as clarifying questions because the child may interpret them as suggesting blame or guilt. Multiple-choice questions may help obtain specific details; however, it is always best to include an open-ended choice as one of the answers. Such questions give the choice of two specific answers plus a third "or something else" option. The child is not forced to select a specific answer if the "or something else" is correct. The questions asked and the answers given should be documented in detail because this information obtained through questioning by health care providers for the purpose of diagnosis and treatment may be admissible in court.[10,11]

THE PHYSICAL EXAMINATION

The physical examination of the child or adolescent who is a victim of acute sexual assault should consist of a complete general examination and a detailed, focused anogenital examination. Some aspects of the general examination to record include the behavior and interaction at the time of arrival and the condition of the victim's clothing. Initial inspection should include observing and documenting foreign material including stains, secretions, grass, and soil on the clothing and body. Collection of these materials may provide useful evidence, as is further described in this chapter. The general examination also allows documentation of injuries outside the anogenital area that may be the best proof of the use of force. The location and pattern of the injuries can be used to support both their inflicted causation and the victim's description of the violence. Nongenital injuries should be photographed or described in drawings and documented in the medical record.

The anogenital examination in prepubertal children is often conducted with the child in a number of examination positions including the supine frog-leg, supine knee-chest, prone knee-chest, lateral knee-chest, and modified lithotomic position (ie, positioned on the lap of a parent or other support person). There is no single examination position or combination of examination positions that combines the best visualization and the best level of comfort and cooperation for the child. The anogenital examination in adolescents is typically conducted in the lithotomic position, but visualization and documentation of genital injuries can sometimes be maximized by using additional positions as with prepubertal children. A moistened swab can be helpful to detect injuries around the hymenal rim in adolescents, and others recommend using the Foley catheter technique. The Foley catheter is inserted into the hymenal opening, the balloon is inflated inside the vagina, and the balloon is positioned so that the hymen is stretched over the surface of the balloon to improve visualization. This technique is not recommended for prepubertal girls.[17,18] Genital injury can indicate both recent sexual contact and the use of force. Genital injury can be described in drawings and documented in the medical record, but photocolposcopy has become the standard in many protocols.[13]

Appropriate preparation should precede the actual process of the examination. Initially the examiner should discuss the process of the examination as well as the limits of confidentiality of the information collected because of the necessary reporting of the results to law enforcement and child protective service investigators when required by law.[3,12] Permission for the physical examination and the collection of forensic specimens should be obtained from the legal guardians of the children. Children and adolescents should be asked to consent or assent to the examination and be allowed to maintain control over the conduct of the examination. Children and adolescents should be allowed to choose whether or not a parent or other support person is present in the examining room.

The child or adolescent should have a thorough physical examination, but the conduct of the examination should not result in additional physical and emotional trauma.[3] A slow, deliberate, nonthreatening approach maximizes cooperation and minimizes trauma. Examination of prepubertal and early pubertal females does not routinely require inclusion of a speculum examination. If there is acute vaginal bleeding and the source of the bleeding is not seen on routine examination, a speculum examination may be required. In all of these cases, the examination should be done under anesthesia by using a small speculum such as the Huffman speculum. In pubertal adolescents, speculum examination to obtain Papanicolaou test results or endocervical swab specimens may be appropriate to maximize collection of spermatozoa (sperm) and seminal fluid. The examiner should take into account the adolescent's willingness and comfort with a speculum examination, and force or coercion should not be used to obtain a speculum examination.[12]

Toluidine blue dye is a vital dye that has been used for sexual assault evaluations because it enhances injuries by staining injured skin or mucous membranes. Toluidine blue dye is not indicated in prepubertal children. There is no reason to use it when a laceration is clearly visible without it. Toluidine blue can cause stinging or burning when applied, limiting the cooperation of young children.[19-21] The use of toluidine blue is controversial because it changes the appearance and enhances injuries; therefore, many centers do not use it in adolescent or adult victims.[16]

Photography of both anogenital injuries and nongenital injuries can be helpful in preserving evidence that is likely to heal completely within a short time. Options involved in photographic documentation include the type of photography preferred (eg, nondigital or digital, video or still photography) and the type of equipment used to aid in the examination and photography of the anogenital area (eg, colposcopy with varying photographic formats attached or other camera systems that can provide lighting and magnification in addition to photographic documentation).[9,11,22-27] Photographic documentation is particularly important when examination findings are being described as abnormal or indicative of injury. Not all sexual assault evaluation programs or legal jurisdictions are in agreement whether photographs should be routinely obtained in all cases of normal anatomy involved in the assault, as well as all detected injuries, or whether photographic evidence should be limited to detected injuries only.[13,16] Regardless of the type of photography and the type of equipment used, certain details are important to obtain useful photographs. The photographs need to be labeled in some manner to identify the patient and the date the photographs were taken. They need to be clear and accurate, which includes proper lighting, focus, and color. A color bar standard in the photographs is helpful to ensure accurate color reproduction and a measurement standard, or ruler, is essential to allow determination of the size of injuries. Obtaining multiple photographs of the same area of injury from varying distances may be helpful in showing the location of the injury; however, obtaining a limited number of high-quality photographs of injuries is much better than collecting numerous low-quality photographs.

FORENSIC EVIDENCE COLLECTION

Two basic types of forensic evidence are sought in sexual assault cases: transfer and identification evidence. Transfer, or associative, evidence includes foreign materials found on the surface of the victim's body or clothing that are transferred to the victim from the abuser or from the crime scene itself. Identification evidence includes biological materials such as sperm, seminal fluid, or other body fluids that contain DNA material that can be used to identify the abuser.[16]

Forensic evidence collection is recommended when the examination occurs within 72 hours of acute sexual assault or sexual abuse.[2-4,13,16] This recommendation is based, at least in part, on research suggesting seminal fluid and other foreign substances are rarely recoverable in adults more than 72 hours following the last sexual contact. There are few new clinical data to support the collection of evidence beyond the 72-hour time frame, but considering that some studies conducted 3 decades ago indicate up to 50% of samples being positive for sperm 72 hours following intercourse in adults, and occasional positives up to 17 days following intercourse,[28] there is substantial historical data that support an expanded time frame. Combined with the increasing sensitivity of DNA analysis and the increasing importance of DNA evidence in the prosecution of acute sexual assault of adults and adolescents, the possibility of finding DNA evidence more than 72 hours following a sexual assault has prompted some centers to set a guideline for evidence collection, some ranging as long as 96 hours after the event and some as long as 168 hours.[16]

Collection of forensic evidence is appropriate to consider in children presenting within 72 hours of a sexual contact that may have involved ejaculation into the vagina; when the child presents with a nonspecific history but has fluorescent material when examined under a Wood's light or blue light; if the child has been kidnapped regardless of the history; if law enforcement requests collection regardless of history; or when parents, older children, or adolescents who have been victimized request evidence collection despite absence of a clear history. The examiner should understand that the aforementioned criteria are not a mandate to collect an evidence kit. Forensic evidence is usually not found in evidence kits from young children who are victims of sexual assault.[29-34] This subject will be discussed in more detail later in this chapter. The reasons that young children do not have evidence as often as adults include differences in the dynamics of the assault and physiological differences. Child sexual abuse is more often coercive or manipulative rather than violent, and semen is less likely to be recovered from prepubertal vaginas because of the lack of estrogen, the smaller volume of the vaginal cavity itself, and the lower probability of deep penile penetration into the vaginal canal occurring during the sexual contact. For health care professionals, it is important to remember to make the medical decisions based on what is medically appropriate for the patient.

Several general guidelines about evidence collection need to be addressed before outlining a specific approach to specimen collection. First, the specific process of collection, labeling, and packaging of specimens should be consistent with the parameters established by the laboratory processing the specimens. Second, a specimen collection protocol should be used to ensure that all appropriate specimens are collected, labeled, and packaged. Third, collection kits should be standardized by providing containers, collection devices, and forms or checklists to ensure proper collection of specimens. These first three guidelines have prompted legal jurisdictions, ranging from individual counties to entire states, to use a common, standardized pre-packaged evidence collection kit for all sexual assault cases.[4,13,16] Fourth, the procedures for collecting specimens should be explained in advance to the child or adolescent and caregivers to ensure the cooperation necessary for proper specimen collection. Fifth, appropriate consent must be obtained from the parent and child before performing the examination and collecting evidence. Finally, the handling of collected specimens should be limited and clearly documented to maintain a "chain of evidence." Documentation includes limiting the number of personnel involved in handling specimens and clearly recording the specimen handlers from the time of collection through the processing of the specimens in the laboratory. Examiners of victims who have been abused should maintain control of evidence beginning with the process of collecting the samples, through the steps of appropriate drying and packaging individual samples, placing individual samples inside and sealing the container for the evidence kit, storage of the kit when necessary, and handing the sealed kit over to an appropriate law enforcement official for processing.[4,13,16]

General guidelines have been established, but the specific evidence collection kit and the process of collection, labeling, and packaging of specimens vary.[4,13] The specific methods used to collect and transport specimens vary, including the use of synthetic rather than cotton swabs or other minor variations in techniques. Any foreign substances introduced or used by the examiner should be documented (eg, lubricating jelly, toluidine dye, or betadine) so their source can be explained if the laboratory analyzing the specimens finds these. Those collecting and handling the specimens should wear gloves to avoid exposure to potentially infectious materials and to prevent contamination of the specimens with the collector's DNA. These individuals should avoid contaminating body sites with secretions from distant sites, by collecting specimens carefully and then removing remaining secretions or stains before sampling another site. Air-drying of wet specimens and packaging them in paper envelopes or paper containers is essential to their preservation. Drying should take place at room temperature to prevent damage from high temperatures and in a clean area to prevent contamination during the drying process. Plastic bags or plastic containers retain moisture, promoting the growth of bacteria and molds that can destroy the samples. Collected "wet" evidence including urine samples, blood samples, wet clothing, tampons, sanitary napkins, diaphragms, and condoms generally should be refrigerated until released to a law enforcement representative. An outline of the basic steps in collecting and documenting forensic evidence follows[4,13,16]; further discussion of the yield of forensic evidence in the clinical setting is included later in this chapter.

Steps in Collecting and Documenting Forensic Evidence

The collection process should follow parameters established by the forensic laboratory processing the specimens and use an established, standardized protocol and evidence collection kit. The procedure for collection should be explained to the child or adolescent and caregivers, and appropriate consents should be obtained. The examiner should ensure a "chain of evidence." All steps should be documented as performed or not performed, and each individual sample should be appropriately packaged, labeled, and sealed. All individual samples should be placed in a sealed container (ie, forensic evidence kit) except for toxicology and medical specimens for infections that are processed separately from the forensic evidence kit. The steps for evidence collection should consist of the following:

1. Collect clothing and foreign material dislodged while the victim is undressing.

2. Collect debris from the victim's body (eg, dirt, leaves, fibers, hair) on a paper collection sheet.

3. Collect foreign materials from the surface of the body.

4. Collect hair combings (eg, pubic, head, facial) when appropriate.

5. Collect hair reference samples as needed.

6. Collect oral and genital swabs and smear.

7. Conduct wet mount evaluation of motile sperm.

8. Collect perianal and anal/rectal samples.

9. Collect known reference sources of DNA.

10. Collect toxicology samples from urine and blood as indicated.

11. Collect medical specimens to identify sexually transmitted infections.

The initial step in evidence collection is the collection of foreign material dislodged while the victim is undressing. Many protocols recommend having the victim undress over a paper collection sheet to catch any foreign material that is dislodged. This material may contain fibers or other substances that can help corroborate where the assault occurred. Routine collection of all clothing is generally not indicated; however, clothing that is stained or damaged can provide important evidence. Torn clothing can be used to support the history of a forced sexual contact. Of particular importance is underwear worn during or subsequent to the assault, because it may contain seminal fluid from the assault.[13] Seminal fluid or other foreign materials might persist longer on clothing than on skin or mucosal surfaces. The importance of collecting clothing in prepubertal victims has been well documented,[14,29,34] but the utility of clothing collection in adolescents is less conclusive.[15]

When collecting debris (eg, dirt, leaves, fibers, hair) during undressing, it should be collected from the victim's body onto a paper collection sheet. Although this evidence is more useful in corroborating the location of the assault, hairs have the potential to enable identification of the assailant.[4,13,35,36] Additional materials should be collected from the body surface as indicated by a history and examination prior to collecting oral, genital, and anal samples. The collection of fingernail evidence is recommended particularly if the victim describes scratching the assailant or if material is visible under the nails. Scraping under the nails with tools included in the kit or clipping of the nails may be used to obtain samples. Fingernail clipping or scraping is not useful in most situations involving young children; however, this process can be valuable when there is evidence of physical force or violence or the child gives a history of scratching the abuser. Foreign materials from the surface of the body might include DNA-containing materials. The highest yield would be expected from any areas with suspicious stains or that fluoresce under long-wave ultraviolet light or short-wave blue light.[5,37] If visible dried secretions are present, they can be gently scraped or "flaked off" or removed with a minimally moistened swab that is air-dried before packaging. When the victim's hair is matted with foreign substances, either "flaking off" the crusted material or cutting out sections of the encrusted hair can be done to collect this material. If bite marks are present, the surface of any bite marks should be swabbed. Swabbing the areas inside and around the arches of the bite mark, rather than from the tooth marks, maximizes the yield of DNA-containing material from sites where the lips and tongue of the biter would touch during the act of biting.[38,39] Tampons or sanitary pads in menstruating females may contain seminal fluid so they should be collected and air-dried completely if possible. If they cannot be dried completely, they may need to be handled as wet evidence requiring separate packaging and alerting law enforcement to its presence and the need for special handling.[16]

Pubic hair combings are typically collected if the assault involved the patient's genital area because of a significant rate of pubic hair transfer from the assailant.[35] Head and facial hair combings should also be considered, particularly if secretions, debris, or other foreign materials are seen on the hair.[16] Experts disagree on routinely collecting any hair reference samples,[13,16] but if they are collected, cut hairs should be adequate for comparison and do not require the pain associated with plucked or pulled hairs. In reality, hair cut or pulled from the victim has become less important in identification of the suspect because of the reliance on DNA technology with much higher specificity. Hair evidence may be important in cases in which no nuclear DNA evidence is found. Although there are some data to suggest an individual's hair characteristics can change over time, there is little scientific support for collecting reference samples from the victim because hair evidence is only important in cases in which hairs are found during forensic examination but no DNA evidence is found. If reference hairs are needed, they can be collected at a later time from the victim.[16]

External genital and perianal samples should be obtained before any internal samples are collected in order to prevent contamination. The female external genitalia should be swabbed initially with at least one dry swab then with a slightly moistened swab. Swabbing the surface of the penis with a slightly moistened swab is reasonable, but obtaining a urethral swab for evidential purposes is not warranted.[13] If dried secretions are present in the perianal area, they can be scraped or flaked off initially, then the area can be swabbed with a slightly moistened swab.

Protocols vary as to whether collection from all 3 sites (ie, oral, genital, and rectal) is done routinely or collection is done from only sites involved according to the history or from all 3 sites when the history is unclear or uncertain.[16] The number of swabs collected from each site, the type of packaging used, whether smears are made on slides in addition to the swabs, and the time frames in which samples are collected vary between protocols. Part of this variation is dependent on the laboratory processing the samples, but protocols are subject to differing interpretation of scientific data, reliance on anecdotal experience, and opinion.

The yield of oral samples is maximized when samples are obtained by swabbing between the gums and cheek and under the tongue. Oral samples only rarely yield positive results more than a few hours after the assault, but early literature suggested occasional positive results were found up to 13 hours later.[40] Internal genital samples in young girls may be limited to samples obtained from the vaginal vestibule and vaginal canal or vaginal pool samples. In older adolescents, cervical swabs should be taken in addition to the vaginal pool sample because sperm persist for a longer time in the cervix than in the vaginal canal itself.[41,42] Some protocols include vaginal washes to collect sperm and DNA evidence, but these are not commonly used because of concerns about diluted evidence and the proper handling of "wet evidence."[13,16] There is little scientific evidence to support obtaining anal/rectal samples unless anal penetration is reported or anal trauma is found in an individual who is unable to provide a clear history; furthermore, these samples must be collected within a limited time frame of less than 24 hours.[13,43]

Some jurisdictions recommend wet mount microscopic examination of vaginal and cervical samples to look for motile and nonmotile sperm, because detection of motile sperm is limited. Sperm can cease movement within 30 minutes and rarely past 3 hours in vaginal specimens, but they may persist for up to 7 days in cervical specimens.[40] Therefore, finding motile sperm in vaginal specimens would be a strong indicator of recent assault, but cervical specimens would be more variable. Some protocols do not rely on examiners to do wet mount evaluations despite this being the only opportunity for such an evaluation, because the experience of the individual viewing the slide is related to the ability to detect motile sperm. Putting a drop of normal saline on the slide and rolling the swab into the drop is the appropriate method to prepare wet mounts. Wet mounts should not result in any loss of evidence. If a wet mount is done, both the slide and the swab should be air-dried and placed in the evidence kit.[16]

Known reference sources of DNA include blood, saliva, and buccal swabs. Buccal swabs should be taken for reference samples after rinsing the mouth. If there has been no reported oral penetration, a buccal swab should be a reasonable reference source for DNA, and blood samples from the victim as a reference are not needed. If there has been recent oral penetration, a blood sample is a more appropriate known source for DNA, and it enables avoidance of a potentially contaminated buccal swab. Considering modern testing protocols, salivary samples are not indicated.[13,36,44,45]

Specimens for toxicology testing and testing for sexually transmitted infections are typically collected during the collection of the evidence kit but are submitted for testing separate from the testing for the evidence kit itself. For suspected drug-facilitated assaults, obtain urine samples if the assault occurred within 96 hours of the examination. Some protocols also recommend obtaining a blood sample if the assault occurred within the last 24 hours, but urine samples will have positive results if the blood test has positive results and may continue to be positive for a longer period of time. The collection and handling of medical specimens used to identify sexually transmitted infections should follow the medical facility's policy for such specimens. A more complete discussion of testing for drugs and sexually transmitted infections is included later in this chapter.

WOOD'S LIGHT AND ALTERNATE LIGHT SOURCE ILLUMINATION

Most forensic evidence protocols recommend a Wood's light or similar blue or ultraviolet light sources as an aid in identifying semen stains on skin or clothing.[2,4,9,13,16] The fluorescing stains can be swabbed for forensic analysis. Semen will exhibit white to yellowish-green fluorescence under a Wood's light. Wood's light examinations have limitations resulting in frequent false-negative and false-positive test results.

False-negative tests are common because the Wood's light has low sensitivity for semen. Santucci et al[46] reported the experience of a group of physicians using a Wood's light on known semen samples and other materials. None of the semen samples fluoresced, whereas a number of ointments fluoresced. In another study, Gabby et al[47] were able to document the fluorescence of known semen samples using an ultraviolet lamp, but they noted the transience of the fluorescence. The fluorescence of semen usually faded within 28 hours, yet semen was still detectable through the use of sensitive forensic DNA tests. Standard Wood's lights produce long ultraviolet light with wavelengths within the range of 320 nm to 400 nm. Maximal semen fluorescence is produced by visible blue light at wavelengths between 450 nm and 490 nm. Ultraviolet lamps with shorter wavelengths including those with old bulbs may not produce fluorescence. Selecting ultraviolet lamps or alternative light sources that produce light with wavelengths of 450 nm to 490 nm will maximize sensitivity and specificity.[37,48] The visibility of fluorescence is also increased by higher concentrations of the semen on the surface inspected and by reducing the distance of the light source from the surface. Visibility is not significantly affected by the angle of the light source with respect to the surface.[49]

False-positive tests are common because many substances fluoresce better than semen. Products commonly found in the perineal area in children such as A & D Ointment, Surgilube, Barrier Cream, and bacitracin will fluoresce under the Wood's light.[46] Other skin creams, lubricants, soaps, and infant formulas have also been shown to fluoresce. Urine and semen may both fluoresce with a white to yellowish-green color, and urine fluorescence persists for considerably longer.[47] Recognizing these limitations (eg, alternate light sources producing short wavelength visible blue light or producing long wavelength, ultraviolet light, including the Wood's light) may be of some help in identifying suspect areas for more definitive testing.[5,37]

Alternate light source illumination is typically provided by a high-intensity, tunable light source. These lighting systems typically include a number of narrow bands of light including visible blue light, and some include infrared light with wavelengths of greater than 700 nm. In addition to providing maximal fluorescence of semen, visible blue light may enhance the cutaneous and subcutaneous tissue changes associated with skin injury. Photographs of injured skin taken with narrow-band blue light may capture more clearly delineated and defined patterns of injury than those taken with broad-band white light. This process may aid in determining the specific object that produced the injury and also in recognizing subclinical injury.[50,51] Others have suggested the use of alternate light sources on the skin, which is of limited value, but its greatest value is in detection of foreign substances including semen on clothing.[52]

RECOMMENDED TESTING FOR SEXUALLY TRANSMITTED INFECTIONS AND PREGNANCY

Routine sexually transmitted infection (STI) testing of pubertal adolescents and adults who are suspected of being sexually abused is generally recommended.[2,3,6,7,15,53] The US Department of Health and Human Services Centers for Disease Control and Prevention (CDC) recommends cultures for *Chlamydia trachomatis* and *Neisseria gonorrhoeae* from all sites of penetration or attempted penetration; however, a US Food and Drug Administration (FDA)–approved nucleic acid amplification test (NAAT) can be substituted for cultures in adolescents and adults, but positive test results should be confirmed with a second NAAT that targets a different nucleotide sequence than the initial test. Wet mount and culture of vaginal specimens for *Trichomonas vaginalis* are recommended, and if vaginal discharge or odor is present, a wet mount for bacterial vaginosis (BV) and vaginal candidiasis should be obtained. A blood sample should be obtained for serologic testing for syphilis, human immunodeficiency virus (HIV), and hepatitis B. Repeat testing should be considered at a 2-week follow-up for *C. trachomatis*, *N. gonorrhoeae*, and *T. vaginalis*. Repeat serologic testing for syphilis and HIV is recommended 6 weeks, 12 weeks, and 24 weeks later.[53]

Sexually active adolescents and adults have a high baseline prevalence of STI; therefore, postassault STI testing may enable the identification of previously acquired STI, incubating STI infection from the assault, or pathogens in the ejaculate itself.[53] Adolescents who deny prior sexual activity should be approached in the same manner as younger children in terms of screening for STIs, considering the significance of STI on an individual with no prior exposure to STIs, except for the sexual assault itself. The high prevalence of preexisting STIs among adults and adolescents significantly limits the forensic value of the identification of an STI in a victim. Some authorities do not recommend routine testing of adolescents and adults who have been victimized who routinely receive prophylactic antibiotics because of the limited forensic value as well as concerns that information about previously acquired STI may undermine the credibility of the victim.[4,13,16] Not obtaining appropriate screening tests for STIs undermines the public health role of assessing or treating sexual contacts for infection while ignoring the fact that identification and treatment of STI among adolescent and adult assault victims is more important from a medical and psychological viewpoint rather than an evidentiary perspective. Prophylactic antibiotics should be offered to all adolescent victims, however, regardless of whether or not STI testing has been performed.

Routine STI testing of all young or prepubertal children who are suspected of being sexually abused or assaulted is not recommended. The decision to test for STIs should be made on an individual basis, weighing the risk of infection against the additional discomfort of obtaining specimens from a young child. A parent's or child's request for testing and living in a high-prevalence region for STI should be considered; otherwise, criteria for screening for STIs include a number of historical and physical parameters associated with increased risk of infection. Historical criteria include assault by multiple perpetrators, history of genital discharge, a sibling or other child in the household with a known STI, or a perpetrator with a known STI or a high risk for STI. Testing for STI is generally recommended if there is a reasonable disclosure by the child of genital-genital, genital-anal, or genital-oral contact. Physical criteria include the presence of genital injury, genital discharge, or genital lesions suggestive of STI.[3,53]

The CDC recommends that selected, high-risk children who were sexually abused be tested for *C. trachomatis*, *N. gonorrhoeae*, syphilis, HIV, and hepatitis B. The preferred method for screening is by using cultures for *C. trachomatis* and *N. gonorrhoeae*, but if NAATs are used, confirmatory testing before initiating treatment should be done. In girls, vaginal secretions should be evaluated for *T. vaginalis* and BV. Children should be assessed for warts and lesions, and any ulcers or vesicles should be cultured for herpes. Follow-up testing should be considered at a 2-week follow-up for gonococcal, chlamydial, and trichomonal infection. Repeat serologic testing for syphilis, hepatitis B, and HIV is recommended 6 weeks, 12 weeks, and 24 weeks later.[53] Samples for STI testing often have higher yields when collected more than 72 hours after sexual contact; however, they are often collected at the same time as the forensic evidence collection kits. When samples for STI testing are obtained at the time of the acute evaluation in children not receiving prophylactic antibiotics, follow-up testing for STI is essential to maximize the identification of infected children.

DRUG-FACILITATED SEXUAL ASSAULT

At least 20 drugs have been used to facilitate nonconsensual sexual activity and drug-facilitated sexual assault, with alcohol being the most commonly used drug. More than 40% of both adolescents who were victimized and adolescents who were assailants have reported drug or alcohol use immediately prior to sexual assault.[2] Of samples obtained from adults and adolescents who were victims of suspected drug-associated sexual assault, 46% to 67% of the samples tested positive for alcohol.[54,55] In addition to alcohol, common "recreational drugs" have been implicated in sexual assault including marijuana, benzodiazepines, cocaine, opiates, barbiturates, and amphetamines. The typical urine toxicology screens can enable detection of recent use of most of these "recreational drugs."[15]

Two drugs have been popularized and studied as so-called date rape drugs, despite being documented less frequently in sexual assault than alcohol and other "recreational drugs." These 2 particular date rape drugs, Rohypnol (ie, flunitrazepam) and gamma hydroxybutyric acid (GHB) have been used by assailants to take advantage of the amnesia and confusion they produce in the victims. Alcohol potentiates their effects and often accompanies their ingestion in sexual assault cases. Rohypnol is a benzodiazepine that is colorless, odorless, and tasteless. Although it is neither manufactured nor legally sold in the United States, it is marketed by Roche Pharmaceuticals in approximately 50 countries, mainly in Europe and Latin America, as a hypnotic sedative for the treatment of sleep disorders, to promote musculoskeletal relaxation, and for use as a preanesthetic or agent for conscious sedation. The drug GHB is known as a behavioral depressant and hypnotic and was previously marketed in a number of health food products, with most of the currently circulating GHB being manufactured in "home-brew" laboratories with ingredients available from chemical supply houses and through recipes from the Internet.[56,57]

Rohypnol comes as small tablets that can be introduced into various drinks. The onset of action is within 30 minutes, with peak action at 1 hour to 2 hours after ingestion and a duration of 8 hours to 12 hours. The long half-life of 23 hours to 33 hours allows symptoms of fatigue, confusion, and inattention to persist for up to 2 days after acute ingestion. Other symptoms include drowsiness, confusion, inability to focus, memory impairment, amnesia, visual problems, urinary retention, and gastrointestinal problems. Periods of lucidity may be interspersed with confusion, and the individual may display excitability or aggressive behavior.[57,58] To reduce Rohypnol's use as a date rape drug, Rohypnol's manufacturer, Roche, introduced a new formulation in 1998 that dissolves very slowly in liquids and releases a blue dye. This new tablet has completely replaced the former rapidly dissolving, colorless formulation.

Usually distributed as a liquid, GHB is often mixed with strong-tasting beverages to cover up its salty taste. The onset of action is within minutes, with peak action at 20 minutes to 60 minutes. The half-life is 20 minutes to 60 minutes, and the duration of action is 4 hours to 5 hours. Most people experience nausea and vomiting, and other symptoms include visual disturbances, amnesia, and reduced inhibitions. Intense intoxication can be manifested in the victim, who appears as either a "happy drunk" or a "mean drunk."[56]

Blood test results may remain positive after Rohypnol ingestion for 5 to 7 hours and for 4 hours to 6 hours after GHB ingestion. Urine test results can remain positive for 36 hours for Rohypnol and for 12 hours for GHB. Only approximately 5% of GHB is excreted in urine. Despite low yields, urine should be collected for up to 72 hours in cases in which the ingestion of date rape drugs is suspected. Urine should be collected, refrigerated, and frozen as quickly as possible. Routine urine toxicologic tests may be positive for benzodiazepines with Rohypnol, and confirmation can be obtained by using gas chromatography or mass spectrometry.[56,57]

In 2005, researchers Scott-Ham & Burton[55] studied 1014 cases of sexual assault thought to have been drug-facilitated. Alcohol was found in 46% of the cases, and 34% had taken illicit drugs, primarily marijuana (112%) or cocaine (11%). In 2% of the cases there was clinically apparent, but hidden and deliberate, spiking of drinks with a sedative or other disinhibiting drug, and 1% reported being forced to drink liquids spiked with these drugs.[55] In 2001, Hindmarch et al[54] reported on the analysis of 3303 urine samples submitted from across the United States for testing because of suspicion of a drug-facilitated sexual assault. The majority of the samples were positive (61.3%) for one or more substances. More than a third of all positive samples contained multiple substances. Of the positive results, alcohol was most common (67%), marijuana was the second most-prevalent drug (30.3%), and benzodiazepines were the third most common (24.8%), followed by cocaine (13.8%), amphetamines (10.8%), and opiates (4.3%). In only 4.9% of the samples was GHB present, and Rohypnol was found in only 0.5%.[54] The data from these and other studies lend support that there is widespread use of alcohol, marijuana, and several illicit drugs, but it does not confirm the widespread use of GHB or Rohypnol to secretly spike drinks in drug-facilitated sexual assault.

Drugs used to facilitate sexual assaults can be difficult to detect because of relatively small doses and rapid clearance from the body. Urine samples are the primary source for detecting the drugs; however, a delay in obtaining urine samples can create negative test results. Hair provides another means for documenting drug-facilitated sexual assault. The drugs are incorporated into the growing hair, and analysis by means of sophisticated analytical techniques of hair collected approximately 1 month after the assault may enable identification of the agent. The advantage of hair testing is its increased sensitivity; that is, the test yields positive results long after the drug has cleared from the blood and urine. A positive blood or urine test result indicates a drug's recent use, and this fact makes it easier to associate the presence of the drug with the timing of the sexual assault, which is not always the case with drug evidence found in hair samples. Hair testing should not be considered an alternative to blood and urine testing, but a complement.[59]

FINDINGS AND INTERPRETATION

PHYSICAL INJURY INTERPRETATION

Nongenital injury might be the best proof of force. The location and pattern of the injuries can be used to support both the inflicted cause and the victim's description of the violence. Nongenital injuries should be photographed, described in drawings, and documented in the medical record. The color of bruises should be noted, but care must be taken in interpreting the timing of injuries because injury healing and color changes in bruises take place at variable rates.[11,60] Genital injury can be used to illustrate both recent sexual contact and the use of force. Genital injury can be described in drawings and documented in the medical record, but photocolposcopy has become the standard in many protocols.[13]

NONGENITAL TRAUMA

Nongenital injury can take many forms, and the absence of nongenital injury does not prove consensual sexual activity. Common injuries include facial bruises, abrasions, and lacerations occasionally accompanied by tympanic membrane ruptures. Neck bruising can occur with choking. Common upper extremity injuries include bruising of the lateral upper arm from punches and defensive bruises of the forearms. Punching and kicking the lateral thighs cause common lower extremity injuries. Other common injuries include whiplike or cordlike bruises on the back, punch bruising on the abdomen, and bruising and bite marks on the breasts.[13,61-64]

Multiple studies have revealed that the rate of nongenital injury in adolescents and adults who were victims of sexual assault ranges from 33% to 67%.[61-65] Rates of nongenital injury tended to be higher in adults who were victims (55%) than in adolescents who were victims (33%)[65]; likewise when strangers committed the assaults, injury rates to victims were higher (61%) than when the assaults were committed by known persons (40%).[62] One explanation for these findings is that assaults involving adults who were victimized and strangers who were assailants are more violent than assaults involving adolescents who are victimized and when known persons committed the assaults. The rates of anogenital injuries were higher than the rates of nongenital injuries in the studies reporting both types of trauma.[61-63,65]

GENITAL TRAUMA

Multiple studies have reported that the rate of anogenital injury in adolescent and adult sexual assault victims ranges from 12% to 83%.[22,61-68] A comparison of rates of anogenital trauma between adolescents and adults who were victims has been inconclusive. Some studies report higher rates of anogenital injury in adolescents,[66,65] whereas others report higher injury rates in adults.[62,67] In 2001, Strickland[67] compared genital findings among adolescents and adults who were victimized. Genital trauma was found in 37% of the adults, but in only 12% of the adolescents. A possible explanation was proposed: that adolescent assault may be less violent because they more frequently know their assailant (65% versus 35%). However, Jones et al[62] reported similar rates of anogenital trauma in sexual assault by strangers (77%) and by known assailants (71%). In an earlier study, Jones et al[65] reported that adolescents had a greater frequency of anogenital injuries than adults (83% versus 64%).

Hilden et al[66] found higher rates of injury among virgins, people aged 12 years to 19 years, and those victims reporting anal penetration. Sugar et al[64] studied 819 victims of acute sexual assault who were 15 years and older and found anogenital injury was more frequent in virgins, victims younger than 20 years, victims older than 49 years, in those examined within 24 hours, and in those experiencing anal assault. Overall, 20% had anogenital injuries.[64] In support of these studies, White and McLean[68] reviewed the injury pattern found during examination of adolescent females who were virgins and nonvirgins and who had experienced acute assault. In this study, only 31% of 81 virgins had genital injury, whereas 53% of 81 nonvirgins had genital injury.[68]

The study by Jones et al[65] revealed anogenital injuries in 83% of 329 cases of acute sexual assault in adolescents; these researchers also noted that anogenital injuries were most frequently located at the fossa navicularis, hymen, posterior fourchette, and labia minora. Adams et al[22] reviewed the medical findings from investigation of acute sexual assault of 214 adolescents and found a correlation between the time since assault and the physical findings. Only 21% had no findings, and the most common finding was tears of the posterior fourchette or fossa (40%). Erythema was found in 32%, and hymenal swelling was seen in 19%. Hymenal tears were more common in self-described virgins (19%) than in nonvirgins (3%), but other injuries were similar in type and location in both groups.[22]

Digital vaginal penetration can also produce injury, although redness or erythema is the most common finding. In 2004, Rossman et al[69] reviewed genital findings in 53 females reporting only digital vaginal penetration. In this study, 81% had genital injuries, with 34% having only erythema, and superficial tears were seen in 29% and abrasions in 21%.

CONSENSUAL SEX

Several studies describe a low rate of genital injury, ranging from 10% to 17.8%, from consensual sexual activity; these studies moreover describe lower injury rates with consensual sex than with sexual assault.[21,70,71] Slaughter et al[71] compared injuries in 311 rape victims with those of 75 females reporting consensual sex. Nongenital trauma was found in 57% of the rape victims. Of the rape victims, 68% had anogenital trauma, usually occurring in multiple sites, and 11% of those reporting consensual sex had genital trauma involving only a single site. The most common sites of injury in the rape victims were the posterior fourchette (70%), labia minora (53%), hymen (29%), and the fossa navicularis (25%). Fraser et al[70] studied 107 sexually active, otherwise healthy adult women over a 6-month period. The following changes, in order of frequency, were found in 56 of 314 (17.8%) colposcopic examinations: petechiae, erythema, abrasions, and edema. These changes were most frequently seen when examinations were done within 24 hours of intercourse or tampon use.[70] Jones et al[72] compared injuries for adolescents reporting acute sexual assault with injuries for those reporting consensual sex; the researchers in this case used toluidine blue dye to enhance the findings. Both groups had a similar high rate of injury overall, with posterior fourchette lacerations the most frequently seen injury in both groups. The injury rate was 85% in the group reporting nonconsensual sex and 73% in the group reporting consensual sex. Therefore, some literature suggests that the pattern of genital injury may be different in females experiencing sexual assault than in those who took part in consensual sexual activity.[70-72] However, Sommers et al[25] concluded in their 2005 study that "we cannot differentiate injuries that occur as the result of consent versus non-consent on the basis of visual inspection, toluidine blue dye, or colposcopy."

ANAL TRAUMA

Anal trauma is less regularly seen among female sexual assault victims than are genital injuries. Slaughter et al[71] reported that 55 of 311 (17.7%) rape victims indicated anal contact and that 31 of the 55 (56.4%) examined through colposcopy had evidence of anal trauma. In their study of acute sexual assault of adolescents, Adams et al[22] found that 61% of the 214 adolescents reporting anal penetration had anal injuries. Sachs and

Chu[73] reported on anal findings from a retrospective review of 548 cases. Although forced anal penetration was found to be less frequent than vaginal rape, there was an increased severity of injury, including anal and rectal tears. Ernst et al[74] reported on anal injuries in 67 males who were sexually assaulted; on gross examination of these victims, 63% were found to have evidence of anal injury. In the study by Ernst et al,[74] the use of anoscopy and colposcopy increased the yield of cases with positive findings to 72%. There are no data comparing the prevalence of anal injury in consensual anal penetration with that in nonconsensual anal penetration.[74]

BITE MARKS

Typical human bite marks are circular- or oval-patterned indentations or injuries composed of 2 opposing *U*-shaped arches separated by open spaces at their bases. Along the edge of the arches one frequently finds a series of small interrupted abrasions, contusions, or lacerations representing injury corresponding to individual teeth. Central bruising might be present between the arches and is caused by crush injury from jaw closure, by sucking, or by tongue-thrusting. Multiple overlapping bite marks and partial bite marks and occasional avulsive bite marks may also occur.[38,75]

Bite marks by adults can often be differentiated from bite marks by children based on size. The intercanine distance in adults ranges from 2.5 cm to 4.0 cm, and in children this distance is less than 3.0 cm. Therefore, a bite mark with an intercanine distance of greater than 3.0 cm is strongly suggestive of an adult bite mark. Animal bite marks tend to be deeper and narrower, and the mechanism of the bite is more ripping or tearing in nature (known as *avulsive*) than the crushing mechanism of a human bite.[76]

Bite-mark identification techniques can be used to determine the source of bite marks on the victim's body. Bite marks are rarely present in child and adolescent sexual assault victims, and accurate sampling and analysis are difficult. High-quality photographs of bite marks can be helpful in identifying the perpetrator, because bite marks can be highly specific for individuals. A forensic odontologist is the best resource for documenting bite-mark evidence. This includes obtaining optimal photographs and preparing bite-mark casts. When a forensic odontologist is not immediately available, a series of high-quality black-and-white and color photographs with assured color balance, showing overall orientation views and a series of close-ups, can be interpreted at a later date, though it is recommended that "the photographic procedures be performed by a forensic odontologist or under the odontologist's direction." The photographs should be taken with and without a measuring scale; when a scale is used, it should be on the same plane as and adjacent to the bite mark. It should be included in the photographs, and the photographs should be taken at 90 degrees to each arch to prevent picture distortion due to the curvature of the skin.[38,75] Swabs from acute bite marks may contain saliva that can be analyzed for DNA.[39]

PHYSICAL INJURY IN PREPUBERTAL CHILDREN

There are limited data on the frequency of acute injuries in sexually abused prepubertal children. Most studies reporting findings among sexually abused prepubertal girls combine data from acute and nonacute evaluations, and these studies indicate the rates of specific positive physical findings are less than 5%.[6,77] Heger et al[77] noted that many of the positive examinations were from acute assaults, but neither the percentage of acute assaults nor specific descriptions of the injuries were reported. Heppenstall-Heger et al[23] reported on the healing of acute anogenital injuries in prepubertal children. Of 6320 children evaluated, only 109 (1.7%) had acute injuries, but the percentage of the total evaluated for acute sexual assault was not reported.[23] The injuries occurred in both accidental and abusive cases, with 62 children providing a specific history of sexual abuse. Twenty-four children described penile-vaginal penetration; 19 described digital-vaginal penetration; and 19 anal penetration. More than half of the anal injuries were anal lacerations and tears; the remainder were hematomas and abrasions. There were also 9 anal injuries found in girls who reported only penile vaginal penetration. Of the 24 girls reporting penile vaginal penetration, many had concurrent injuries in more than one site; posterior fourchette (18; 14 tears), hymen (17; 12 complete tears and 2 partial tears), perihymenal area (7), and labia minora (2). Of the 19 girls reporting digital-vaginal penetration, many had injuries in more than one site; posterior fourchette (6; 4 tears), hymen (7; 4 partial tears), perihymenal area (13), and labia minora (3).[23] This study helps to describe the types of acute injuries seen in prepubertal victims of sexual abuse, but it does not allow a determination to be made of the frequency of injuries among prepubertal victims examined acutely.

Two of the three studies evaluating forensic evidence findings in prepubertal children describe injuries found during medical evaluations of acute injuries.[29,32] Christian et al[29] reported that 62 (22.7%) of the 273 children under 10 years of age in their study had anogenital injuries; after the exclusion of those with erythema, 13.9% were found to have injuries that were more serious. One fourth of the injuries involved the anal tissues, and half were almost equally distributed between the posterior fourchette, labia minora, and hymen. Of those children with injuries, 88% were examined within 24 hours of their assault.[29] Palusci et al[32] reported that 25 (13.2%) of the 190 children under 13 years of age in their study had anogenital injuries. More than two thirds of the injuries were hymenal lacerations, abrasions, and bruises, and one quarter of the injuries were anal lacerations and bruises. Of those children with injuries, 56% were examined within 24 hours of their assault.[32] Prepubertal children evaluated for acute sexual abuse within the first 72 hours have a significant rate of acute injuries, although the majority will have no injuries and the frequency of injury is much lower than reported among adult and adolescent victims of acute sexual assault. Many acute injuries heal rapidly and completely,[23,78] suggesting that the lower rates of injuries in nonacute evaluations is in part due to the delay of more than 72 hours in seeking medical evaluation. Immediate medical examination of prepubertal children within 72 hours of suspected sexual abuse is appropriate for detecting injury; however, the limited data on forensic evidence in prepubertal children support a more selective approach for forensic evidence kit collection.[29,32,34]

EXAMINATION FINDINGS INDICATIVE OF ABUSE

Most physical findings on anogenital examination of children and adolescents seen during evaluation for suspected sexual abuse or assault are nonspecific.[1,3,9,66,78-82] Only a limited number of findings provides support for a disclosed history of sexual abuse and, even in the absence of a disclosure, are highly suggestive of abuse unless the child or the child's caregiver provides a clear, plausible description of accidental injury. Evidence of acute trauma to external genital and anal tissues includes acute lacerations or extensive bruising of the labia, penis, scrotum, perianal tissues, or perineum. These acute injuries can be the result of physical abuse, sexual abuse, or unwitnessed accidental trauma. In addition, a fresh laceration of the posterior fourchette, not involving the hymen, can be the result of sexual abuse, consensual sexual activity in adolescents, or accidental trauma.

Other injuries are indicative of blunt-force penetrating trauma or abdominal/pelvic compression injuries. These injuries include acute laceration, a partial or complete tear of the hymen, and perianal laceration extending deep to the external anal sphincter. In the absence of known coagulopathy or infectious process, bruising of the hymen is also indicative of penetrating trauma.[1,79] When hymenal bruising is suspected, it is important to reexamine the child within a few days or weeks to be certain the bruiselike area has resolved, which will allow differentiation of a bruise from a hemangioma or nevus, neither of which would resolve.

During evaluation for acute sexual assault, additional findings may be discovered that represent healing injuries from prior sexual abuse or anogenital trauma. Evidence of residual healing injury to the external genital and anal areas include scars of the posterior fourchette, fossa navicularis, or perianal tissue. A detailed history is important, because these findings may be attributable to medical conditions, sexual abuse, accidental injuries, or previous medical procedures. Other healing hymenal injuries indicative of blunt-force penetrating trauma or abdominal/pelvic compression injury are missing segments of hymenal tissue or healed hymenal transection in the posterior or inferior half of the hymen. The missing segment of hymenal tissue, a healed hymenal transection, or a complete cleft—a cleft that is located posteriorly between 4 o'clock and 8 o'clock on the hymenal rim and in which the hymen appears either to be torn through or nearly severed to the base in a way that there appears to be virtually no remaining hymenal tissue at that location—should be confirmed by prone knee-chest positioning or use of a swab or water to maximize visualization of any remaining tissue.[1]

SEXUALLY TRANSMITTED INFECTIONS AS EVIDENCE

Sexually active adolescents and young adults have the highest rates of STIs, and they are more commonly identified in pubertal adolescents than in prepubertal children being evaluated for suspected sexual assault or abuse. The presence of STIs in the pubertal adolescent may represent an infection acquired through the abuse or prior sexual activity. The risk of acquiring an STI through sexual assault or abuse is directly related to the prevalence of STI found in the adult and adolescent population from which the abuser comes.[2,53,83-85] One study showed that 43% of the adults and adolescents who were victims of sexual assault had at least one preexisting STI, but relatively few developed new chlamydial (2%) or gonococcal (4%) disease. However, 12% had developed trichomoniasis and 19% had developed BV as a result of their assault.[83] Several studies suggest that approximately 5% of prepubertal children evaluated for sexual abuse will have an STI.[3,9,86] The incubation periods for the organisms and the timing of the examination in relation to the abuse are critically important in detecting infections.[87]

The strength of the association between STI and child sexual abuse is variable. Several factors must be considered when evaluating the strength of association between STI and child sexual abuse, particularly the age of the child and the specific disease identified. The physician should consider the possibility that the identified organism represents a perinatally acquired infection or an infection spread by fomites or nonsexual contact; however, the fact that an explanation of perinatal or nonsexual transmission for a specific disease is plausible does not mean that it is correct. Children with an STI may be unable or unwilling to disclose sexual abuse, and the inability to document a specific STI in a possible or suspected perpetrator does not exclude the possibility that this individual was the source of the child's infection.[3,9]

There are 4 STIs that provide strong forensic evidence in prepubertal children. Infections caused by *C. trachomatis*, *N. gonorrhoeae*, *Treponema pallidum*, and HIV in prepubertal children are primarily sexually transmitted, and in the absence of perinatal transmission (or contaminated needles or blood transfusion for HIV), they are strong evidence of sexual abuse. Cultures are considered the "gold standard" for the diagnosis of *C. trachomatis* and *N. gonorrhoeae* in children; however, positive results from 2 sequential NAATs targeting different genetic sequences may be acceptable.[3,53] Syphilis should be diagnosed by using standard nontreponemal serologic testing such as the Venereal Disease Research Laboratory test and the rapid plasma reagin test, confirmed by specific antibody serology for *T. pallidum* such as the fluorescent treponemal antibody absorption test or the microhemagglutination–*Treponema pallidum* test.[9,53] The forensic significance of other STIs in prepubertal children is not as strong. *T. vaginalis* infections in prepubertal children beyond the first months of life are strongly suggestive of sexual abuse; however, nonsexual transmission is possible theoretically. *T. vaginalis* infection can be reliably diagnosed by using a wet mount preparation, but specific culture media have higher sensitivity. Herpes simplex virus (HSV) infection, either type 1 HSV (HSV-1) or type 2 HSV (HSV-2) by culture, in the genital area of a child or adolescent should be considered as possible evidence of sexual abuse or sexual contact. Commercially available, type-specific serologic tests have acceptable accuracy in adults, but these tests have not been standardized in children—even in adults, these tests cannot with regularity enable a researcher to accurately distinguish HSV-1 from HSV-2. The evidence suggests that, except for transmission at birth, most HSV-2 genital infections are sexually transmitted. The source and mode of transmission in many cases of childhood human papillomavirus (HPV) infection is difficult to identify because of the lengthy and variable incubation period of HPV, the contradictory data on perinatal transmission, and the general prevalence of subclinical infection. The diagnosis of HPV infection is usually made clinically, but biopsy and polymerase chain reaction (PCR) testing can be used to confirm diagnosis. When there are no data that clearly indicate perinatal transmission, every prepubertal child with genital *T. vaginalis* infection, genital HSV infection, or anogenital HPV infection should have a complete medical evaluation for sexual abuse.[3,9,87]

Specimens used in the analysis of STIs have forensic significance in children, but such specimens are often not considered important forensically in older adolescents and adults.[3,13] Sexually abused children and adolescents are at risk for acquiring infections prevalent among sexually active adolescents and adults. Prepubertal children do not commonly experience STIs. Some STIs have much stronger association with sexual abuse; however, children can acquire some STIs through vertical transmission at birth and through nonsexual contact. The discovery of an STI in a child might prompt an evaluation for child sexual abuse and can be the only physical evidence of sexual abuse in some cases.[3,9,53]

FORENSIC EVIDENCE INTERPRETATION

SPERMATOZOA

Spermatozoa (sperm) detected in specimens taken from body orifices provide strong evidence of recent sexual contact. Live, motile sperm are detected by using a saline wet mount and are the most tangible proof of recent ejaculation into the orifice. The survival time of motile sperm is variable, depending on the body orifice in which it was deposited. Sperm motility may be present for only 30 minutes and rarely persists for more than a few hours. The mouth presents a particularly hostile environment because of the cleansing and digestive action of saliva, whereas motile sperm can persist occasionally up to 5 days in the cervix. Prepubertal girls do not produce cervical mucus, so the prepubertal female genital tract may be more destructive to semen and sperm.[14,88]

Nonmotile sperm (ie, dead sperm) are detectable for a longer time than are live sperm. Several studies suggest that sperm are often present for 24 hours but rarely up to 48 hours to 72 hours in the vagina after voluntary intercourse.[40] Other studies have found higher rates of positive samples, particularly in cervical samples. One study reported that sperm may be found in the endocervical canal in adults 6 days after intercourse,[89] and another study, by Soules et al,[28] involved 15 couples after voluntary intercourse and had the conclusion that sperm persists for up to 17 days. At 72 hours, sperm were still present in 50% of the vaginal specimens of the women.[28] Using vaginal and cervical scrapings for the presence of sperm, Silverman and Silverman[88] screened women who reported varying intervals between their last vaginal intercourse and their evaluation. Two thirds of the women with a history of intercourse within that last day had sperm present, and one third of those reporting intercourse 1 week before had sperm present.[88]

Some studies have revealed high rates of identification of sperm in samples of adolescent and adult sexual assault victims, but the researchers involved didn't specifically address the timing of samples. Riggs et al[63] described findings in 1076 victims of acute sexual assault. Sperm or seminal fluid was found in 48% of the 612 samples taken. Gray-Eurom et al[61] described findings in 801 victims examined for acute sexual assault. Sperm or seminal fluid was found in 31% of the 355 cases in which samples were processed.[61] Although other researchers did not rigorously evaluate the relationship between the timing of sexual assault and the examination findings, the Tucker et al[90] study provided details on the interval between the assault and the examination. The study reported the timing of samples in 1007 adult rape victims. A total of 919 vaginal specimens were collected and 344 (37.4%) were positive for sperm; however, 97% of the positive specimens were from women examined within 20 hours of the assault. Oral and anal specimens were rarely positive. Only 1% of the oral rape cases had positive sperm results, and all positive results were examined within 3 hours of the rape. Only 2% of the anal rape cases had positive results for sperm, and all positive specimens were obtained within 4 hours of the rape. Of specimens obtained from skin surfaces, 19% yielded positive results for sperm and only 2 of 12 positive specimens were obtained more than 4 hours after the rape.[90]

Sperm are rarely present more than 24 hours in rectal specimens.[43] Persistence of nonmotile sperm in rectal sites, however, has been documented for up to 113 hours.[40] Sperm may be found for longer periods of time in vaginal and rectal sites in dead bodies than in samples taken from these sites in live bodies.[91] Dry specimens from any site are quite stable, and sperm can be detected in stains on clothing for 12 months or longer.[40,88,92]

ACID PHOSPHATASE AND OTHER SEMINAL FLUID MARKERS

Acid phosphatase is an enzyme secreted by the prostate gland. The concentration in semen is high, 130 IU/L to 1800 IU/L, but it is present in only very low levels (ie, less than 50 IU/L) in vaginal secretions. Acid phosphatase is often considered a more sensitive indicator of recent intercourse than sperm, but it should be considered complementary to the identification of sperm.[74] In the study by Tucker et al[90] of 1007 adult rape victims, 37.4% of vaginal specimens were positive for sperm, but only 1% of the oral samples, only 2% of the anal samples, and 19% of skin specimens were positive for sperm. However, tests for prostatic acid phosphatase yielded positive results more frequently: that is, positive results were found in 62% of vaginal specimens, 11% of oral specimens, 12% of anal specimens, and 42% of skin specimens. Of samples positive for acid phosphatase, all were collected within 36 hours, with 88% collected within 12 hours and 68% collected within 5 hours of the sexual assault. This study supports the concept of the increased sensitivity of acid phosphatase as an indicator of recent intercourse over that of sperm.[90] In individual cases acid phosphatase levels may remain elevated longer than sperm can be visualized or sperm might be detected in the absence of significant elevation of acid phosphatase levels.

Enzyme levels return to normal within 72 hours, so significantly elevated acid phosphatase levels in vaginal secretions usually indicate intercourse within 24 hours to 48 hours. Half of all specimens will have negative levels within 24 hours of vaginal intercourse with ejaculation, but levels can return to normal as soon as within 3 hours of ejaculation. The level of acid phosphatase remains elevated for an even shorter duration in the mouth (perhaps only 6 hours) and in the rectum (less than 24 hours), but limited data are available regarding these sites.[40] Anecdotal evidence supports the stability of acid phosphatase in dried seminal fluid stains on clothing for at least 3 years after the deposition of the semen, and the enzyme may persist indefinitely.[40,88,92,93]

Two other tests, the p30 test and the MHS-5 antigen detection test (which evaluates MHS-5 antigen, a seminal vesicle–specific protein), have been developed to detect the presence of seminal fluid residues by identifying male-specific proteins. p30, or semen glycoprotein of prostatic origin, is a protein manufactured in the prostate gland that is secreted in the seminal fluid. Any amount of the male-specific p30 protein found in the vaginal fluid, urine, or saliva of females is indicative of recent sexual contact, because the amount of p30 declines to undetectable levels within 48 hours of ejaculation into the vagina. The p30 test is a more sensitive test for the presence of seminal fluid than acid phosphatase in the first 48 hours, but acid phosphatase remains detectable in some vaginal specimens for longer than 48 hours. p30 protein is extremely stable when dried, and therefore it may be detectable for up to 12 years in dried seminal stains on clothing.[94] The MHS-5 test uses a monoclonal antibody probe technique for the detection of seminal fluid. The MHS-5 protein is produced only in a male's seminal vesicles and found only in semen.[95] Standardized laboratory kits are available for this test, but the test has not yet come into general usage.[9]

Laboratory tests for the presence of seminal fluid can be interpreted properly only if certain limitations are recognized. First, tests for sperm will yield negative results, but the acid phosphatase test, p30 test, and MHS-5 test may provide positive results if the alleged perpetrator has aspermia or has had a vasectomy, because seminal fluid is still produced and released. Chronic alcohol or drug abuse, chemotherapy, cancer, infection, or congenital conditions may suppress semen production.[16] Second, the tests for sperm, acid phosphatase, p30, and MHS-5 will give negative results if ejaculation has not occurred or if a condom has prevented deposition of the ejaculate. Third, all tests may yield negative results, despite rapid collection of specimens, because of inadequate sampling; problems in the handling or processing specimens; or if bathing, washing, or toileting activities have removed the ejaculate. Finally, all tests are very likely to provide negative results if they are conducted more than 48 hours to 72 hours after intercourse, because all levels fall rapidly. Clothing worn during or immediately after the abuse may test positive more than 72 hours later, however, because sperm and the seminal fluid products in dried stains can persist for a longer time.

TRACE EVIDENCE

Trace evidence pertains to the analysis of foreign materials found on the bodies of sexual assault victims, including hairs, fibers, and epithelial cells. The Locard exchange principle states that when two objects come into contact, material is exchanged between these objects. This principle is the scientific basis of fingerprint and trace evidence collection. Sweat and oil produced in the skin also aid in the transfer and adhesion of epithelial cells from one person's body to objects or to another person's body with physical contact.[96]

It has been estimated that the detectible primary transfer actually involves a small number of epithelial cells, approximately 20 to 1000 cells. A secondary transfer theoretically could take place, transferring some of those cells to a third individual or third object. A detectible secondary transfer, however, is very unlikely. Only a small amount of the primary transfer's small number of cells would be secondarily transferred, and the individual involved in the theoretical secondary transfer would be likely to leave behind a primary transfer of her own cells in a larger number than through secondary transfer. Therefore, the trace DNA identified on a surface is very likely to have come from the last individual who had contact with that surface.[96]

The average human sheds approximately 400 000 skin cells every day.[96] In addition, the secretions of the sweat glands and the oil glands carry additional cells to the surface of the body daily as they pass through the ducts and pores. Each nucleated skin cell contains approximately 5 pg of nuclear DNA. Multiplex PCR DNA analysis can produce full DNA profiles to identify individuals at or below 100 pg of purified DNA, so as few as 20 cells may be a sufficient source from which to produce an individual's DNA profile.[96]

The amount of DNA transferred during handling or touching is independent of the duration of contact, because the transfer would be instantaneous. The amount of DNA is dependent, however, on the individual doing the transfer and the surface to which the transfer is made. Some individuals slough more epithelial cells and are better exchangers, and any exchanged cells are more likely to adhere to a porous surface than to a smooth surface.[96]

The type of DNA-containing material that is exchanged also affects the likelihood of detectible DNA transfer. Solid tissue such as skin scrapings from under victims' fingernails and seminal fluid contain the highest density of DNA. Blood is a relatively good source of DNA, but it is lower in density because only the white blood cells are nucleated. Saliva has an even lower density of DNA, and the number of epithelial cells transferred by handling or touching represents the smallest reservoir of DNA-containing material.[96]

Epithelial cell transfer during sexual contact has been documented between individuals. Dziegelewski et al[97] demonstrated male epithelial cells in vaginal samples up to 7 days after sexual contact by using a fluorescence in situ hybridization (FISH) Y chromosome probe. Collins et al[98] were able to identify female genital cells from penile smears by using a FISH technique between 1 hour and 24 hours after sexual contact in a group of men who had not bathed since the incident. The application of this technology to child and adolescent cases of sexual assault has not been reported.

HAIR AND FIBER ANALYSIS

Body or scalp hair from the perpetrator occasionally can be found on the victim's body. Exline et al[35] studied the transfer of pubic hair during consensual sexual contact. Pubic hair combings were done immediately after intercourse, and at least one transferred hair was found in 17.3% of the 110 combings. Transfers to males (23.6%) were more common than transfers to females (10.9%).[35]

Collection of "foreign" hairs, human or non-human, from a victim's body might provide a link of the perpetrator to the victim. Hair analysis requires the collection of any "foreign" hair from the body of the victim, hairs collected from the alleged perpetrator directly, and the victim's own hair as a control. Multiple specimens from the alleged abuser and the victim must be collected from multiple sites because of the variability of hair types from different sites in one individual. Neutron activation analysis is a precise technique that can enable identification of 18 variable components common in human hair, but the instruments to perform this analysis are expensive and not widely available.[9,99] Microscopic analysis has limited specificity, and the laboratory can conclude in the majority of cases only that the sample is consistent with, inconsistent with, or inconclusive when compared with the perpetrator's hair. Similar microscopic comparison of foreign fibers found on the victim's body with known fibers from the perpetrator's house can help confirm the location of the abuse. Appropriate handling of fiber evidence maximizes the value of fiber analysis.[16,100]

CLOTHING EVIDENCE

Clothing evidence has 3 purposes: (1) torn clothing may help provide physical proof of force, (2) stained clothing (eg, grass-stained) may suggest victim resistance or struggle, and (3) stains may provide evidence of seminal fluid or DNA of the assailant. Although some protocols suggest collection of all clothing from the victim, most recommend only selective collection of clothing with suspected stains or tears.[13] Protocols often recommend collection of underwear worn at the time of the assault and underwear worn since the assault.[16]

ROLE OF FORENSIC EVIDENCE IN PROVING THE IDENTITY OF THE PERPETRATOR

Semen, blood, saliva, body hair, bite marks, and other materials occasionally found on or in the body of the victim may help to identify the perpetrator. Proper analysis of these materials requires the expertise of a forensic pathologist or a specialized crime laboratory.

Before the development of DNA analysis, serologic genetic markers were the primary method for identifying the likely origin of body fluids. The basis of the conventional serologic identification system is the fact that approximately 80% of humans are "secretors," and all bodily fluids of secretors, including blood, semen, saliva, vaginal secretions, and perspiration, will contain genetic markers that are specific to certain individuals and, thus, enable differentiation and identification. The commonly assayed genetic markers are the ABO blood group antigens, the Lewis blood group system, the subtypes of the enzyme phosphoglucomutase, and the peptidase A enzyme system. Some subtypes of individual genetic markers are common, whereas others are rare and the frequency of particular combinations of subtypes of the genetic markers in the general population can be estimated. From this estimate, the chances of the body fluid being from a specific individual can be calculated. Although perhaps more helpful for excluding suspects, analysis using seralogic genetic markers could be precise enough to provide a high probability of the perpetrator's identity. However, approximately 20% of the population consists of "nonsecretors," and genetic marker analysis provides little help in further characterizing the nonsecretor. Control samples of the victim's saliva and blood are required to determine which genetic markers represent the victim and which represent the perpetrator. Body secretions or blood found on clothing or on the body of the victim may represent blood from the victim or assailant and can be analyzed for genetic markers by using the same procedures to determine their likely source.[9,36]

The typing of DNA is the most specific and important development in the identification of the perpetrator of sexual assault and has largely replaced conventional serologic testing.[36,44,45] The typing of DNA has 2 main features that make it superior to conventional serologic evaluation: better stability and higher specificity. There is greater stability in DNA than in protein and enzyme genetic markers used in conventional serologic testing. DNA is more resistant to degradation than are proteins. There is very high specificity in DNA, exceeding the specificity of a battery of tests that make use of conventional serologic techniques. In principle, DNA typing can enable the differentiation of one individual from all others except for an identical twin.[36]

The forensic application of DNA analysis is based on research data identifying regions of human DNA that are extremely variable among individuals. These regions, or loci, have been dubbed **restriction fragment length polymorphisms** (RFLP). One particular subgroup of these RFLPs is called **variable number of tandem repeats** (VNTR) loci. A comparison of these loci in samples was the initial application of DNA typing in forensic medicine. The major advantages of VNTR loci use for DNA typing are in the large number of alleles per locus and in the fact that combining several loci provides high discrimination power among compared DNA samples. The major limitations are that a relatively large amount of high-quality (ie, not degraded) DNA is required for analysis and the process is very time-consuming.[36]

PCR amplification techniques provide the second major tool for forensic DNA typing because they allow amplification of a tiny amount of DNA into virtually any amount. Techniques of PCR amplification greatly increase the sensitivity of DNA testing because a higher number of degraded samples can be tested. This process can take advantage of considerably smaller variable areas of DNA known as **short tandem repeat** (STR) units, rather than the larger VNTR units. The smaller size makes them more amenable to PCR amplification, thereby increasing sensitivity, because specimens with very small amounts of DNA can be analyzed. Specificity is also increased because STR loci are more numerous than VNTR units, so comparisons can be made between larger numbers of variable DNA sequences. In addition, multiple STR loci can be analyzed simultaneously or multiplexed, which results in increased efficiency, speed, and power of analysis. The Federal Bureau of Investigation has identified 13 specific STR loci as a core set for use in matching crime scene materials to previously typed individuals. This core set forms the basis of the **C**ombined **D**NA **I**ndex **S**ystem (CODIS).[36]

Even smaller areas of DNA variation, or segments shorter (smaller) than STR loci, hold some potential for use in forensic DNA testing. Single nucleotide polymorphisms (SNPs) represent alterations in DNA sequence at a single nucleoside position due to changes, insertions, or deletions. These SNPs are very numerous, with millions occurring in each individual, but they typically produce only 2 alleles and, less commonly, 3 or 4 alleles. Therefore, to be of discriminating forensic value, a relatively large number of SNPs would have to be analyzed. As a result, although SNP may be more helpful in excluding suspects, ongoing research is still necessary to improve the utility of SNP testing.[36]

Mitochondrial DNA and Y chromosomal DNA may also have forensic application. Mitochondria contain their own small DNA genomes known as mitochondrial DNA (mtDNA). Normally, only maternal mtDNA is transmitted to children. Each cell contains only one nucleus, but it can contain hundreds to thousands of mitochondria. Specimens with degraded DNA or that lack nuclear DNA but contain mtDNA can be analyzed forensically. For example, a sample of hair without a root ball lacks nuclear DNA, but it still contains large amounts of mtDNA for comparison with known samples from a suspect. The limitations of mtDNA are its relatively low discriminating power and the lack of available databases compared with those available for nuclear DNA.[36]

The Y chromosome has hundreds of recognized STR loci that can be used for identification. The Y chromosome is transmitted in a single copy only from father to son, whereas mtDNA is transmitted in multiple copies from a mother to all of her children. Therefore, Y chromosomal analysis can be useful in resolving mixtures of DNA from different males, but its overall discriminating power is limited by the size of the database. Also, Y chromosomal STR analysis (Y-STR) may be useful in cases in which sperm are no longer present but some seminal fluid remains. Johnson et al[101] reported that of 45 samples that were negative for spermatozoa but positive for seminal fluid, a Y-STR profile was obtained in 86.2%. Sibille et al[102] analyzed 104 samples from 79 females testing negative for sperm. In the samples, Y-STR was present in 30% of the cases greater than 48 hours after their assault.[102] Delfin et al[103] in 2005 described 112 children and adolescents (aged 2-17 years) testing positive for seminal fluid but negative for sperm. All were negative for autosomal DNA, but Y-STR was positive in 92.3%.

In testing, DNA is more stable than other conventional serologic testing, but degradation can occur. Factors producing degradation include exposure to sunlight and ultraviolet light, time, temperature, humidity, chemicals, and biological contamination. Mixed samples present some difficulty, but this situation is expected in sexual assault cases because both victim and assailant DNA is expected to be present. Contaminated specimens are more problematic, because the addition of soaps, chemicals, bacteria, and fungi can cause degradation of the samples. Stability is improved by preventing contamination and drying, then freezing, the samples.[36]

The analysis of DNA can result in 3 determinations regarding identity: exclusion, inconclusive, and match. Exclusion means that the 2 DNA samples are different, and inconclusive means that the results do not allow a determination as to whether the DNA samples are the same or different. A match means the DNA types are similar and there are no significant differences, so the DNA samples could have the same source. The current technology for DNA typing has progressed to the point at which the reliability and validity of properly collected, properly preserved, and properly analyzed DNA data should not be in doubt.[36,104]

FORENSIC EVIDENCE IN CHILDREN

Most children evaluated for sexual abuse do not have forensic evidence. Studies focusing on highly selected groups of children and adolescents who were victims reported 14% to 30% had positive test results for sperm or acid phosphatase.[105-107] Enos et al[105] reviewed 162 cases of children who were victimized for less than 14 years, and 29 (17.9%) had positive tests for sperm or acid phosphatase. Sperm was found in 16, sperm and acid phosphatase in 11, and acid phosphatase in only 2. These tests were most commonly positive in the 11- to 13-year-olds evaluated, but no specific age breakdown was provided.[105] Rimsza and Niggemann,[106] in a study conducted by them, performed forensic tests on 50 of the 311 children and adolescents they evaluated. Sperm was found in 15 (30%), and all positives were collected within 24 hours of the sexual contact. There were no data reported that would enable a determination of whether different rates of positive tests were found among prepubertal and pubertal victims.[106] Spencer and Dunklee[107] evaluated 140 boys (aged 1 to 17 years) who were sexually abused and found that 8 of 30 boys (112.6%), examined within 72 hours, had positive forensic test results. Fluorescence with ultraviolet light alone, however, was considered a positive test result.[107]

Authors of other studies suggest that only 2% to 9% of all sexually abused preteen or prepubertal children evaluated have positive test results for sperm or acid phosphatase.[14,29-34] However, Dahlke et al[30] reported positive test results in 28% of 132 children younger than 15 years; in addition, in their study the percent of rape victims with positive test results increased as the age of the victims increased. Although 73% of all victims older than 14 years had positive test results, 36% of children 11 years to 14 years and only 3% of children younger than 11 years had positive tests for sperm or acid phosphatase.[30] Three additional studies focus on the results of forensic evidence collection for prepubertal children who were sexually abused.[14,29,34] All 3 of these studies had as a conclusion that guidelines for evidence collection for adolescents and adults who were sexual assault victims might not be appropriate for prepubertal victims.

Christian et al[29] retrospectively studied 273 children younger than 10 years who selectively had evidence collection kits obtained for suspected acute sexual abuse. Some form of evidence was found in 24.9%, but only 9% had evidence found in samples from body sites. Evidence samples were most often positive for blood; moreover, only 18 (6.6%) had sperm or seminal fluid detected. All children with positive forensic evidence were seen within 44 hours, and more than 90% were examined within 24 hours of the assault. Furthermore, no swabs from any child's body were positive for blood longer than 13 hours or sperm or semen longer than 9 hours after the assault. Almost two thirds of all evidence was found on clothing or linens, and all evidence with the exception of one pubic hair was found on clothing or linens when the examination was completed more than 24 hours after the sexual contact. The authors suggested that swabbing the child's body for evidence might be unnecessary after 24 hours. Because clothing and linens yielded the majority of evidence and retained the evidence for longer periods following the assault, they should be vigorously pursued for analysis.[29]

Young et al[34] retrospectively reviewed forensic evidence collected from 80 children taken to the emergency department with a history of sexual abuse or assault with genital contact occurring within the last 72 hours. The subjects were 49 children younger than 12 years and 31 children aged 12 to 16 years. Sperm or seminal fluid was found in 16 (20%) of the 80 evidence kits collected. Positive samples were correlated with the age of the victim and the length of the interval between the sexual act and evaluation in the emergency department. Only 3 of the 49 younger children (aged 11 years or younger) had positive results, and none had positive test results from samples taken from body sites. The 3 positive samples came from underwear, and one child's washcloth was also positive. In contrast, 13 of the 31 adolescents had positive results, and all 13 tested positive from samples taken from body sites. In addition, the clothing of 8 of these 13 adolescents also tested positive. Ten of these positive kits were from children who were evaluated within 6 hours, and all 16 positive kits were from children evaluated within 24 hours of the sexual contact. The authors concluded that forensic evidence collections from body sites in children and adolescents who were sexual assault victims are unlikely to yield positive results for sperm or seminal fluid more than 24 hours after the sexual contact or when taken from prepubertal children.[34]

Palusci et al[32] retrospectively studied 122 children younger than 13 years who had evidence collection kits done within 72 hours of suspected acute sexual abuse. Specimens were initially evaluated for acid phosphatase, and positive results were further assessed with microscopic examination for sperm and immunoassay for p30 antigen. Of the children, 69% were evaluated within 24 hours of sexual contact. Only 9% of the children had positive forensic evidence from body sites or from clothing. Pubertal children, or those having physical injury at the time of evaluation, were more likely to have positive forensic results. Children who bathed, changed clothing, or who were examined later within the 3-day period were less likely to have positive test results. Nearly twice as many positive results were obtained from clothing as from samples from body sites. Semen or sperm was identified from body swabs only from unbathed, female children older than 10 years of age or on clothing and other objects.[32]

All three of the immediately aforementioned studies emphasize the importance of the collection of clothing, and all underscore the limited yield from specimens collected from the bodies of prepubertal victims. All 3 studies also have a similar limitation: they all used microscopic examination for the detection of sperm and assays for either prostatic acid phosphatase or p30 to identify seminal fluid. These studies use the microscopic examination and chemical analysis approach, rather than emerging DNA analysis, to assist in the detection of very small quantities of male DNA. Unfortunately, there are no published data assessing the usefulness of these highly sensitive technique assays for DNA in prepubertal or young pubertal children.

Sperm and acid phosphatase are usually not detected in children who were sexual abuse victims, and the frequency of detection is likely to be lower in unselected samples. Other forms of forensic evidence such as hairs, fibers, or other foreign substances are reported in fewer cases than are sperm or seminal fluid.[29] Certainly, the collection of clothing and linens should be performed. The questions remain, however, whether forensic specimens should be collected from the body cavities of all prepubertal children, unless we are absolutely certain the tests will be negative, or whether we should consider the absence of data in support of this approach while remembering that the primary goal is to provide sensitive, supportive clinical care to these children.

RELATIONSHIP OF PHYSICAL AND FORENSIC EVIDENCE TO SUCCESSFUL PROSECUTION

Tintinalli and Hoelzer[108] reviewed the legal outcomes of 67 prosecuted cases involving adult and adolescent victims and found no correlation between physical and forensic evidence and legal outcome. In contrast, Rambow et al[109] reviewed cases of 182 victims who had forensic examinations performed and concluded that forensic findings were significantly associated with successful prosecution. Three more recent studies of adult and adolescent victims sought association between physical evidence of sexual contact and the filing of charges and successful prosecution.[61,110,111] Gray-Eurom et al[61] reviewed 801 forensic evaluations; in 355 cases a suspect was identified. Evidence of trauma was found in 202 (57%) and sperm was found in 110 (31%) of cases in which a suspect was identified. When the authors looked for correlation between evidence and successful prosecution, the presence of trauma was correlated but the presence of sperm was not. Victims younger than 18 years of age and the use of a weapon were factors also associated with successful prosecution. The successful prosecution was related to evidence of force or lack of consent (ie, trauma), rather than the evidence of a sexual act itself (eg, sperm).[61] In the second study,[110] the extent of injury was associated with the filing of charges and rates of conviction. McGregor et al[110] also reported greater than a threefold increase in filing charges in the presence of forensic specimens being collected, irrespective of the test results. This suggests that the victim's willingness to submit to forensic evaluation appears to provide some validation of the victim's reported sexual assault.[110] The third study[111] reported that only 15% of the 888 girls and women older than 15 years evaluated for sexual assault had charges filed. Characteristics positively associated with prosecution were examination within 24 hours of the assault, assault by a partner or spouse, oral assault, and anogenital trauma.[111]

Studies of features related to prosecutorial outcome in child sexual abuse cases generally include more nonacute cases than cases of acute sexual assault. The likelihood of cases being accepted for prosecution has been associated with perpetrator confessions and physical injury. Cross et al[112] reviewed 431 cases referred for prosecution and found that confessions and medical evidence were the strongest predictors of prosecution. Stroud et al[113] reported that slightly more than half the cases involving 1043 children completing a forensic interview were accepted for prosecution. Cases with children who had mild to no injury were more likely to result in acceptance, but cases with children who had the injuries that were most severe were less likely to be prosecuted for some unknown reason.[113] Brewer et al[114] reviewed 200 cases and found prosecution was more likely when the perpetrator abused multiple victims or was not a nuclear family member or when the abuse involved older children or acts that were more serious with the presence of physical evidence. Most cases involved nonacute sexual abuse, and prosecutorial outcomes were not discussed in these studies.

Kerns and Ritter[115] compared the frequency of abnormal genital findings in 83 girls examined following perpetrator confessions and 583 girls who reported abuse but whose cases did not have perpetrator confessions. There was no significant difference in the likelihood of abnormal genital findings between the 2 groups. Neither the number of girls evaluated for acute assault nor the prosecutorial outcomes were reported.[115] Muram[89] reviewed 31 cases with perpetrator confessions of sexual abuse. Significant examination findings were observed in 11 of 18 (61%) of girls with admitted vaginal penetration but were also found in 3 of 13 (23%) of girls when penetration was denied. Hymenal or vaginal tears were reported in 9 of 17 girls evaluated within 72 hours of the sexual abuse. The prosecutorial outcomes were not reported.[89]

De Jong and Rose[31] reviewed 115 cases of child sexual abuse prosecuted for felony charges. Medical evidence of injury or seminal fluid was present in only 23% of cases that resulted in felony convictions, but the overall conviction rate was 76%. Convictions occurred in 67 of 85 cases (79%) without medical evidence, whereas only 20 of 30 cases (67%) with medical evidence resulted in convictions. The felony conviction rate was significantly lower among 23 children who were younger than 7 years of age (52%), despite a higher rate of physical evidence (56%). This study suggests that the verbal evidence may have been more critical than physical evidence in many cases.[31] Adams et al[116] analyzed 236 cases in children younger than 18 years of age with perpetrator conviction for sexual abuse. Most of the legal cases were decided by guilty pleas, only 14% by trials. Abnormal genital findings were present in 14%, and abnormal anal findings were present in 1%. Only 10% of the children were examined acutely within 72 hours of sexual contact, and they had a significantly higher rate of abnormal examinations.[116] Palusci et al[117] studied the relationship of physical findings and prosecution outcome in 497 children having nonacute examinations for sexual abuse. Overall, 17% of the children had significant physical findings. Those cases involving positive findings were 2.5 times more likely to result in successful prosecution; however, 67% of children with positive physical findings had either no prosecution or unsuccessful prosecutorial outcomes. Positive physical findings were better than disclosure of abuse to predict acceptance for prosecution and successful prosecution, but a lack of disclosure was the best predictor of not seeking prosecution and unsuccessful prosecution.[117] Therefore, most of the data on prosecuted cases involving children of sexual abuse focus on nonacute sexual abuse rather than acute sexual assault. These authors[31,116,117] emphasize the importance of verbal evidence, history, or disclosure in studies primarily reporting nonacute sexual abuse. Verbal evidence is expected to be important in acute cases, based on the reported rates of documentation of specific injuries, STIs, and forensic evidence in acute child sexual assault cases.

MEDICAL MANAGEMENT CONSIDERATIONS

The major medical interventions required for children and adolescents who are sexual assault victims involve therapy for STIs, emergency contraception, treatment of injuries, certification of physical health, and recommendations for counseling. These interventions are often initiated at the first medical evaluation, but medical follow-up is recommended to maximize the effect of the interventions.

Prophylactic antibiotic therapy for children who were sexually abused is a controversial subject, but routine prophylaxis is not generally recommended for prepubertal children.[3,9,53] Routine prophylaxis is commonly offered to adolescents and adults for *C. trachomatis*, *N. gonorrhoeae*, *T. vaginalis*, and BV as follows: ceftriaxone 125 mg intramuscularly in a single dose, plus metronidazole 2 g orally in a single dose, plus either azithromycin 1 g orally in a single dose or doxycycline 100 mg orally twice a day for 7 days.[53] Other cephalosporins can be substituted for ceftriaxone, but they do not offer any advantage over ceftriaxone. Fluoroquinolone antibiotics (eg, ciprofloxacin, ofloxacin, levofloxacin) are no longer recommended for the treatment of gonorrhea.[118] If the individual is not previously immunized for hepatitis B, a first dose of vaccine is recommended, with follow-up doses to be given 1 to 2 months and 4 to 6 months after the initial dose. Routine prophylactic use of hepatitis B immune globulin (HBIG) is not recommended, but HBIG is recommended as an adjunct to initiating hepatitis B immunization when the perpetrator of the sexual assault is known to be positive for hepatitis B surface antigen.[53] Selective testing should be done for STIs in younger children as outlined previously. An individually tailored therapy should be initiated if this testing reveals specific infections.

Conducting HIV **p**ost**e**xposure **p**rophylaxis (PEP) for victims of all ages who were sexually assaulted is a controversial subject. The CDC states that there is a lack of data on the efficacy of antiretroviral agents to reduce HIV transmission after a possible nonoccupational exposure. The CDC recommends considering the use of PEP for HIV in sexual abuse or assault cases when the perpetrator is known to be HIV-infected, the exposure event presents a substantial risk of transmission, and treatment can be initiated within 72 hours. If the perpetrator's HIV status is unknown, PEP should be considered on a case-by-case basis. If there is "negligible exposure risk," HIV PEP is not recommended.[53,119] Examiners should discuss the risk of acquiring HIV, the potential benefits of PEP and its unknown efficacy in this setting, and known toxicity of PEP with the victim and parents, in the case of children. Many clinicians prefer a three-drug combination of two nucleotide analog reverse transcriptase inhibitors (NRTIs), zidovudine and lamivir for example, and one protease inhibitor, such as nelfinavir for children and adolescent PEP.[120] The regimen used with these three drugs might suppress virus replication better, but multiple-drug regimens are likely to increase potential toxicity and decrease compliance with the required 28-day PEP course. Some clinicians recommend regimens with only two NRTI drugs because they have lower toxicity. Clinicians involved in acute sexual abuse evaluations of children and adolescents should establish a protocol that includes the approach to discussing PEP for HIV, the immediate availability of a 3-day starter kit of the PEP drugs, and follow-up in consultation with a pediatric infectious disease specialist.[120]

Pregnancy risk and pregnancy prevention should be considered in all postmenarcheal girls. The chance of pregnancy after a single instance of unprotected intercourse is 20% to 30% during the midcycle and 2% to 4% anywhere else in the cycle. The actual risk for many adolescents is difficult to determine because many have irregular cycles and few can pinpoint their ovulation days. Therefore, all postmenarcheal girls should have a pregnancy test and be offered pregnancy prophylaxis.[14,121] Emergency contraception should be discussed with the adolescent if she is not pregnant and if less than 120 hours has elapsed since the assault. Although prophylaxis is most effective if initiated within 72 hours, it appears to be moderately effective up to 120 hours after unprotected intercourse. Emergency contraception will prevent approximately 80% of expected pregnancies if taken appropriately. The FDA has approved two specific regimens for emergency contraception, Plan B and Preven. Plan B is a regimen containing only progestin, with a total dose of 1.5 mg of levonorgestril in 2 pills. Initially, 1 pill is given and 12 hours later 1 more pill is given. Preven is an estrogen-progestin combination containing a total dose of 200 μg of ethynyl estradiol and 1.0 mg of levonorgestril in 4 pills. Initially, 2 pills are given and then 12 hours later 2 more pills are given. The Preven regimen is similar to an established regimen for emergency contraception combining estrogen and progestin, known as the Yuzpe method, prescribing a total dose of 200 μg of ethinyl estradiol plus 2.0 mg of dl-norgestril (equivalent to 1.0 mg of levonorgestril) in 2 divided doses given 12 hours apart. A regimen of 2 doses of a number of combined oral contraceptives can also be used as emergency contraception.[121] Nausea (50%) and vomiting (17% to 22%) are common side effects. Oral antiemetics, including meclizine and metoclopramide, can be helpful when given 1 hour before the initial dose. Although Preven was removed from the US market in 2006, the Yuzpe method is still recommended, and a number of other combination oral contraceptives (estrogen-progestin combinations) are utilized. The progestin-only regimen is associated with a lower incidence of nausea and vomiting, as well as a lower pregnancy rate, than the estrogen-progestin regimens.[121] Menstruation occurs within 21 days in more than 95% of patients receiving emergency contraception. If menstruation does not occur, both physiologic and psychological factors should be assessed.[14,121]

Most acute genital and perianal injuries do not require surgical intervention. The primary therapy for acute injuries is maintaining proper hygiene in the anogenital area. Sitz baths can be initiated, after specimens for evidence and culture are collected, to promote healing and to prevent secondary infections. Prophylactic broad-spectrum antibiotics are not generally indicated in wound care. Topical or oral antibiotics may be recommended for extensive injuries, but few data support their efficacy. Lubricating ointments or diaper creams may be helpful to reduce irritation. Nonstick dressings or absorbent pads may be considered in individual cases, but frequently changed cotton underwear may be sufficient. Small vulvar or perianal hematomas may be treated with pressure and ice packs. Large hematomas or lacerations may require a surgical or gynecologic consultation, with surgical repair done, when necessary, with the patient under general anesthesia.[9]

A mental health professional should evaluate all children and adolescents who have been sexually abused or assaulted.[3] This assessment is both to determine the need for counseling for both the child who has been victimized and the parents and to evaluate the level of family support for the child. Sexual assault can trigger significant acute and chronic emotional trauma. One must remember that the role of the medical provider is primarily promoting the child's physical and emotional well-being; with that said, the management of both the physical and emotional trauma begins at the time of the acute medical evaluation of the child or adolescent who has been sexually abused. The parents and child need reassurance regarding physical and emotional concerns. When the child's examination reveals no trauma, both need reassurance that the child is physically normal now and can grow and develop into a physically normal adult despite this experience. If the child has injuries, reassurance can be given that most injuries heal rapidly and completely and, once healed, should have no physical effects on the functioning of the genital and anal areas. Acknowledge that the child and the parents may experience a number of emotional reactions, including anger, humiliation, guilt, blame, and sadness. Reassure the child and parents that, regardless of events leading to the abuse or assault itself, the child is not responsible for being sexually assaulted; the assailant is responsible for abusing the child.[3,12]

The physical and emotional needs of the child should be coordinated, whenever possible, with the child's medical primary care provider.[12] Girardet et al[122] found that 8% of children who had been victimized had significant unmet health care needs that could result in patient morbidity unrelated to sexual abuse identified during their medical evaluation that needed intervention. All children should have a follow-up appointment whether or not an acute injury or infection is present. In children without initial injury or infection or with minor acute injury, this examination can be a time to reassure the child and the parents that no permanent physical damage has occurred. This "certification of physical wellness" may help some of the children avoid the "damaged goods" feelings commonly experienced by abused children. The unmet health care needs can also be addressed at this time. Children with injury that is more severe should be carefully followed up until healing is complete. They need assurance that any residual scarring should not affect their health and functioning as adults.

SUMMARY

All children and adolescents being evaluated for suspected acute sexual assault or abuse should have a medical evaluation that incorporates the major objectives of providing appropriate medical care while collecting and documenting evidence of sexual contact. The medical history or interview can help direct the medical care of the child and provide a unique opportunity to obtain important evidence in the form of the history of the sexual assault. The majority of acute examinations in prepubertal children will not disclose physical trauma, STIs, or positive forensic medical evidence that sexual contact has occurred. Many physical examinations in adolescents will yield some physical injury evidence or positive forensic evidence, with higher rates reported when evaluations occurred within the first 24 hours to 48 hours after the assault. Identification of certain STIs in prepubertal children is forensically important, but the forensic value of these infections is more limited in adolescents. The quality of forensic evidence is maximized by following an appropriate protocol for evidence collection and the documentation of proper handling of all evidence. Analysis of DNA provides a more sensitive and more specific approach to the identity of the offender than conventional serologic testing, but there are few published data about the performance of DNA analysis in child and adolescent sexual assault cases. The history of the abuse or assault is the most important evidence in victims of prepubertal sexual assault. Physical evidence of force, injury, or sexual contact is helpful, but it is neither necessary nor sufficient for conviction of the perpetrator of acute sexual assault. The major medical interventions required involve prophylactic and therapeutic antibiotics for STIs, emergency contraception, treatment of injuries, certification or reassurance of physical health, and recommendations for counseling.

REFERENCES

1. Adams J. Medical evaluation of suspected child sexual abuse. *J Pediatr Adolesc Gynecol.* 2004;17:191-197.

2. Kaplan DW, Feinstein RA, Fisher MM, Klein JD, Olmedo LF, Rome ES, et al. Care of the adolescent sexual assault victim. *Pediatrics.* 2001;107:1476-1479.

3. Kellogg N. American Academy of Pediatrics Committee on Child Abuse and Neglect: Clinical Report: The evaluation of sexual abuse in children. *Pediatrics.* 2005;116:506-512.

4. American College of Emergency Physicians. *Evaluation and management of the sexually assaulted or sexually abused patient.* Dallas: American College of Emergency Physicians; 1999;1-134.

5. Atabaki S, Paradise JE. The medical evaluation of the sexually abused child: lessons from a decade of research. *Pediatrics*. 1999;104(1 pt 2):178-186.

6. Bechtel K, Podrazik M. Evaluation of the adolescent rape victim. *Pediatr Clin North Am*. 1999;46:809-823, xii.

7. Cantu M, Coppola M, Lindner AJ. Evaluation and management of the sexually assaulted woman. *Emerg Clin North Am*. 2003;21:737-750.

8. Danielson CK, Holmes MM. Adolescent sexual assault: an update of the literature. *Curr Opin Obstet Gynecol*. 2004;16:383-388.

9. Finkel MA, De Jong AR. Medical findings in child sexual abuse. In: Reece R, Ludwig S, eds. *Child Abuse: Medical Diagnosis and Management*. 2nd ed. Philadelphia: Lippincott Williams & Wilkins; 2001.

10. Frasier LD. The pediatrician's role in child abuse interviewing. *Pediatr Ann*. 1997;26:306-311.

11. Giardino AP, Finkel MA. Evaluating child sexual abuse. *Pediatr Ann*. 2005;34: 382-394.

12. Laraque D, DeMattia A, Low C. Forensic child abuse evaluation: a review. *Mt Sinai J Med*. 2006;73:1138-1147.

13. Ledray LE. *Sexual Assault Nurse Examiner Development and Operation Guide*. Washington, DC: Office for Victims of Crime, US Department of Justice; 1999.

14. Paradise JE. The medical evaluation of the sexually abused child. *Pediatr Clin North Am*. 1990;37:839-862.

15. Poirier MP. Care of the female adolescent rape victim. *Pediatr Emerg Care*. 2002;18:53-60.

16. US Department of Justice. A national protocol for sexual assault medical forensic examinations: adults/adolescents [NCJ 206554]. Washington, DC: US Department of Justice, Office on Violence Against Women; 2004.

17. Ferrell J. Foley catheter balloon technique for visualizing the hymen in female adolescent sexual abuse victims. *J Emerg Nurs*. 1995;21:585-586.

18. Starling SP, Jenny C. Forensic examination of adolescent female genitalia: the Foley catheter technique. *Arch Pediatr Adolesc Med*. 1997;151:102-103.

19. Jones JS, Dunnuck C, Rossman L, Wynn BN, Nelson-Horan C. Significance of toluidine blue positive findings after speculum examination for sexual assault. *Am J Emerg Med*. 2004;22:201-203.

20. McCauley J, Gorman RL, Guzinski G. Toluidine blue in the detection of perineal lacerations in pediatric and adolescent sexual abuse victims. *Pediatrics*. 1986;78:1039-1043.

21. McCauley J, Guzinski G, Welch R, Gorman R, Osmers F. Toluidine blue in the corroboration of rape in the adult victim. *Am J Emerg Med*. 1987;5:105-108.

22. Adams JA, Girardin B, Faugno D. Adolescent sexual assault: documentation of acute injuries using photo-colposcopy. *J Pediatr Adolesc Gynecol*. 2001;14:175-180.

23. Heppenstall-Heger A, McConnell G, Ticson L, Guerra L, Lister J, Zaragoza T. Healing patterns in anogenital injuries: a longitudinal study of injuries associated

with sexual abuse, accidental injuries, or genital surgery in the preadolescent child. *Pediatrics.* 2003;112:829-837.

24. Ricci L. Photodocumentation of the abused child. In: Reece R, Ludwig S, eds. *Child Abuse: Medical Diagnosis and Management.* 2nd ed. Philadelphia: Lippincott Williams & Wilkins; 2001.

25. Sommers MS, Fisher BS, Karjane HM. Using colposcopy in the rape exam: health care, forensic, and criminal justice issues. *J Forensic Nurs.* 2005;1:19, 28-34.

26. Teixeira WR. Hymenal colposcopic examination in sexual offenses. *Am J Forensic Med Pathol.* 1981;2:209-215.

27. Woodling BA, Heger A. The use of the colposcope in the diagnosis of sexual abuse in the pediatric age group. *Child Abuse Negl.* 1986;10:111-114.

28. Soules MR, Pollard AA, Brown K, Verma M. The forensic laboratory evaluation of evidence in alleged rape. *Am J Obstet Gynecol.* 1978;130:142-147.

29. Christian CW, Lavelle JM, De Jong AR, Loiselle J, Brenner L, Joffe M. Forensic evidence findings in prepubertal victims of sexual assault. *Pediatrics.* 2000;106(1 Pt 1):100-104.

30. Dahlke MB, Cooke C, Cunnane M, Chawla J, Lau P. Identification of semen in 500 patients seen because of rape. *Am J Clin Pathol.* 1977;68:740-746.

31. De Jong AR, Rose M. Legal proof of child sexual abuse in the absence of physical evidence. *Pediatrics.* 1991;88:506-511.

32. Palusci VJ, Cox EO, Shatz EM, Schultze JM. Urgent medical assessment after child sexual abuse. *Child Abuse Negl.* 2006;30:367-380.

33. Tilelli JA, Turek D, Jaffe AC. Sexual abuse of children: clinical findings and implications for management. *N Engl J Med.* 1980;302:319-323.

34. Young KL, Jones JG, Worthington T, Simpson P, Casey PH. Forensic laboratory evidence in sexually abused children and adolescents. *Arch Pediatr Adolesc Med.* 2006;160:585-588.

35. Exline DL, Smith FP, Drexler SG. Frequency of pubic hair transfer during sexual intercourse. *J Forensic Sci.* 1998;43:505-508.

36. National Commission on the Future of DNA Evidence. The future of forensic DNA testing: predictions of the Research and Development Working Group. Washington, DC: US Department of Justice, National Institute of Justice; 2000.

37. Nelson DG, Santucci KA. An alternate light source to detect semen. *Acad Emerg Med.* 2002;9:1045-1048.

38. Sweet DJ. Bitemark evidence: Human bitemarks: examination, recovery, and analysis. In: Bowers CM, Bell GL, eds. *Manual of Forensic Odontology.* Colorado Springs: American Society of Forensic Odontology; 1995.

39. Sweet D, Lorente JA, Valenzuela A, et al. PCR-based DNA typing of saliva stains recovered from human skin. *J Forensic Sci.* 1997;42:447-451.

40. Allard JE. The collection of data from findings in cases of sexual assault and the significance of spermatozoa on vaginal, anal and oral swabs. *Sci Justice.* 1997; 37:99-108.

41. Nicholson R. Vitality of spermatozoa in the endocervical canal. *Fertility and Sterility*. 1965;16:758-764.

42. Sharpe N. The significance of spermatozoa in victims of sexual offences. *Can Med Assoc J.* 1963;89:513-514.

43. Enos WF, Beyer JC. Spermatozoa in the anal canal and rectum and in the oral cavity of female rape victims. *J Forensic Sci*. 1978;23:231-233.

44. Annas GJ. Setting standards for the use of DNA-typing results in the courtroom— the state of the art. *N Engl J Med*. 1992;326:1641-1644.

45. Gill P, Jeffreys AJ, Werrett DJ. Forensic application of DNA "fingerprints." *Nature*. 1985;318:577-579.

46. Santucci KA, Nelson DG, McQuillen KK, Duffy SJ, Linakis JG. Wood's lamp utility in the identification of semen. *Pediatrics*.1999;104:1342-1344.

47. Gabby T, Winkleby MA, Boyce WT, Fisher DL, Lancaster A, Sensabaugh GF. Sexual abuse of children. The detection of semen on skin. *Am J Dis Child*. 1992;146:700-703.

48. Santucci KA, Hsiao AL. Advances in clinical forensic medicine. *Curr Opin Pediatr*. 2003;15:304-308.

49. Lincoln CA, McBride PM, Turbett GR, Garbin CD, MacDonald EJ. The use of an alternative light source to detect semen in clinical forensic medical practice. *J Clin Forensic Med*. 2006;13:215-218.

50. West M, Barsley RE, Frair J, Stewart W. Ultraviolet radiation and its role in wound pattern documentation. *J Forensic Sci*. 1992;37:1466-1479.

51. West MH, Barsley RE, Hall JE, et al. The detection and documentation of trace wound patterns by the use of an alternative light source. *J Forensic Sci*. 1992; 37:1480-1488.

52. Wawryk J, Odell M. Fluorescent identification of biological and other stains on skin by the use of alternative light sources. *J Clin Forensic Med*. 2005;12:296-301.

53. Centers for Disease Control and Prevention, Workowski KA, Berman SM. Sexually transmitted diseases treatment guidelines, 2006. *MMWR Recomm Rep*. 2006;55(RR-11):1-94. [erratum in: *MMWR Recomm Rep*. 2006 Sep 15;55 (36):997.]

54. Hindmarch I, ElSohly M, Gambles J, Salamone S. Forensic urinalysis of drug use in cases of sexual assault. *J Clin Forensic Med*. 2001;8:197-205.

55. Scott-Ham M, Burton FC. Toxicological findings in cases of alleged drug-facilitated sexual assault in the United Kingdom over a 3-year period. *J Clin Forensic Med*. 2005;12:175-186.

56. Li J, Stokes SA, Woeckener A. A tale of novel intoxication: seven cases of gamma-hydroxybutyric acid overdose. *Ann Emerg Med*. 1998;31:723-728.

57. Schwartz RH, Milteer R, LeBeau MA. Drug-facilitated sexual assault ("date rape"). *South Med J*. 2000;93:558-561.

58. Anglin D, Spears KL, Hutson HR. Flunitrazepam and its involvement in date or acquaintance rape. *Acad Emerg Med*. 1997;4:323-326.

59. Kintz P. Bioanalytical procedures for detection of chemical agents in hair in the case of drug-facilitated crimes. *Anal Bioanal Chem.* 2007;388:1467-1474.

60. Schwartz AJ, Ricci LR. How accurately can bruises be aged in abused children? Literature review and synthesis. *Pediatrics.* 1996;97:254-257.

61. Gray-Eurom K, Seaberg DC, Wears RL. The prosecution of sexual assault cases: correlation with forensic evidence. *Ann Emerg Med.* 2002;39:39-46.

62. Jones JS, Wynn BN, Kroeze B, Dunnuck C, Rossman L. Comparison of sexual assaults by strangers versus known assailants in a community-based population. *Am J Emerg Med.* 2004;22:454-459.

63. Riggs N, Houry D, Long G, et al. Analysis of 1076 cases of sexual assault. *Ann Emerg Med.* 2000;35:358-362.

64. Sugar NF, Fine DN, Eckert LO. Physical injury after sexual assault: findings of a large case series. *Am J Obstet Gynecol.* 2004;190:71-76.

65. Jones JS, Rossman L, Wynn BN, et al. Comparative analysis of adult versus adolescent sexual assault: epidemiology and patterns of anogenital injury. *Acad Emerg Med.* 2003;10:872-877.

66. Hilden M, Schei B, Sidenius K. Genitoanal injury in adult female victims of sexual assault. *Forensic Sci Int.* 2005;154:200-205.

67. Strickland JL. Adolescent acute sexual assault: contrasting with adult experiences. *Obstet Gynecol.* 2001;(4 Suppl 1):S6.

68. White C, McLean I. Adolescent complainants of sexual assault; injury patterns in virgin and non-virgin groups. *J Clin Forensic Med.* 2006;13:172-180.

69. Rossman L, Jones JS, Dunnuck C, et al. Genital trauma associated with forced digital penetration. *Am J Emerg Med.* 2004;22:101-104.

70. Fraser IS, Lähteenmäki P, Elomaa K, et al. Variations in vaginal epithelial surface appearance determined by colposcopic inspection in healthy, sexually active women. *Hum Reprod.* 1999;14:1974-1978.

71. Slaughter L, Brown CR, Crowley S, et al. Patterns of genital injury in female sexual assault victims. *Am J Obstet Gynecol.* 1997;176:609-616.

72. Jones JS, Rossman L, Hartman M, Alexander CC. Anogenital injuries in adolescents after consensual sexual intercourse. *Acad Emerg Med.* 2003;10:1378-1383.

73. Sachs CJ, Chu LD. Predictors of genitorectal injury in female victims of suspected sexual assault. *Acad Emerg Med.* 2002;9:146-151.

74. Ernst AA, Green E, Ferguson MT, et al. The utility of anoscopy and colposcopy in the evaluation of male sexual assault victims. *Ann Emerg Med.* 2000;36:432-437.

75. Arheart KL, Pretty IA. Results of the 4th ABFO Bitemark Workshop—1999. *Forensic Sci Int.* 2001;124:104-111.

76. Barsley RE. Forensic and legal issues in oral diagnosis. *Dent Clin North Am.* 1993;37:133-156.

77. Heger A, Ticson L, Velasquez O, et al. Children referred for possible sexual abuse: medical findings in 2384 children. *Child Abuse Negl.* 2002;26:645-659.

78. McCann J. The appearance of acute, healing, and healed anogenital trauma. *Child Abuse Negl.* 1998;22:605-622.

79. Adams JA, Kaplan RA, Starling SP, et al. Guidelines for medical care of children who may have been sexually abused. *J Pediatr Adolesc Gynecol.* 2007;20:163-172.

80. Berenson AB, Chacko MR, Wiemann CM, et al. A case-control study of anatomic changes resulting from sexual abuse. *Am J Obstet Gynecol.* 2000;182:820-834.

81. McCann J, Voris J. Perianal injuries resulting from sexual abuse: a longitudinal study. *Pediatrics.* 1993;91:390-397.

82. McCann J, Voris J, Simon M. Genital injuries resulting from sexual abuse: a longitudinal study. *Pediatrics.* 1992;89:307-317.

83. Jenny C, Hooton TM, Bowers A, et al. Sexually transmitted diseases in victims of rape. *N Engl J Med.* 1990;322:713-716.

84. Risser WL, Bortot AT, Benjamins LJ, et al. The epidemiology of sexually transmitted infections in adolescents. *Semin Pediatr Infect Dis.* 2005;16:160-167.

85. Schwarcz SK, Whittington WL. Sexual assault and sexually transmitted diseases: detection and management in adults and children. *Rev Infect Dis.* 1990;12(Suppl. 6):S682-S690.

86. Ingram DL, Everett VD, Lyna PR, et al. Epidemiology of adult sexually transmitted disease agents in children being evaluated for sexual abuse. *Pediatr Infect Dis J.* 1992;11:945-950.

87. Woods CR. Sexually transmitted diseases in prepubertal children: mechanisms of transmission, evaluation of sexually abused children, and exclusion of chronic perinatal viral infections. *Semin Pediatr Infect Dis.* 2005;16:317-325.

88. Silverman EM, Silverman AG. Persistence of spermatozoa in the lower genital tracts of women. *J Am Med Assoc.* 1978;240:1875-1877.

89. Muram D. Child sexual abuse: relationship between sexual acts and genital findings. *Child Abuse Negl.* 1989;13:211-216.

90. Tucker S, Claire E, Ledray LE, et al. Sexual assault evidence collection. *Wis Med J.* 1990;89:407-411.

91. Collins KA, Bennett AT. Persistence of spermatozoa and prostatic acid phosphatase in specimens from deceased individuals during varied postmortem intervals. *Am J Forensic Med Pathol.* 2001;22:228-232.

92. Ricci LR, Hoffman SA. Prostatic acid phosphatase and sperm in the post-coital vagina. *Ann Emerg Med.* 1982;11:530-534.

93. Paul DM. The medical examination in sexual offences against children. *Med Sci Law J.* 1977;17:251-258.

94. Graves HC, Sensabaugh GF, Blake ET. Postcoital detection of a male-specific semen protein. Application to the investigation of rape. *N Engl J Med.* 1985;312:338-343.

95. Keil W, Bachus J, Tröger HD. Evaluation of MHS-5 in detecting seminal fluid in vaginal swabs. *Int J Legal Med.* 1996;108:186-190.

96. Wickenheiser RA. Trace DNA: a review, discussion of theory, and application of the transfer of trace quantities of DNA through skin contact. *J Forensic Sci.* 2002;47 442-450.

97. Dziegelewski M, Simich JP, Rittenhouse-Olson K. Use of a Y chromosome probe as an aid in the forensic proof of sexual assault. *J Forensic Sci.* 2002;47:601-604.

98. Collins KA, Cina MS, Pettenati MJ, et al. Identification of female cells in postcoital penile swabs using fluorescence in situ hybridization. *Arch Pathol Lab Med.* 2000;124:1080-1082.

99. Taupin JM. Hair and fiber transfer in an abduction case—evidence from different levels of trace evidence transfer. *J Forensic Sci.* 1996;41:697-699.

100. Grieve MC, Wiggins KG. Fibers under fire: suggestions for improving their use to provide forensic evidence. *J Forensic Sci.* 2001;46:835-843.

101. Johnson CL, Giles RC, Warren JH, et al. Analysis of non-suspect samples lacking visually identifiable sperm using a Y-STR 10-plex. *J Forensic Sci.* 2005;50:1116-1118.

102. Sibille I, Duverneuil C, Lorin de la Grandmaison G, et al. Y-STR DNA amplification as biological evidence in sexually assaulted female victims with no cytological detection of spermatozoa. *Forensic Sci Int.* 2002;125:212-216.

103. Delfin FC, Madrid BJ, Tan MP, et al. Y-STR analysis for detection and objective confirmation of child sexual abuse. *Intl J Legal Med.* 2005;119:158-163.

104. National Academy of Science. The evaluation of forensic DNA evidence. Excerpt from the Executive Summary of the National Research Council Report. *Proc Natl Acad Sci USA.* 1997;94:5498-5500.

105. Enos WF, Conrath TB, Byer JC. Forensic evaluation of the sexually abused child. *Pediatrics.* 1986;78:385-398.

106. Rimsza ME, Niggemann EH. Medical evaluation of sexually abused children: a review of 311 cases. *Pediatrics.* 1982;69:8-14.

107. Spencer MJ, Dunklee P. Sexual abuse of boys. *Pediatrics.* 1986;78:133-138.

108. Tintinalli JE, Hoelzer M. Clinical findings and legal resolution in sexual assault. *Ann Emerg Med.* 1985;14:447-453.

109. Rambow B, Adkinson C, Frost TH, Peterson GF. Female sexual assault: medical and legal implications. *Ann Emerg Med.* 1992;21:727-731.

110. McGregor MJ, Du Mont J, Myhr TL. Sexual assault forensic medical examination: is evidence related to successful prosecution? *Ann Emerg Med.* 2002;39:639-647.

111. Wiley J, Sugar N, Fine D, Eckert LO. Legal outcomes of sexual assault. *Am J Obstet Gynecol.* 2003;188:1638-1641.

112. Cross TP, De Vos E, Whitcomb D. Prosecution of child sexual abuse: which cases are accepted? *Child Abuse Negl.* 1994;18:663-677.

113. Stroud DD, Martens SL, Barker J. Criminal investigation of child sexual abuse: a comparison of cases referred to the prosecutor to those not referred. *Child Abuse Negl.* 2000;24:689-700.

114. Brewer KD, Rowe DM, Brewer DD. Factors related to prosecution of child sexual abuse cases. *J Child Sexual Abuse.* 1997;6:91-111.

115. Kerns DL, Ritter ML. Medical findings in child sexual abuse cases with perpetrator confessions. *Am J Dis Child*. 1992;146:494.

116. Adams JA, Harper K, Knudson S, Revilla J. Examination findings in legally confirmed child sexual abuse: it's normal to be normal. *Pediatrics*. 1994;94:310-317.

117. Palusci VJ, Cox EO, Cyrus TA, et al. Medical assessment and legal outcome in child sexual abuse. *Arch Pediatr Adolesc Med*. 1999;153:388-392.

118. Centers for Disease Control and Prevention. Update to CDC's sexually transmitted diseases treatment guidelines, 2006: fluoroquinolones no longer recommended for treatment of gonococcal infections. *MMWR Morb Mortal Wkly Rep*. 2007;56:332-336.

119. Smith DK, Grohskopf LA, Black RJ, et al. Antiretroviral postexposure prophylaxis after sexual, injection-drug use, or other nonoccupational exposure to HIV in the United States: recommendations from the U.S. Department of Health and Human Services. *MMWR Recomm Rep*. 2005;54(RR-2):1-20.

120. Havens PL; American Academy of Pediatrics Committee on Pediatric AIDS. Postexposure prophylaxis in children and adolescents for nonoccupational exposure to human immunodeficiency virus. *Pediatrics*. 2003;111(6 Pt 1):1475-1489.

121. American Academy of Pediatrics Committee on Adolescence. Emergency contraception. *Pediatrics*. 2005;116:1026-1035.

122. Girardet R, Giacobbe L, Bolton K, et al. Unmet health care needs among children evaluated for sexual assault. *Arch Pediatr Adolesc Med*. 2006;160:70-73.

Chapter 12

DISTANCE LEARNING AND IMAGING TECHNOLOGY

Lori Frasier, MD
Kathi L. Makoroff, MD
Rich Kaplan, MSW, MD, FAAP

The following questions commonly face those who diagnose and treat children who have been sexually abused: (1) How does one overcome the relative isolation inherent in such a specialized practice? and (2) What is the optimal imaging technology for a given practice setting? It is incumbent upon medical providers to stay current in their fields. This is much more challenging in a field in which there are so few practitioners and only limited educational resources. Although there are several publications dedicated to scientific issues in child maltreatment, it is often extremely useful to supplement these journals with other educational materials. Many providers are in geographically isolated settings and are often unable to attend regional or national meetings focused on maltreatment. The first section of this chapter is dedicated to distance-learning strategies with the hope that an individual plan can be crafted from the various alternatives presented.

The second section of this chapter is dedicated to digital imaging technology. High-quality photographic imaging is a requisite for medical evaluations of sexual abuse. Accurate imaging has the potential to obviate the need for multiple examinations of an already traumatized child. Equally important is the ability to engage in peer review and mentoring activities—both of which are essential elements of any medical practice dealing with the medical evaluations of possible victims of sexual abuse. To that end, options for peer review and mentoring will also be presented.

DISTANCE LEARNING STRATEGIES

Distance learning or distance education is an area of education and instructional systems design that delivers learning opportunities to participants who are not necessarily in the same location. Through distance learning, participants can communicate in real time or staggered times. In a distance-learning scenario, participants can meet and they can also share printed materials and electronic media. Strategies for distance learning include Internet, or World Wide Web, conferencing; online learning tools; and videoconferencing.

These strategies have many advantages. Participants can have access to peers in different parts of the world, and users from diverse backgrounds can be brought together. Ideas are more readily shared. Time and money can be saved through distance learning, but the costs and time that need to be put into setting up systems are considerable.

Some strategies used for distance learning, such as Internet conferencing and video-conferencing, have applications beyond education; these uses extend to research collaboration, peer review, quality initiatives, and case-sharing.

INTERNET, OR WEB, CONFERENCING

Internet conferencing, also known as *Web conferencing*, can be used to hold meetings or presentations over the Internet. These meetings are held live and are therefore considered "synchronous"; that is, all the members of the meeting are seeing the same information at the same time. With a Web conference, each participant needs a computer. The meeting site is reached by either downloading an application or by accessing a Web site. Web seminars (also called *Webinars*) or Web broadcasts (also known as *Webcasts*) are a form of Web conferencing in which speakers are usually giving a lecture to an audience. A Webinar can take the form of a meeting, involving audience interaction, *pooling*, and question-and-answer features that are available with many of the Web-conferencing applications.

With some Web-conferencing applications, participants speak through their telephones or speakerphones over a standard telephone line. Some Web-conferencing technologies also incorporate the use of Voice over Internet Protocol (VoIP), which is an audio technology that transmits voice over the Internet; this alleviates the need for any external devices outside of the computer. One advantage of VoIP is that a cost savings is realized through the use of a single network to carry voice and data.

Some considerations in choosing conferencing software include price, technological support, and compatibility with other environments. Web-conferencing technologies can be used for many purposes such as peer review, lectures, visual presentations, case-sharing, mentoring, meetings, and quality initiatives. Researchers can collaborate with colleagues at other institutions.

Web-conferencing technologies carry many advantages. For instance, the Web offers a relatively inexpensive way to conference or to meet without having to travel. Only a computer or a computer and a telephone are needed. Technologically speaking, it is very easy to connect to a meeting; one need only download an application or connect to a Web site.

One consideration with the use of Web-conferencing technologies is maintaining privacy; after all, potentially sensitive information is being transmitted over the Internet. Web meetings should be password-protected so that only the invited members can join. Some Internet meeting sites will encrypt the Web meeting to add another layer of protection. There are also technological considerations such as institutional firewalls that could make joining an Internet meeting difficult.

ONLINE LEARNING TOOLS

Software applications and online applications that are designed to aid and enhance teaching and learning can be used as online learning tools. With these tools that are accessible through the Internet, teachers can design and build courses that can be used by students worldwide. The applications can be used to entirely teach a course online or to enhance or expand a "traditional" course. Online learning tools can also encourage learners to work together and to share ideas and projects. Many applications also have a testing system that would allow a pretest and posttest to be given along with a course or tutorial.

One advantage of online learning tools is that they can easily have a wide distribution. Some barriers include the cost and time to build a computer-based curriculum. Programmers and designers are often needed to build good programs, and they need to work with medical professionals. Once a course is built, course material needs to be updated as well.

Videoconferencing

Videoconferencing uses audio and visual telecommunication to bring people in different locations together. It differs from Internet, or Web, conferencing by the addition of video so the groups can actually see each other. Videoconferencing can include only 2 groups (ie, point-to-point), or it can involve several sites (ie, multipoint). The latter type of conferencing can accommodate large groups at the individual sites. Besides audio and video transmission of people's images and voices, videoconferencing can be used to share documents, pictures, videos, computer-displayed information, and whiteboards.

Videoconferencing can occur over digital telephone lines or Integrated Services Digital Network (ISDN) lines, or can occur over the Internet, referred to as *Internet Protocol (IP) lines*. The use of ISDN lines may give better video quality than the use of IP lines because the quality of the IP line transmission may depend on the amount of Internet traffic. However, the use of ISDN technology is costlier than the use of IP lines.

Videoconferencing has many potential uses. Point-to-point meetings can be set up for research meetings and for mentoring purposes. Researchers can collaborate with colleagues at other institutions on a regular basis without the loss of time or the expense of travel. Educational forums and meetings that integrate guest lecturers, conferences, case-sharing, and literature reviews can be held. Images and videos can be shared among many different sites and institutions as a form of peer review. Quality initiatives involving patient care or research can more readily occur among different groups and institutions. Videoconferencing also allows groups from all over the world to come together to share information. It is also a particularly important tool for smaller programs and for programs that are geographically isolated.

If videoconferencing is used to share cases, patient privacy must always be at the forefront of choosing a type of videoconferencing system. Greater security is achieved by using ISDN technology, but some videoconferencing devices use encryption on the outgoing information, which makes either technique secure.

One advantage to the use of videoconferencing is that medical professionals get to see the other parties. For some, this adds greatly to the experience, almost like being in the same room. The quality of this experience will depend on the quality of the equipment used. Room layouts, cameras, and lighting at the individual sites will also affect the quality. The use of videoconferencing can reduce travel time and the costs associated with travel. It can also allow a greater number of meetings to take place because time and costs are reduced. In addition, it can increase collaboration, sharing, and quality initiatives.

A disadvantage of videoconferencing is the cost of the systems. The use of IP technology will cost less than the use of ISDN technology, but the money saved by not having to travel may make videoconferencing a less-expensive alternative. However, videoconferencing is costlier than communicating by Internet, or Web, conferencing because each site needs to purchase a system, and, in the case of ISDN lines, there is a monthly rental fee as well as a per-call fee. Another disadvantage of videoconferencing is that it requires a great deal of technical support, at least initially, to set up the system.

Digital Imaging

Documentation of physical findings in child abuse through photography has long been a standard practice. Images are especially important from a medicolegal point of view in child physical abuse cases or when such images demonstrate specific genital injuries. In child sexual abuse cases, the colposcope, which was adapted from gynecologic applications, was the initial device used for the documentation of genital images. The colposcope basically provided an excellent light source, magnification, and a stable base for a camera. Attached to colposcopes were 35-mm cameras, followed by video cameras, connected through the optics of the scope. Computer capture devices were used to digitize a single frame of an analog video image. Telephone consulting (teleconsulting) was accomplished by using telephone lines to transfer an image directly from computer to computer via modem. The Picasso Still Image Phone by AT&T was one of the first devices to connect to colposcopes for image transfer. However, each user had to have this device in order for images to be transferred or received. The rapid expansion of the Internet, initially through institutional networks, then through dial-up connections from more remote sites, facilitated the ability to transfer images. High-speed Internet access from nearly anywhere, via broadband or Digital Subscriber Line (DSL), added ease and rapidity to this process. Two companies, Second Opinion Software, LLC— makers of Second Opinion Software—and CooperSurgical/Leisegang, makers of the ImageQUEST Digital Imaging System, developed proprietary software that captured analog video and integrated it directly into their programs. The images could be sent initially "modem-to-modem" over telephone lines and eventually as encrypted electronic-mail (e-mail) attachments. The encryption required that each user have the same or a compatible version of the proprietary software. The captured images could be printed digitally and stored on either secure networks or the hard drive of an individual computer. Such images were of significantly lower resolution than a 35-mm print or slide film. As digital cameras advanced, images could be captured directly as a digital file rather than through converting analog video into digital files.

The first digital cameras provided rather low resolution images. The resolution of a digital image is often described in terms of pixels. The word *pixel* was taken from the phrase "pix [an abbreviation for "pictures"] element" and is now the term used to define the smallest piece of information in a digital image. Pixels are normally arranged in a two-dimensional grid. The more pixels that are used to represent an image, the closer the result will resemble the original. For example, an image that is displayed as 640 pixels by 480 pixels on a display is a 307 200-pixel image (approximately 0.3 megapixels). This is called the resolution of an image. These early digital images of less than 1-megapixel resolution appear adequate at 3 inches–by–5 inches medium, but as the image is expanded, the digital information becomes spread out into small squares representing each pixel and is therefore "pixelated." In the late 1990s, digital still-camera technology allowed the capture of images of increasingly higher resolution. Consumer cameras that capture 10 million pixels per image (10 megapixels) are common and economical today. Digital still cameras were quickly adapted for use with colposcopes. Newer, single-lens reflex (SLR) cameras could be directly attached to the scope, whereas in the past, a 35-mm camera had been used. High-resolution digital images, from colposcopes or freestanding cameras, have become standard for image capture. These images lend themselves to rapid electronic transfer through e-mail, proprietary "store and forward" programs, or Web-based programs, where images are uploaded to a secure server for storing, accessing, and consultative viewing.

DIGITAL VIDEO

Digital video (DV), or the ability to capture the video signal and process it directly into a digital format, became commercially available in 1986, but because of its expense it was used mostly by large television networks. Consumer DV appeared in a crude form in approximately 1990 with Apple Inc.'s QuickTime multimedia software, but the footage derived from this software was of poor resolution and necessitated significant computer knowledge to upload and edit. The first commercially available playback standards were compression methodologies by the Moving Pictures Experts Group (MPEG), known as MPEG-1 and MPEG-2, followed by DV tape format. This allowed for recording directly to digital data and simplified the editing process. Most clinicians preferred analog video, especially when captured in Super–Video Home System (S-VHS) format and found it far superior to any DV capture available at the time. It was not until the early 2000s that the capture of genital images directly with DV recording devices came into clinical use. As these devices improved in resolution and became less expensive, clinicians began to recognize that a high-quality digital image, video or still, could be obtained without the use of a colposcope. As zoom capabilities also improved on consumer cameras, the magnification required to see important anatomic and traumatic findings began to satisfy most examiners. DV technology has been enhanced through the advent of high-definition (HD) video, which generally refers to any video system taking advantage of resolutions higher than that of standard definition (SD) video, or 420 vertical lines. The display resolutions common for HD video are as follow: 1280 horizontal by 720 vertical lines or 1920 horizontal by 1080 vertical lines. One important factor is that the monitor must also be HD-compatible for such images to be viewed in optimum resolution. Many computer monitors are capable of HD resolution. Optical systems found on colposcopes may provide better true magnification of a finding; however, DV and high-resolution still images can be more than adequate, with nearly colposcopic quality. The examiner must pay attention to camera stability and have adequate lighting to obtain acceptable images. Many resourceful examiners have adapted still-photography tripods and other types of stands and mounts to assist in this area.

Because it consists of thousands of image frames of images, DV is very data-intensive. In its raw form, HD video will consume huge amounts of computer memory and be difficult to transmit via most network or high-speed Internet connections. Video-editing software can be used to limit the video size or capture individual frames as still images, but its use requires specialized computer skills. Many new HD DV camcorders also have the ability to capture 5- to 10-megapixel still images, save them onto standard memory devices, and easily upload them onto a computer.

Storage of any type of digital images should be carefully considered. Ideally, images and video are stored on a networked server that is backed up on a daily basis. Restricting access of images to those have a clinical need to have access is important. Storage on optical media or secure external hard drives may be an alternative for those without extensive network support.

Traditional colposcopy with a 35-mm SLR camera allowed examiners to obtain photographic findings and either seek consultation by sending prints or slides of their patient through the mail or by convening at meetings to discuss cases. The ability to send high-quality digital images rapidly and securely has revolutionized peer review of cases. As electronic communication has advanced, concerns about the security of protected health information and sensitive images have also increased. These concerns are acutely felt in the field of child abuse, where the capture of highly sensitive genital images is standard practice. Many hospitals and other large institutions with well-developed information technology (IT) departments have established protocols and guidelines for the use and transmission of such information. The US Health Insurance Portability and Accountability Act (HIPAA) has added additional protections to such information. For example, HIPAA now requires that technical security services be implemented to guard data integrity, confidentiality, and availability.

E-MAIL ATTACHMENTS

Attachments of images with identifiable information sent by e-mail may not be secure, and such e-mail may require protected health information (PHI) safeguards under HIPAA. Many institutions have instituted a PHI policy with regard to tele-communications such that when the word *PHI* is placed into the subject line of an e-mail, the e-mail server automatically encrypts that e-mail, which requires the recipient to be an internal user of the network or to log into a secure Web portal that allows the viewing of the e-mail. However, smaller entities such as satellite offices of the National Children's Advocacy Center and independent clinics may not have this level of security available and will instead prohibit PHI from being included in any e-mail message. It is unadvisable to routinely use nonencrypted e-mail systems for reviewing child abuse images. Any identifiable patient information should be carefully stripped from images, if they are to be sent in this manner.

PROPRIETARY SOFTWARE PROGRAMS

As mentioned previously, there are already established proprietary software programs that capture images in encrypted formats. Only computers with the specific programs can open these images. For teleconsulting, this requires that both parties involved in the consultative process have access to the same or a compatible version of the program. Such programs often come as bundled packages (eg, a colposcope, camera, computer, and the software). A user who is not technologically adept may find such programs useful if they have limited IT support. Second Opinion and ImageQUEST are two such commercially available programs that are HIPAA-compliant.

WEB-BASED PROGRAMS

The concept of Internet-based applications is not new, but the term Web 2.0, coined by O'Reilly Media, describes how the World Wide Web enhances collaboration among users. Applications that allow image-sharing and collaboration via a secure Internet-based server are examples of Web-based technology. Teleconsulting in Child Abuse Medicine (TeleCAM) by VisualShare is a commercially available application that allows real-time or staggered collaboration around images and clinical information. One major advantage to this form of collaboration is that neither the program nor the images reside on any individual computer. In addition, an administrator familiar with the users controls access to the program, and data about each interaction can be collected and analyzed. The server can be accessed via a virtual private network (VPN) or reside within a secure server center that uses a standard uniform resource locator (URL) and is password-protected. TeleCAM was designed for health care applications and was built to be HIPAA-compliant. TeleCAM also accepts any standard digitally formatted images (video and still), regardless of the device or camera used to capture images. All that is required to use such a program is a computer with Internet access and uploadable digital images. A new program has been initiated using TeleCAM technology. The TeleHealth Institute for Child Maltreatment (THICM) is a peer review program using VisualShare technology, which allows for anonymous peer review regardless of provider location. For more information, one can access http://www.thicm.org.

Clinicians considering any program or application should choose based upon their technical skills and needs. The following represent some considerations:

— How shall the program be used? Shall it be used for archiving and storing images, case collaborations, or peer reviews only?

— What level of technological skill is required to use the program?

— How cost-efficient is the program (ie, number of cases)?

— What technical support is provided by the company that sells the program?

— What is the policy regarding program upgrades?

— Is there adequate initial training for users of the program?

— Is the manual for end-users easy to understand? Is it electronic or printed? Is it available on the Internet?

Many applications and programs have been purchased with enthusiasm only to remain unused because of lack of technical skill or because the product does not meet the needs of the end-users. The main purpose of any program is to help the medical professional work efficiently and competently. This includes making accurate diagnoses in a timely manner. Obtaining second opinions and the peer review of images are only pieces of the whole body of clinical work, yet they become exceedingly important if medical professionals have limited experience or training or if they are geographically remote from higher levels of expertise. The process of capturing images, reviewing them, reaccessing them, and obtaining assistance in the interpretation of findings should not be overly difficult or time-consuming. Any program that is being considered should have a demonstration (demo) version with which medical professionals can practice to determine whether it meets their clinical and technological needs. Careful research and understanding of one's own specific clinical needs will result in more satisfaction with any program or application. The ultimate goals are to facilitate clinical efficiency and to integrate technology seamlessly into the workflow.

Chapter 13

DEVELOPING STANDARDS FOR EDUCATION AND QUALIFICATIONS OF THE CHILD SEXUAL ABUSE MEDICAL EXAMINER

Suzanne P. Starling, MD, FAAP

Child abuse medicine is a highly integrated discipline requiring the ability to identify or exclude abuse as well as knowledge of the social and legal aspects of abuse. A diagnosis of child abuse is multifaceted. Child abuse affects the child's health and may impact the child's social situation as well. Following a diagnosis of child abuse, the child and family may have interactions with social services, police, and the legal system. A medical finding of abuse may lead to the incarceration of a family member and disruption of the child's family life. An error may lead to prosecution of an innocent person. Failure to make a correct diagnosis of abuse may leave the child in an unsafe environment and potentially place other children at risk. An accurate medical evaluation is critical to the well-being of the child and the multidisciplinary assessment of child abuse.

Child sexual abuse examiners come from a diverse group of medical practitioners and bring with them the views and values of their fields. All of the examiners, regardless of training and expertise, share a common goal: an accurate assessment and diagnosis capable of meeting both the needs of the child and requirements of the legal system. Physicians, nurse practitioners (NPs), physician assistants (PAs), and nurses bring different skill levels and training to the examination room. Within the different fields, a great diversity of expertise is found. Although each examiner has varying levels of expertise, it is imperative that consistent and accurate knowledge and abilities are developed and maintained by all examiners.

Medical providers who examine children for suspected sexual abuse must be well trained, knowledgeable, and comfortable performing a specialized genital examination. They must be astute at diagnosing findings related to abuse and findings that only mimic abuse. Each of the many medical disciplines involved in the medical evaluation of child abuse has different training and skills. As of 2008, no national consensus exists on the appropriate levels of training for medical providers examining children for suspected sexual abuse. This important examination should be provided by the most qualified person available; however, a clear idea of what constitutes medically qualified for such a diverse group of providers is not well defined.

As the field of child abuse medicine has matured, many researchers have studied how medical providers' training and experience have affected the diagnostic process. In

1987, Ladson and colleagues surveyed pediatricians and family practitioners who were asked to identify genital structures on a photograph of female genitalia.[1] Only 59% of the physicians could correctly identify the hymen on the photograph. In a follow-up study published in 2000, Lentsch, using the same photograph, surveyed 166 pediatricians, family practitioners, and emergency medicine physicians.[2] Only 61.7% of physicians correctly identified the hymen. When shown a photograph of a hymen with normal findings, 64% of the physicians believed the photograph depicted abnormal findings and 62% believed the photograph depicted signs of possible sexual abuse, even in the absence of a history concerning for abuse. The authors specifically noted that physicians seeing more than 25 patients per week for sexual allegations were more likely to correctly identify genital structures, highlighting the importance of clinical experience in the diagnostic process. A subsequent study of NPs yielded similar results: less than 60% of NPs could correctly identify 2 genital structures (the hymen and vaginal opening) on a photograph.[3]

Many authors have studied examiner agreement on physical examination findings. In 1993, Adams showed 170 colposcopic photographs to examiners who were blinded to the history of the allegation.[4] Examiners with more experience (based on the number of cases an examiner had seen in a month) agreed more with the expert than those examiners with less experience. The less-experienced examiners overstated the findings more often, diagnosing a normal examination as an abnormal one. Similarly, in 1997, Paradise and colleagues measured diagnostic agreement among physicians who identified themselves as skilled in child sexual abuse examinations, and compared their opinions to those of an expert panel.[5] The opinions of the physicians with the most experience resembled those of the experts more closely than did the opinions of the less-experienced physicians. In a subsequent study, Paradise and colleagues found that the history could influence the examination findings of less-experienced physicians.[6] Inexperienced physicians asked to evaluate a photograph depicting normal findings accompanied by a normal history diagnosed the examination as normal. However, when later presented with the same photograph coupled with a history of trauma, they would often reinterpret the examination as abnormal, reflecting the history. In 2002, Makoroff and colleagues studied the diagnostic accuracy of emergency medicine physicians.[7] They found that in 79% of the female genital examinations diagnosed as abnormal and indicative of sexual abuse by pediatric emergency medicine physicians, 70% were diagnosed as normal and another 9% as nonspecific when reviewed by physicians trained in child abuse.

Diagnostic acumen in child abuse can be a reflection of the decade during which a physician trained. Child sexual abuse research did not become prevalent until the late 1980s. Physicians trained during or before that time who have not had updated training may be basing their knowledge on obsolete and incorrect information. It may be assumed that more recently trained physicians would be better trained, more comfortable, and more knowledgeable about sexual abuse. Dubow and colleagues tested this assumption in 2005 by surveying all the pediatric chief residents in the United States to determine their ability to recognize prepubertal female anatomy. They found that 30% incorrectly identified the hymen on a photograph. These chief residents indicated that the child sexual abuse training in their residencies varied widely. Half felt their training was inadequate; however, the authors did not correlate the amount of training with the residents' scores. A 2006 national study of residents' child abuse training, knowledge, and comfort found that only 13% of residents could identify 3 genital structures (the hymen, labia minora, and urethra) on a photograph.[8] Residents in that study also reported that they were uncomfortable performing a genital examination. As seen in earlier studies, increased training and increased patient exposure led to higher comfort levels and higher knowledge scores in these residents.

The conclusion that must be drawn from the summary of the literature to date is that the majority of medical providers remain inadequately trained to examine children for sexual abuse. Although research has identified pediatricians as the best trained and most experienced in examinations, they still are not well trained. Many examiners are unfamiliar with prepubertal genital anatomy and the range of anatomic findings that can be considered normal. An untrained or undertrained medical provider should not provide an expert opinion in a case of child sexual abuse. Inexperienced examiners tend to overstate positive examination findings, which can lead to inappropriate legal consequences in the investigation of potential child abuse. A national call to action to identify the requisite knowledge and skills of the trained examiner and to improve the education and qualifications of medical providers in the evaluation of child sexual abuse is needed.

PURPOSE OF THE MEDICAL EXAMINATION FOR SEXUAL ABUSE

The purposes of a medical examination for sexual abuse should be clearly delineated in order to determine the qualifications for the examiner. Although collection of evidence necessary for a legal proceeding may be one goal of the examination, issues related to the child's well-being and safety are of primary importance.

The health care provider must help ensure the safety and well-being of the child. An appropriate diagnosis can assist in the adjudication of a civil or criminal court case and the protection of the child. Assessment of the child for developmental, emotional, or behavioral concerns may reveal the need for further evaluation and treatment. In addition, the child and family may benefit psychologically from assurance that the child's examination findings are normal. Referrals for appropriate mental health counseling, if not in place, can be initiated by the medical provider.

The medical provider should be able to fully diagnose, document, and address medical conditions resulting from abuse. When an abnormal finding is present, the family can be assured that it will heal and can be advised of any further medical treatment that may be necessary. An examiner must differentiate medical findings indicative of abuse from those that may be explained by other medical conditions or injuries. Conditions such as urethral prolapse, lichen sclerosus, or genital hemangiomas may be mistaken for abuse by an inexperienced examiner.[9] Accidental mechanisms such as straddle injuries also may be mistaken for abuse and must be diagnosed and appropriately treated. Untrained examiners may make 2 types of diagnostic errors. First, physical findings may be misinterpreted, eg, an examiner may see a case of lichen sclerosis and misdiagnose it as sexual trauma. Another diagnostic error occurs when examiners overlook findings that may be diagnostic. Providers who cannot identify a hymen on a photograph will not be able to identify injury to a hymen.

The provider must also be able to diagnose, document, and address health conditions unrelated to abuse. Many children have limited contact with health care providers after infancy and may not have had recent contact. At the time of their examinations they may have unmet health needs. Children arrive in child sexual abuse clinics with serious untreated heart conditions, undiagnosed diabetes and other endocrine disorders, and dermatologic problems needing immediate referrals. The provider should be able to assess the health needs of the child and make referrals as necessary. Linkage to a tertiary care center or specialized medical assessment facility allows isolated examiners and those with less training in general pediatric diagnosis to properly care for these children.

Often the most important aspect of the child sexual abuse evaluation is the history. A health care provider may be the first professional a child has contact with after a disclosure of sexual abuse. Some children may share a special bond with a health care provider and may disclose information to the provider that they might not share with investigators. Although all health care providers learn diagnostic history taking in their general training, interviewing a child for suspected sexual abuse requires specific skills and knowledge not normally possessed by a nontrained provider. The provider must have the ability to gather a history that is both forensically sensitive and medically relevant. Untrained examiners may mistakenly ask leading questions or misinterpret a child's statements. Formal training in interviewing in suspected child sexual abuse cases is recommended.[10,11]

The history provided by the patient and family should be documented in direct quotations whenever possible. An accurate history and diagnosis must be accompanied by detailed documentation. A health care provider must document the history, physical examination findings, and interpretation of the examination accurately and in detail. This type of documentation can be learned from extensive training and from mentors. Comfort with this level of documentation usually develops over time.

Another aspect of documentation in child abuse cases is photodocumentation. Examination findings should be captured photographically for peer review, second opinion consultation, and potential use by the court system. An examiner should remain open to the scrutiny involved in peer review of photographs. The ability to obtain still or video images is mandatory. Photographic systems vary widely; although photographic technique can be learned in a training session, ongoing experience with the equipment is necessary to adequately obtain high-quality documentation of examination findings. The examiner must have policies in place for safe storage and distribution of the images.

A health care provider must interact effectively within a multidisciplinary team. The examiner will be a member of a team that may consist of law enforcement, child protective services, prosecutors, and mental health providers. Accurate and timely information must be conveyed to other professionals to assist in the protection of the child and/or the adjudication of a criminal proceeding. The provider should be willing to share information and cooperate with various agencies to provide the best outcome for a child. Often the health care provider will provide court testimony regarding the medical findings. As with many of the skills necessary for child abuse evaluations, the more experience an examiner has testifying in court, the more comfortable the process becomes. The multidisciplinary team is discussed in more detail in Chapter 15.

Children who are victims of sexual abuse may also be victims of physical abuse and neglect. Although physicians, NPs, and PAs typically are trained to evaluate all aspects of the medical care of a child, most nurses who are trained as sexual assault examiners are trained to evaluate only acute sexual assault. Such providers will need written procedures for medical intervention when there are physical injuries present or when a child needs a referral for emergency medical care.

WHO EXAMINES CHILDREN FOR SEXUAL ABUSE?

Many different medical disciplines are involved in the evaluation of child sexual abuse. The examiner may be a physician, a NP, PA, or sexual assault nurse examiner (SANE). The training and experiences of each of these groups vary.

There is no national standard for training medical residents in child abuse. Physicians often have little, if any, exposure to abuse training in their residencies. Even programs that offer educational rotations and education in sexual abuse may not offer acute sexual assault training to students and residents. Pediatricians receive the most training on abuse-related topics, but they are still undertrained.[8,12] Other physicians such as gynecologists, emergency medicine physicians, and family medicine physicians who may see child sexual abuse victims may receive little, if any, training in sexual assault and abuse of children.

The American Board of Pediatrics (ABP) established the subboard of Child Abuse Pediatrics in 2006. Prior to the availability of fellowship training, physicians were largely self-trained, and their expertise was dependent upon their years of experience in the field. It was only in the early 1990s that fellowship training in child abuse became widely available as a means to obtain expertise in the field. As the process has developed, pediatricians will be able to become board certified in this subspecialty beginning in 2009. Although many physicians will elect to continue to evaluate child abuse without subspecialty certification, all eligible pediatricians who wish to become board certified will be required to apply to the ABP to sit for the Child Abuse Pediatrics certifying examination. After an initial grandfathering period ends in 2013, fellowship training will become the entry point for all pediatricians desiring to specialize in the field. The curricula across the training programs will be more standardized as the Accreditation Council for Graduate Medical Education accredits qualified programs offering 3-year fellowships in Child Abuse Pediatrics.

Training for providers other than pediatricians varies widely. Physicians in other fields such as emergency medicine, family medicine, or gynecology, although they may practice in the field of child abuse, are not eligible to be certified through the ABP. As of 2008, no medical specialty other than pediatrics has formal subspecialty certification in child abuse.

Practitioners other than physicians are active in the field of child abuse. Physician assistants may specialize in pediatrics, but as of 2008 there is no formal certification process for PAs to specialize in child abuse. Training can be obtained under the guidance of an experienced mentor, and typically the PA will work closely with an experienced child abuse physician to further refine skills and develop expertise. Similarly, although NPs may specialize in pediatrics, no child abuse certification specifically for NPs is available as of 2008. Nurse practitioners are required to practice with a medical director, and most who specialize in child abuse work closely with a child abuse physician.

Sexual assault nurse examiners may be advanced- or nonadvanced-degree nurses. Since nursing school curricula do not cover sexual assault in great detail, nurses must seek additional training. Registered nurses may be trained and certified both in adult/adolescent assault as well as pediatric assault evaluation in courses that range from a few days to several weeks in length. The International Association of Forensic Nurses offers nurses certification in sexual assault nursing and outlines the clinical training and the hours of patient contact needed to receive the certificate. Although ongoing patient contact and continuing education is necessary to maintain skills, no national governing body monitors the quality of the training or continuing education of nurses. Because the training times for SANEs can be as little as a few days, SANEs should seek the most qualified medical director available to them.

TRAINING AND EDUCATION

Since 2002 there has been a national consensus effort to establish standards for training and education of child abuse professionals. In 2006, a group of expert pediatricians and nurses met in Ely, Minnesota, to establish the minimum standards for child sexual abuse examinations.[13] In attempting to develop minimum standards, this consensus group recommended that a health care provider should have a minimum of 16 hours of formal competency-based medical training in child sexual abuse evaluation taught by experts in the field. However, 16 hours of training is not enough to make a provider an expert in the field of child sexual abuse, and may not be sufficient to make an examiner comfortable with the evaluation. In order to become more competent and comfortable, examiners need to pursue more intensive courses taught over a longer period. These courses may include hands-on experience with patients as well as intensive didactic presentations. Since remaining up-to-date is important in any specialty, ongoing training and more patient contact make an examiner more comfortable with the subject.[2,4,8]

As the field of child abuse pediatrics grows, and as research continues to show the inadequacy of resident training in abuse, efforts toward standardized curriculum for pediatric residency training are beginning to emerge. Similarly, pediatric fellowships are developing standardized curricula, ensuring that fellowship-trained pediatricians enter the field with a well-defined knowledge base. However, these education efforts will be directed primarily at pediatricians, not at the family doctors, emergency physicians, and gynecologists also involved in the evaluation of these children. Given the diversity of professionals who provide child abuse examinations, these efforts to train pediatricians will not be sufficient.

Most medical skills and knowledge require long-term commitment to develop and maintain. A health care provider who does not see sexual abuse cases on a regular basis may not be able to maintain a comfort level with the examination process. The inexperienced and/or low-volume examiner needs access in many instances to an expert second medical opinion. Since inexperienced examiners are more likely to make a diagnostic error suggesting that a finding is present when it is not, second opinions should be obtained in cases where a medical finding diagnostic of sexual abuse is being considered.[7,8]

EXPERTS

For the courts, an expert is defined as someone who is qualified through expertise, training, and special knowledge regarding a subject. What qualifies an expert in a courtroom is not what qualifies an expert in the examination room. Although physicians are readily acknowledged as experts in the interpretation of human physical and physiological processes, there is tremendous variability in their knowledge in any specific area. An expert general pediatrician or family physician may have limited training or knowledge of child sexual abuse.

An expert medical consultant in child sexual abuse is generally a physician, PA, or NP with considerable experience in the medical evaluation and photodocumentation of children suspected of being abused. This person ideally should be involved in scholarly pursuits in the field of child sexual abuse, including conducting original research studies, publishing, and speaking at regional or national conferences on topics involving the medical evaluation of children with suspected abuse. Experts typically have a large clinical practice and often practice at academic medical centers. Their medical knowledge base is broad and encompasses all aspects of sexual abuse including evaluation of chronic cases and knowledge of the differential diagnosis of mimics of abuse.

In many cases the qualifications of an NP or other provider may exceed the qualifications of local physicians, and the most qualified expert in the area may not be a physician. SANEs, although experts in sexual assault nursing, may have very little training in or knowledge of broader aspects of nonacute sexual abuse and evaluation of nonabuse-related medical concerns. Nonadvanced practice nurses also may be limited in the scope of their practice by their state Nurse Practice Acts. SANEs should practice with a qualified expert medical director.

Every medical provider, regardless of expertise, should have a method for oversight and review in order to increase accuracy and validity of findings and ensure continued refinement of skills. Some professional settings will have expert examiners as full- or part-time staff. In these settings, internal review among all the medical providers can play an important role in the quality review process as well as the continuing education of the providers. Some programs must obtain this expertise through affiliation with local hospitals or other facilities. Programs in smaller or more rural communities may not have direct access to qualified examiners and may develop mentoring or consultative relationships with experts in other communities. The use of telemedicine technologies can play a valuable role in this form of consultation.

Programs with geographically isolated examiners, programs with inexperienced examiners, and nonadvanced practice SANE programs should have a system in place for continuing review. At a minimum, these examiners should seek secondary review of all cases considered to be abnormal or diagnostic of abuse. The ongoing mentorship of an expert is beneficial and provides both support and ongoing education to the more inexperienced examiner. The Ely, Minnesota, consensus group has plans to establish and disseminate a national resource for mentoring and peer review that will assist isolated examiners in establishing a mentorship with national experts.

ONGOING EDUCATION

The field of child sexual abuse medicine is evolving and knowledge can quickly become obsolete. The examiner should obtain continuing education on a routine basis in order to stay abreast of new developments. A health care provider who trained many years ago may have incomplete or inaccurate knowledge and need an update to remain current and consistent with standards of best practice. Dedication to remaining current in the field is mandatory to maintain a current knowledge base. Minimum national standards have not been developed, but the Ely, Minnesota, consensus group has suggested a minimum of 3 hours of continuing education specific to child sexual abuse every 2 years.[13] These minimum education requirements will provide a foundation on which to expand and reinforce knowledge, but this is not adequate to maintain expertise in child sexual abuse. It is mandatory for health care providers to interact with local and national experts in order to become apprised of updates in the field. In addition to this formal continuing education, providers should be able to demonstrate that they have kept up-to-date with published research studies on findings in abused and nonabused children as well as sexual transmission of infections in children. Current guidelines and recommendations for the evaluation of sexually abused children are available from national professional organizations such as the American Academy of Pediatrics and the Centers for Disease Control and Prevention.

CONCLUSION

There are a variety of health care professionals trained to examine children for sexual abuse, each with individual training and talents in the field. It is imperative to continue to strive for the best-educated, most-qualified, and best-trained individuals to provide medical services to child victims of abuse. Examinations by unqualified professionals are a disservice to both the children and their families. Although communities differ in the types of professionals they have in place, the common goal is the health and well-being of the children. To that end, national standards are necessary to ensure abused children receive the quality of care they deserve.

REFERENCES

1. Ladson S, Johnson CF, Doty RE. Do physicians recognize sexual abuse? *Am J Dis Child.* 1987;141(4):411-415.

2. Lentsch KA, Johnson CF. Do physicians have adequate knowledge of child sexual abuse? The results of two surveys of practicing physicians, 1986 and 1996. *Child Maltreat.* 2000;5(1):72-78.

3. Hornor G, McCleery J. Do pediatric nurse practitioners recognize sexual abuse? *J Pediatr Health Care.* 2000;14(2):45-49.

4. Adams JA, Wells R. Normal versus abnormal genital findings in children: how well do examiners agree? *Child Abuse Negl.* 1993;17(5):663-675.

5. Paradise JE, Finkel MA, Beiser AS, Berenson AB, Greenberg DB, Winter MR. Assessments of girl's genital findings and the likelihood of sexual abuse: agreement among physicians self-rated as skilled. *Arch Pediatr Adolesc Med.* 1997;151(9):883-891.

6. Paradise JE, Winter MR, Finkel MA, Berenson AB, Beiser AS. Influence of the history on physicians' interpretations of girls' genital findings. *Pediatrics.* 1999; 103(5):980-986.

7. Makoroff KL, Brauley JL, Brandner AM, Myers PA, Shapiro RA. Genital examinations for alleged sexual abuse of prepubertal girls: findings by pediatric emergency medicine physicians compared with child abuse trained physicians. *Child Abuse Negl.* 2002;26(12):1235-1242.

8. Heisler KW, Starling SP, Edwards H, Paulson JF. Child abuse training, comfort, and knowledge among emergency medicine, family medicine and pediatric residents. *Med Educ Online* [serial online]. 2006;11. Available at: www.med-ed-online.org/pdf/Res00202.pdf. Accessed March 1, 2010.

9. Bernard D, Peters M, Makaroff K. The evaluation of suspected pediatric sexual abuse. *Clin Pediatr Emerg Med.* 2006;7:161-169.

10. Cronch LE, Viljoen JL, Hansen DJ. Forensic interviewing in child sexual abuse cases: current techniques and future directions. *Aggression and Violent Behav.* 2006;11:195-207.

11. Westcott HL, Kynan S. Interviewer practice in investigative interviews for suspected child sexual abuse. *Psychol Crime Law.* 2006;12(4):367-382.

12. Dubow SR, Giardino AP, Christian CW, Johnson CF. Do pediatric chief residents recognize details of prepubertal female genital anatomy: a national survey. *Child Abuse Negl.* 2005;29(2):195-205.

13. The 2006 Ely National Consensus Conference on Medical Care for the Possible Victim of Child Sexual Abuse- written report submitted to the NCA. Ely, MN: Medical Standards Consensus Group; 2006.

Chapter 14

COLLABORATIVE PRACTICE AND PEDIATRIC CARE

Robert W. Block, MD, FAAP
Kathy Bell, MS, RN, SANE-A, SANE-P

There have been significant advances in best practice guidelines for performing health assessments for children who may have been sexually abused. In 1975, Sgroi described child sexual abuse as the "last frontier in child abuse."[1] In 1989, Year Book Medical Publishers released the first pictorial Color Atlas of Child Sexual Abuse.[2] By 1990 an increasing number of physicians were trained or experienced in child sexual abuse examinations. Heger reported that, "The true value of the medical examination for possible sexual abuse is for the protection, the treatment, and the reassurance of the child."[3]

During these early years, most child sexual abuse physical examinations were conducted by a small number of physicians and advanced practice nurses. Following the development of educational and certification programs for sexual assault nurse examiners (SANE), registered nurses (RN) became increasingly involved in child sexual abuse examinations, especially in more rural areas and in association with children's advocacy centers (CAC). As more hospitals developed programs for the evaluation of maltreated children, and as CACs increased in number, it became easier to find resources for the medical examination of these children. Best practice guidelines for all health professionals who evaluate children who may have been sexually abused are the focus of this chapter.

PURPOSE OF THE EXAMINATION

Sexual abuse examinations are sometimes labeled forensic examinations. Physical evidence is collected and a description of the examination findings may be introduced in subsequent legal proceedings. The results of child sexual abuse examinations have the potential to be used as evidence in subsequent legal proceedings and should therefore include all the requirements necessary to face court challenges. However, health care professionals must never lose sight of the most important aspects of a medical encounter for children who may have been sexually abused: reassurance, protection, treatment, and mental health support. The definitions of *doctor*, *nurse*, and *practices*, and the different levels of medical evaluations, are pertinent to a discussion about professionals practicing with a wide variety of education and training.

EDUCATION AND TRAINING

MEDICINE

A physician is, "a person who has successfully completed the prescribed course of studies in medicine in a medical school officially recognized by the country in which it is located, and who has acquired the requisite qualifications for licensure in the practice of medicine."[4] After graduating from college, and an additional 4 years in medical school, students are awarded a doctor of medicine (MD) or doctor of osteopathy (DO).

Following their medical education, physicians complete further training in a residency, typically lasting 3 years for primary-care specialties like pediatrics or family practice. Successful completion of that training and a board certification examination leads to certification in the specialty.

Beginning in late 2006, the American Board of Pediatrics initiated the development of a certification program for pediatricians with additional training and/or experience in the subspecialty of child abuse pediatrics. The program will eventually require an additional 3 years of fellowship training for physicians who will be board certified in this subspecialty.[5]

NURSING

Nurses engage in the practice of nursing, which can be defined as "the performance of services provided for purposes of nursing diagnosis and treatment of human responses to actual or potential health problems consistent with educational preparation." The definition describes how the nursing process is applied through knowledge and skill. "Practice is based on understanding the human condition across the human lifespan and understanding the relationship of the individual within the environment."[6] A more contemporary definition of nursing is available on the American Nurses Association Web page: "Nursing is the protection, promotion, and optimization of health and abilities, prevention of illness and injury, alleviation of suffering through the diagnosis and treatment of human response, and advocacy in the care of individuals, families, and populations." (From Nursing's Social Policy Statement, 2nd ed., 2003, p. 6. and Nursing: Scope and Standards of Practice, 2004, p. 7)[7]

Although a voluntary program, the National League for Nursing is responsible for accrediting all schools of nursing to assure consistency in curriculum and outcome criteria. Basic education requirements for entry into nursing practice have been controversial for many years. As of 2010, a professional nurse can enter the field with an associate degree (AD), diploma, or bachelor of science in nursing (BSN). Typically the AD is completed in 2 years, the diploma in 3 years, and the BSN in 4 years. An RN who receives an associate degree or diploma may take additional coursework to obtain a BSN. Nurses may then decide to further their education and clinical practice by becoming advanced practice registered nurses (APRN). They are subsequently licensed to provide primary and specialized care, including the ability to prescribe medications and treatments. APRNs include nurse practitioners, clinical nurse specialists, nurse anesthetists, and nurse midwives. Nurse Practice Acts vary widely among states, defining specifically what APRNs can do. The APRN uses advanced skills in assessment, analytical thinking, and evaluation.[6] Many career choices are available with options in academics, research, patient care, industry, and others.

Individual state Nurse Practice Acts regulate and hold nurses accountable for their actions. Each state has a Board of Nursing empowered by the state legislature to ensure compliance with the Nurse Practice Acts for that state. Most state Boards of Nursing grant and revoke licenses, accredit programs, and write specific regulations related to the practice of nursing. A state's Nurse Practice Acts define the scope of practice and are available to anyone seeking an understanding of role definitions for all nurses practicing in that state.

A model for evaluating the scope of practice for RNs may be useful as a template for making decisions about nursing practices in various locations. In 1993, the Oklahoma Board of Nursing endorsed a model originally developed by the Kentucky State Board of Nursing with input from other Nursing Boards in Florida, North Carolina, South

Dakota, Pennsylvania, and the National Council of State Boards of Nursing. Revised in 2010, the model is available on the Web at http://www.ok.gov/nursing. A synopsis, based on 7 decision points, follows. First, an act (examination and assessment of a child for suspected sexual abuse) is described. **Figure 14-1** illustrates the questions guiding the nurse's decisions.

In 1997, the International Association of Forensic Nursing (IAFN), in conjunction with the American Nurses Association (ANA), published *The Scope and Standards of Forensic Nursing Practice*. This document describes the specialty of forensic nursing with regard to the core practice arenas, dimensions of practice, and the wide variety of groups that intersect with forensic nursing. *The Scope and Standards of Forensic Nursing Practice* describes standards of care for assessment, diagnosis, outcome identification, planning, and evaluation. It also includes standards of professional performance that describe a competent level of behavior in quality of care, performance appraisal, education, collegiality, ethics, collaborative research, and resource utilization.[8]

In 1996, the SANE Council of the IAFN developed SANE standards of practice. These standards provide a basis for the objective evaluation of the care provided and describe what can be expected when a patient is examined by an RN educated as a sexual assault examiner.[9] The education of a SANE begins with one of the previously described entry levels, including RN, advanced practice, or doctorate. In 1998, the IAFN published guidelines for recommended education of a SANE. Pediatric education guidelines were published in 2002 and address both the didactic and clinical education necessary to perform examinations.[10] A certification examination was developed in 2007 by the IAFN for the specialty of pediatric sexual assault nurse examiners. Successful completion of the certification process acknowledges objective validation of nurses' expertise. The process also enhances professional development and opportunities for professional growth.[11]

COLLABORATION AMONG HEALTH PROFESSIONALS

In some cases, nonmedical investigators make decisions about which children should receive a medical evaluation. However, it is important that all children suspected of being victims of sexual abuse receive medical evaluations. At some point during the development of new programs, parameters should be set for selecting the most appropriate type of evaluation needed to provide the level of care that is in the best interest of the child. It is important to define, on a case-by-case basis, the type of physical examination needed for a child who may have been sexually abused. The purpose of a pediatric examination may be limited (eg, an acute illness, a distinct problem, or—for the purpose of this chapter—a report of suspected sexual abuse). The child sexual abuse examination may, at times, be described as an examination for the collection of forensic medical evidence, best performed within 24 hours but commonly performed within 72 hours after an alleged abuse event (a disclosure of abuse).[12-14] As DNA techniques evolve, it is important to reevaluate the best timing for evidence collection. In more than 2000 cases of suspected child sexual abuse in Tulsa, Oklahoma, less than 10% of all cases were referred within a 72-hour time frame. Although child sexual abuse examinations performed within 72 hours focus on forensic evidence collection, nursing assessments done at later times may include "a systematic collection of data to determine the patient's health status and to identify any actual or potential health problems. Components of this assessment include nursing history, including an incident history and health history, physical examination, review of other sources of assessment data, and analysis and synthesis of data collected."[15] The data collected is helpful in addressing changes in the patient's health status; recognizing alterations from the previous state or condition; synthesizing the biological, psychological, and social

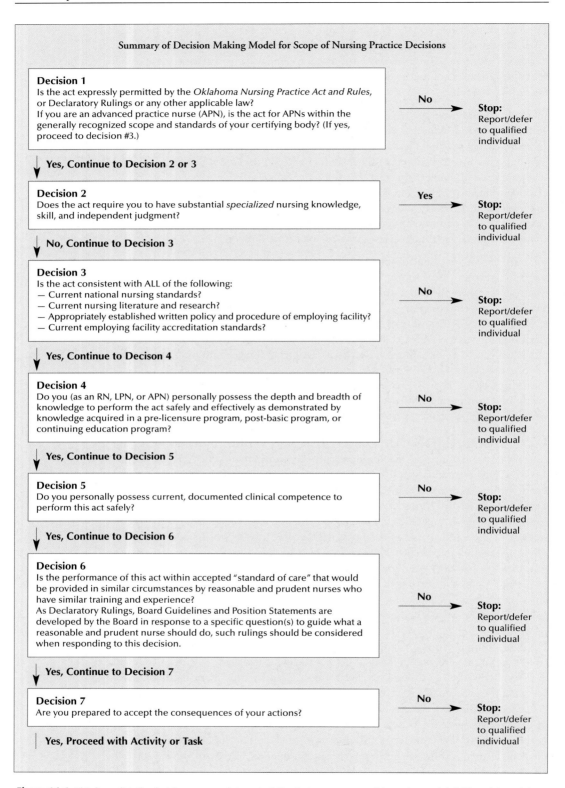

Summary of Decision Making Model for Scope of Nursing Practice Decisions

Decision 1
Is the act expressly permitted by the *Oklahoma Nursing Practice Act and Rules*, or Declaratory Rulings or any other applicable law?
If you are an advanced practice nurse (APN), is the act for APNs within the generally recognized scope and standards of your certifying body? (If yes, proceed to decision #3.)

No → **Stop:** Report/defer to qualified individual

↓ **Yes, Continue to Decision 2 or 3**

Decision 2
Does the act require you to have substantial *specialized* nursing knowledge, skill, and independent judgment?

Yes → **Stop:** Report/defer to qualified individual

↓ **No, Continue to Decision 3**

Decision 3
Is the act consistent with ALL of the following:
— Current national nursing standards?
— Current nursing literature and research?
— Appropriately established written policy and procedure of employing facility?
— Current employing facility accreditation standards?

No → **Stop:** Report/defer to qualified individual

↓ **Yes, Continue to Decison 4**

Decision 4
Do you (as an RN, LPN, or APN) personally possess the depth and breadth of knowledge to perform the act safely and effectively as demonstrated by knowledge acquired in a pre-licensure program, post-basic program, or continuing education program?

No → **Stop:** Report/defer to qualified individual

↓ **Yes, Continue to Decision 5**

Decision 5
Do you personally possess current, documented clinical competence to perform this act safely?

No → **Stop:** Report/defer to qualified individual

↓ **Yes, Continue to Decision 6**

Decision 6
Is the performance of this act within accepted "standard of care" that would be provided in similar circumstances by reasonable and prudent nurses who have similar training and experience?
As Declaratory Rulings, Board Guidelines and Position Statements are developed by the Board in response to a specific question(s) to guide what a reasonable and prudent nurse should do, such rulings should be considered when responding to this decision.

No → **Stop:** Report/defer to qualified individual

↓ **Yes, Continue to Decision 7**

Decision 7
Are you prepared to accept the consequences of your actions?

No → **Stop:** Report/defer to qualified individual

| **Yes, Proceed with Activity or Task**

Figure 14-1. *This figure lists the decisions one needs to make following an assessment of the patient and definition of the activity or task. Adapted with permission from the Oklahoma Board of Nursing.*

aspects of the situation; evaluating the impact of nursing care; and using this broad and complete analysis to develop the nursing plan of care.

Children who disclose abuse beyond the time frame compatible with a forensic evaluation require at least an examination focused on medical history and a physical examination of the oral, anal, and genital areas. In addition, most children are best served by a more comprehensive pediatric medical evaluation, which may be conducted by a licensed physician, certified and licensed advanced practice nurse, or licensed physician assistant. A comprehensive medical evaluation can be defined as a thorough medical history, a complete physical examination, an assessment of behavior and development, a diagnosis, and a treatment plan. If the child has an established medical home the evaluation is part of the child's primary care. If the child does not have a primary care provider, the comprehensive evaluation can be performed at the time of the sexual abuse evaluation, or later, and should be performed by a provider with training in and knowledge of child development, normal prepubertal and pubertal anatomy, interpretation of physical findings, and differential diagnoses with abuse and other medical conditions considered. Careful consideration of differential diagnoses is important, especially among children with physical or behavioral symptoms but no clear disclosure of abuse. Although many physicians and nurses have most of the requisite skills, not all have more than a basic understanding of child abuse, forensic interviewing, and physical examination for abuse. Collaboration with or referral to a physician, physician assistant, or advanced practice nurse specializing or experienced in child abuse pediatrics is helpful in those situations.

The purpose of the medical evaluation should be in the best interest of the child. The evaluation should follow a best practice model with findings that are evidence based.[15] Determining who should be allowed to do what to whom should optimally be based on the knowledge, education, training, and experience of the examiner. In fairness to the child, the child's family, and the systems depending on medical findings (or lack of findings), examinations beyond forensic evidence collection are optimally performed by health care professionals who have specific education and training in the field of child sexual abuse medicine, a knowledge of child physical and emotional development, and other appropriate pediatric care areas. Training in child sexual abuse evaluations should include a component of closely supervised experience performing and interpreting examinations.

Three broad areas of preparation should be evaluated prior to deciding who is best able to provide medical evaluations for sexually abused children. These areas are (1) education, training, certification, and licensing, (2) supervision and case review experience, and (3) ongoing peer review of findings and opinions after examinations. Not all physicians and nurses have the necessary education and training to be skilled in child sexual abuse examination techniques, interpretation of findings, laboratory testing, diagnosis, and management. Consequently, to guarantee best practice models for the medical care of possibly sexually abused children, both doctors and nurses must meet certain advanced skill levels through education, continuing education, supervised experience, and peer review of opinions and findings prior to working independently.

Supervision and peer review are different processes, but both are important to practitioners in the field of child abuse. Supervision requires knowledgeable and experienced mentors to observe the health care professionals as they work with children, and to review, discuss, and refine the health care professionals' assessments and opinions. Often supervisors are responsible for the consequences associated with the work of the people they are supervising. Collaborative practice implies 2 or more professionals working together without a hierarchy. This type of practice is the optimal way to bring complementary skill sets together. Peer review is a process of continually presenting findings and opinions before a group of health care professionals of varying skill levels for the purpose of confirmation of findings, discovery of new ideas, and discussion of controversial issues. All health care professionals who engage in child sexual abuse evaluations should avail themselves of opportunities for peer review.

There are several challenges involving child sexual abuse medical evaluations. The first is the importance of an examiner's ability to perform an appropriate examination. The skilled examiner will pay particular attention to:

— Proper positioning of the patient precluding adequate visualization and interpretation.

— Avoiding overstating a finding by indicating pathology for a finding better described as a variant of normal.

— Correctly diagnosing a finding indicative of a condition mimicking abuse, but not a sign of abuse.

— Correct interpretation of tenderness, pain, or erythema.

— Knowing that introduction of a finger or speculum through a prepubertal hymen is contraindicated.

— Complying with standards for appropriate photographic or video documentation.

Competency in examination techniques is not conferred by any degree, but rather by advanced knowledge, training, and experience. All examinations must be free from personal bias. Examiners must resist the lure of "making the case" for investigators or prosecutors by overinterpreting a normal or nonspecific finding.

Two examples of successful collaborative programs follow.

Example 1

The management of the SANE program in Fort Wayne, Indiana, involves a forensic nurse as chief nursing officer (CNO) and a medical director who is an emergency department physician. Acute and nonacute examinations are available to all ages and genders. Direct patient care is provided by RNs who have completed extensive education. All records are reviewed by the CNO. With the knowledge and consent of parents or guardians, a phone call is made to the child's primary care provider. In addition, a referral form outlining the episode of care is provided so that ongoing medical needs associated with the incident can be addressed. When necessary, 18 pediatric subspecialists including dermatology, radiology, gynecology, and gastroenterology are available as consultants. Photodocumentation of the initial examination and follow-up examination is evaluated in bimonthly case review. Case review participants include nursing, law enforcement, prosecution, family and children services, and mental health specialists.

Example 2

In Tulsa, Oklahoma, nurses who complete pediatric education are already skilled adult and adolescent examiners. They attend an education program that complies with the IAFN pediatric educational guidelines. Following completion of the didactic portion of the education, the nurse completes a clinical component with experienced SANEs, physicians, and advanced practice nurses. The clinical component consists of:

— Observing and performing examinations with an experienced SANE.

— Observing and discussing forensic interviews.

— Observing and discussing well-child examinations.

— Observing physicians and a pediatric nurse practitioner, all members of the University of Oklahoma–Tulsa pediatric faculty, perform examinations at the local advocacy center.

— Observing a wide range of child development stages at an early childhood learning center and a school.

— Performing examinations at the local advocacy center with supervision from the pediatric faculty or established SANEs.

Tulsa SANEs generally perform examinations for children presenting within 72 hours of a suspected event. The patient is examined at a location specifically equipped for forensic evaluations in 1 of the 5 hospitals located in the Tulsa area. Typically, patients come to the location from a radius of about 75 miles. Law enforcement, rape advocacy, and child welfare personnel are often at the examination site. All cases are reviewed by the nursing administrator. In addition, the nurses meet bimonthly to review cases. **Figure 14-1** illustrates the case review protocol. Any case thought to have findings of injury or other abnormal findings is reviewed in a timely manner by the University of Oklahoma pediatricians or advanced practice nurse, and follow-up examinations are performed by those reviewers as well. The pediatricians are board certified in pediatrics by the American Board of Pediatrics, and all were eligible for Child Abuse Pediatrics subspecialty certification when the first certifying examination was offered in 2009.

Both of these programs are based in metropolitan areas. However, with the use of technology, cases from rural areas can be reviewed in a timely manner by a consultant. In some cases, children would have to travel for a confirmatory examination, a small inconvenience compared to the consequences of an erroneous assessment.

Not all communities have a clinical practice setting similar to the 2 examples. All health care professionals are encouraged to work toward best practice solutions for the real world, where physician knowledge of or interest in child sexual abuse may be absent, or where access to subspecialty care is limited. Physicians and nurses can work together to develop a consistent, standardized curriculum that is required of all persons prior to performing examinations on children. Content for education and training curricula are available from the IAFN, the American Board of Pediatrics, and other sources. After initial education, health care professionals learning to perform sexual abuse examinations for children should work under direct supervision until both mentor and examiner are comfortable with examination techniques and interpretation of findings. Photographic and video documentation are very useful for case reviews and consultations. Supervisor review of cases performed by relatively inexperienced examiners is essential, especially for cases initially judged to have findings indicating abuse. That review should occur prior to an impression being shared with investigators.

CONCLUSION

In many health care settings, communication and collaboration among health care professionals can bring excellent outcomes to the assessment and care of a child and family. Different professionals bring different, often complementary, skill sets to a particular situation. Allowed to work in unison, the skill sets can be additive, resulting in optimal communication with child welfare workers, law enforcement personnel, prosecutors and defense lawyers, and others in a community system, as well as a best outcome for the patient and family.

REFERENCES

1. Sgroi SM. Sexual molestation of children; the last frontier in child abuse. *Child Today*. 1975 May-June;4(3):18-21, 44.

2. Chadwick DL, Berkowitz CD, Kerns D, McCann J, Reinhart MA, Strickland S. *Color Atlas of Child Sexual Abuse*. Chicago, IL: Year Book Medical Publishers; 1989.

3. Heger AM. Making the diagnosis of sexual abuse: ten years later. In: Heger AM, Emans SJ, Muram D, eds. *Evaluation of the Sexually Abused Child*. 2nd ed. New York, NY: Oxford University Press; 2000:1-10.

4. Taber's Online. Available at: http://www.tabers.com/. Accessed March 1, 2010.

5. Block RW, Palusci VJ. Child abuse pediatrics: a new pediatric subspecialty. *J Pediatr*. 2006;148(6):711-712.

6. Okla Stat tit 59, §569.3a

7. American Nurses Association, http://nursingworld.org. Accessed December 3, 2008.

8. International Association of Forensic Nurses. Scope and standards of forensic nursing practice. Available at: http://www.iafn.org. Accessed March 1, 2010.

9. International Association of Forensic Nurses. Sexual assault nurse examiner standards of practice. Available at: http://www.iafn.org. Accessed March 1, 2010.

10. International Association of Forensic Nurses. Pediatric sexual assault nurse examiner education guidelines. Available at: http://www.iafn.org. Accessed March 1, 2010.

11. International Association of Forensic Nurses. http://www.iafn.org. Acessed March 1, 2010.

12. Christian CW, Lavelle JM, De Jong AR, Loiselle J, Brenner L, Joffe M. Forensic evidence findings in prepubertal victims of sexual assault. *Pediatrics*. 2000;106(1 pt 1):100-104.

13. Young KL, Jones JG, Worthington T, Simpson P, Casey PH. Forensic laboratory evidence in sexually abused children and adolescents. *Arch Pediatr Adolesc Med*. 2006;160(6):585-588.

14. Kellogg N, American Academy of Pediatrics Committee on Child Abuse and Neglect. The evaluation of sexual abuse in children. *Pediatrics*. 2005;116(2):506-512.

15. Oklahoma Board of Nursing. www.ok.gov/nursing/pracl.html. Accessed November 21, 2008.

Chapter 15

THE MULTIDISCIPLINARY TEAM AND CHILD SEXUAL ABUSE

Rich Kaplan, MSW, MD, FAAP

Child sexual abuse is a medically and socially complex phenomenon. The child victim, the victim's family, and the community all have a stake in a successful evaluation and intervention. The success of such an effort is dependent on effective collaboration by a variety of professionals both in and out of the health care milieu. Health care providers need to have a clear understanding of their own role as well as the practice parameters and competencies of the other professionals. The role of the health care provider within the professional team, the roles of other key members, and the teaming process are addressed in this chapter.

BACKGROUND AND RATIONALE

The concept of an interdisciplinary approach to medical care is certainly not novel. It has traditionally meant the bringing together of several medical and ancillary specialties in response to medically complex diagnoses such as *spina bifida* or craniofacial malformations. With respect to child abuse in general and sexual abuse specifically, the concept of a multidisciplinary team (MDT) is significantly broader. In 1962, in their landmark article "The Battered-Child Syndrome," Kempe and colleagues noted that the physician should be acquainted with "facilities available in private and public agencies that provide protective services for children."[1] They go on to recommend "an evaluation of the psychological and social factors in the case." There is also reference to law enforcement and the courts. In 1976, Fontana and Robison described a system that utilized nonmedical community services to treat and prevent child abuse.[2]

MEMBERS OF THE MULTIDISCIPLINARY TEAM

The MDT concept in child maltreatment cases goes far beyond the traditional interdisciplinary treatment model. It is often considered a vehicle for performing investigations and arresting and incarcerating sexual perpetrators. The MDT concept goes beyond this as well. It has the potential to involve professionals from child protective services (CPS), law enforcement, the courts, and the mental health sector in a process that ideally minimizes trauma to the child victim and creates a synergy that meets the professional mandates of all constituents and, above all, the complex needs of young victims.

CHILD PROTECTIVE SERVICES

The notion that the protection of children is a government responsibility is relatively new. In the eighteenth and much of the nineteenth centuries, maltreated children were placed in institutions known as almshouses. Mainly for orphaned, abandoned, or unwanted children of the poor, these facilities generally provided crowded, chaotic, and unwholesome environments for these vulnerable youngsters.[3] In the late nineteenth century there was a more evolved social apparatus for the protection of animals than for the protection of child victims. In 1874, the Society for the Prevention of Cruelty to Animals (SPCA) filed a writ of habeas corpus to secure the removal of 9-year-old Mary Ellen Wilson from her abusive home. At that time, there was no private or governmental agency to act on behalf of abused children.

Although the Wilson case is widely known, it was not an isolated event. There is an account of a previous attempt by the SPCA to protect an abused child 3 years earlier.[4] Following the case involving Mary Ellen Wilson, the New York Society for the Prevention of Cruelty to Children was formed. Ultimately, quite a number of these societies were formed as part of the American Humane Society. As the child welfare movement evolved into government-provided child protection programs, a healthy dialectic developed between the at-times disparate approaches of investigation/placement and family service/support. This conflict has been generally helpful, with the strongest agencies achieving a dynamic balance between the two poles.

Child protective services play a role in the evaluation and the response phases of child sexual abuse cases. Their primary expertise lies in the assessment of risk to the child who may have been abused and the child's siblings. This assessment is often performed in concert with the law enforcement investigation but may be undertaken separately. Rather than being directed toward criminal prosecution, the CPS evaluation often leads to a juvenile or civil legal proceeding involving protection, placement, and long-term disposition. Additionally, a service or program component of CPS is often involved in the provision of long-term services and support to a victim's family. It should be noted that CPS involvement is often predicated on the abuse being intrafamilial, perpetrated by a caregiver, or the result of inadequate parental supervision.

LAW ENFORCEMENT

The role of law enforcement is central in the evaluation of cases of child sexual abuse. From the community perspective, law enforcement is charged with maintaining public safety. This is usually perceived as the apprehension of criminals. From the MDT perspective, the role of law enforcement is much broader and more complex. In nearly all jurisdictions, law enforcement personnel have the statutory authority to immediately protect children who are in imminent danger. From the standpoint of gathering a history, the police may have exclusive access to the scene of the abuse. In acute cases they can gather material that may contain biologic or physical evidence that may be diagnostically significant. In nonacute cases they can identify details at the scene, such as computer data, photographs, or physical details, that may add to or reduce a possible victim's credibility.

It is simplistic to characterize law enforcement in a one-dimensional manner. As in the field of health care, there are varied roles and competencies. The uniformed officer is often the first contact and is responsible for stabilizing the scene and, at times, taking an initial statement from a possible child victim. This role is extremely sensitive and ideally requires specialized training. In a growing number of communities this initial interaction is protocol driven by various interagency agreements. There are also clear differences among child sexual abuse investigators, including the perception of their roles and the techniques they utilize.[5] There are also clear differences in preparation and specialized training.[6]

There are broad social variables as well. The degree of specialization varies depending on police department size as well as the police and municipal administration's commitment to the support of child abuse services. It is not uncommon for services to children to be cut when budgets are tight, which means that the investigator primarily responsible for a child sexual abuse case may lack the time or experience to perform optimally. Given the lack of physical or corroborative evidence in the vast majority of cases of child sexual abuse, the investigator's skill and ability to obtain an admission of responsibility from an offender may be the most important element in the protection of a child and the community.

THE COURTS

With respect to child maltreatment, the court system has 2 different and often quite separate systems. One, the criminal court, is geared toward the charging and trying of individuals believed to be child abusers. The other, the civil or child protection court, is involved with the determination of abuse or neglect by caregivers or custodians of the child and with decisions regarding parental rights and guardianship. Although the most visible element in child abuse cases is the criminal prosecution of offenders, with the exception of extrafamilial sexual assaults, this aspect is unlikely to have the most impact on the child victim or the family. It is the child protection court that often has the most profound effect on the future well-being of the child.

The milieu of the child protection court is much more amenable to the assimilation of medical and scientific material into the decision-making process for several reasons. First, in most jurisdictions the proceeding is held only in front of a judge, which generally limits polemics and drama. In addition, there is usually more opportunity for a medical provider to provide complex medical answers to complex legal questions. Finally, the standard of proof is different. Civil decisions are more likely to be determined by a preponderance of evidence or clear and convincing evidence, both of which are less stringent than the "beyond a reasonable doubt" standard held in criminal court.*

This is not to imply that there is little or no value in criminal justice. The community has a stake in the status of potentially dangerous pedophiles in their midst. There is also strong evidence that recidivism is high among sexual offenders; therefore, separating them from the community protects children. What is not known is the impact the criminal proceedings have on the child victim. The most ambitious attempts to examine this issue had mixed results and did not provide a clear answer.[7,8] There were multiple variables, such as the age of the child when the child testified, multiple testimonies, and severity of abuse, that have proved difficult to sort out. Nonetheless, inquiries of this nature need to continue. Regardless of the relative impact of the legal proceedings on the patient, it is incumbent on the child abuse medical provider to have complete knowledge of the system.

MENTAL HEALTH

Mental health professionals are involved in the evaluation and treatment of possible child sexual abuse victims. The possible behavioral consequences and emotional impact of abuse on the child are evaluated. This evaluation is useful in assessing the possible therapy needs for the victim and the victim's family. It is also helpful in developing an understanding of a child's behavior relative to a disclosure or lack of disclosure. In 1983, Roland Summit described common behavioral manifestations of sexual maltreatment in children.[9] There have been more formal attempts to categorize the behavioral effects of sexual abuse. With the development of the Child Sexual Behavioral Inventory (CSBI), the late Dr. William Friedrich and colleagues provided a remarkable tool for the interpretation of sexualized behaviors and their relationship to a history of sexual abuse.[10] Although there are a number of causes of sexualization in children, abuse is one

---

* Physicians should learn the specific legal parameters for the jurisdiction(s) in which they practice. They should also be aware of special situations that may impact the procedural rules. For instance, the Indian Child Welfare Act mandates additional procedures and different standards of proof.

of them and the data derived from the CSBI remain extremely useful. For a child who is demonstrating behavioral signs of abuse or for whom there are other reasons to be concerned about abuse although the child has not disclosed abuse, therapy may provide a safe environment in which to discuss abuse issues or may provide reassurance that there is no indication of abuse.

If the collective goal is the well-being of the child who has been abused, it follows that referral to effective psychotherapy is a critical element in the response to sexual abuse. The notion of efficacy is critically important. To refer a child to counseling without having details about or outcome data is somewhat akin to referring a child to an intensive laetrile therapy center for ALL. There is a growing collection of data supporting the fact that specialized trauma therapy is effective in treating child victims of sexual abuse (see Chapter 19).[11-13] There have also been attempts to assess the efficacy of crisis and family therapies with victims of nonfamilial assault.[14-16] These data are promising but more work is necessary.

The greatest barrier to effective therapy may be the availability of a trained therapist. The limited number of skilled practitioners and the restrictive third-party payor environment make it difficult to secure appropriate mental health therapy.

THE HEALTH CARE PROVIDER

The health care provider's role in cases of child sexual abuse is also multifaceted. First and foremost is the provision of skilled, compassionate health care. This care is similar to the care provided to other patients; however, special skills and competencies along with a specialized knowledge base need to be acquired, updated, and subjected to peer review. This care includes a careful diagnostic assessment utilizing history and physical examination data and, when needed, laboratory and imaging studies. In some settings the health care provider will rely on some of the historical data obtained by another team member during the forensic interview. In other settings the health care provider does the entire history taking. Either way the history serves as a basis for guiding the physical examination and determining the need for laboratory or other testing. This includes the development of a differential diagnosis that includes possible mimics of abuse.

The medical professional is also responsible for providing other team members with an understandable assessment of the medical and scientific issues specific to each case (eg, an explanation to an inexperienced team member about the lack of diagnostic utility of a normal genital examination or the lack of probative clarity of a human papillomavirus infection). This means that the health care provider must be available to the MDT for consultation on medical issues. The health care provider is also responsible for providing necessary referrals for follow-up primary and specialty care as well as participating in the referral to appropriate mental health resources. Finally, the health care provider needs to act as a liaison between the nonmedical team members and the medical/hospital community. The child sexual abuse medical provider must educate the rest of the health care team regarding the legal and social issues involved in these cases and must also work within the health care system to develop procedural guidelines that minimize trauma to possible child victims. Systems need to be developed that will prevent examinations by inexperienced practitioners, obviate the need for multiple evaluations, and provide a safe and child-friendly setting for the physical examination.

MULTIDISCIPLINARY TEAM FUNCTION

In order for an MDT to function in a productive manner, several requisite conditions need to be in place. First, team members must clearly articulate their areas of professional competence, the mandate under which they function, and their perception of their role on the team. Second, these perceptions need to be addressed in light of other team member expectations. For example, the medical team member needs to explain why it is necessary to gather a medical history that may overlap with a previous interview or explain the reasons for doing a genital examination in addition to discovering physical evidence. This need for a clear understanding of disciplinary competencies and mutual expectations provides the basis for the trust that is the cornerstone of effective teaming. Team functioning is, however, certainly not static. All of the constituent agencies are fluid and change is inevitable (eg, an experienced investigator is promoted, a new DA is elected, or budget cuts devastate CPS). Changes are to be expected. As long as the fundamental articulation of expectations and roles is continued and trust is maintained, the team can function effectively.

That being said, there will be conflicts that occur for a variety of reasons. The following issues are sources of team conflict:

— Who is most suited to do the interview?[17]

— How will law enforcement and CPS work together?[18]

— Why are some cases not referred for charging?[19]

— Why wasn't the child informed of the need for an examination?[20]

Maintaining a productive and effective MDT is not easy. It takes patience, energy, and an unflagging commitment to the safety and well-being of child victims.

CONCLUSION

The MDT evaluating and intervening in cases of child abuse may include professionals from medicine, nursing, mental health, CPS, and law enforcement. Each member of the team contributes unique knowledge and expertise. Flexibility and an understanding of each others' roles on the team are essential to functioning effectively to minimize trauma and meet the complex needs of young victims.

REFERENCES

1. Kempe CH, Silverman FN, Steele BF, et al. The battered-child syndrome. *JAMA*. 1962;181(1):17-24.

2. Fontana VJ, Robison E. A multidisciplinary approach to the treatment of child abuse. *Pediatrics*. 1976;57(5):760-764.

3. Schene PA. Past, present, and future roles of child protective services. *Future Child*. 1998;8(1):23-38.

4. Lazoritz S, Shelman EA. Before Mary Ellen. *Child Abuse Negl*. 1996;20(3):235-237.

5. Froum AG, Kendall-Tackett KA. Law enforcement officers' approaches to evaluations of child sexual abuse. *Child Abuse Negl*. 1998;22(9):939-942.

6. Portwood SG, Grady MT, Dutton SE, et al. Enhancing law enforcement identification and investigation of child maltreatment. *Child Abuse Negl*. 2000; 24(2):195-207.

7. Quas JA, Goodman GS, Ghetti S, et al. Childhood sexual assault victims: long-term outcomes after testifying in criminal court. *Monogr Soc Res Child Dev*. 2005;70(2):vii.

8. Haugaard JJ. Implications of longitudinal research with child witnesses for developmental theory, public policy, and intervention strategies. *Monogr Soc Res Child Dev*. 2005;70(2): 129-139.

9. Summit RC. The child sexual abuse accommodation syndrome. *Child Abus Negl.* 1983;7(2): 177-193.

10. Friedrich WN, Fisher JL, Dittner CA, et al. Child Sexual Behavior Inventory: normative, psychiatric, and sexual abuse comparisons. *Child Maltreat.* 2001;6(1): 37-49.

11. Cohen JA, Deblinger E, Mannarino AP, et al. A multisite, randomized controlled trial for children with sexual abuse-related PTSD symptoms. *J Am Acad Child Adolesc Psychiatry.* 2004;43(4): 393-402.

12. Cohen JA, Mannarino AP, Knudsen K. Treating sexually abused children: 1 year follow-up of a randomized controlled trial. *Child Abuse Negl.* 2005;29(2):135-145.

13. Cohen, JA. Treating traumatized children: current status and future directions. *J Trauma Dissociation.* 2005;6(2):109-121.

14. Roesler TA, Savin D, Grosz C. Family therapy of extrafamilial sexual abuse. *J Am Acad Child Adolesc Psychiatry.* 1993;32(5):967-970.

15. Grosz CA, Kempe RS, Kelly M. Extrafamilial sexual abuse: treatment for child victims and their families. *Child Abuse Negl.* 2000;24(1):9-23.

16. Stevenson, J. The treatment of the long-term sequelae of child abuse. *J Child Psychol Psychiatry Allied Disciplines.* 1999;40(1):89-111.

17. Wood JM, Garven S. How sexual abuse interviews go astray: implications for prosecutors, police, and child protection services. *Child Maltreat.* 2000;5(2): 109-18.

18. Newman BS, Dannenfelser PL. Children's protective services and law enforcement: fostering partnerships in investigations of child abuse. *J Child Sex Abuse.* 2005; 14(2):97-111.

19. Stroud DD, Martens SL, Barker J. Criminal investigation of child sexual abuse: a comparison of cases referred to the prosecutor to those not referred. *Child Abuse Negl.* 2000;24(5):689-700.

20. Muram D, Aiken MM, Strong C. Children's refusal of gynecologic examinations for suspected sexual abuse. *J Clin Ethics.* 1997;8(2):158-164.

Chapter 16

The Medical Professional's Guide to Court Process and Procedures

Craig L. Barlow, JD

Medical professionals who treat children who have been sexually abused face many challenges. Treatment of children and diagnosis of other injuries and conditions are activities for which medical professionals are prepared and well trained; furthermore, in these situations, they are functioning in a setting of familiarity. However, when allegations of child sexual abuse become part of the legal system, the nature of the challenges changes. Most medical professionals engaged in cases of suspected child sexual abuse will be involved in aspects of the legal system. At some point in their careers, most medical professionals engaged in cases of suspected child sexual abuse will be involved in some aspect of the legal system, whether as an expert witness or otherwise. It is, therefore, vital that these professionals prepare for the experience by having at least a rudimentary understanding of how the legal system works. It is even more important that medical professionals learn to function comfortably and competently in the courtroom setting. This chapter will give an overview of the legal system and provide a practical guide for medical professionals who testify in court.

The Legal System

Law is a complex body of knowledge, process, and application. Most of the concepts presented here are simplified in the interest of the reader's time; after all, it is important that medical professionals who appear in court train their focus on the essentials. As such, the information contained here is abridged and streamlined, with no mention of areas of the law that have no bearing on the issue of child sexual abuse. In addition, the focus here focuses on so-called common law court systems such as those in the United States, Canada, and the United Kingdom, as opposed to civil law systems such as those found in Europe and other regions. Cases in which medical professionals evaluate child victims of sexual abuse can be either civil or criminal. Cases in juvenile court involving abuse, neglect, or dependency are considered part of the civil law system. In almost every American jurisdiction, a judge is the sole fact-finder in juvenile court. The parties in juvenile court are the petitioner and the respondent, and the case is generally referred to as "in the matter of (juvenile's initials)," or "In re: (juvenile's initials)." The party bringing a petition in juvenile court, which is almost always the state's or local government's family services agency, must prove its case by a standard of "clear and convincing evidence." This level of proof is greater than a "preponderance of the evidence," which is the usual standard in other civil cases, but less than the standard of "beyond a reasonable doubt," which must be met in criminal cases. This may not pertain in cases involving Native American children, where "beyond a reasonable doubt" is often invoked.

In criminal cases, the state, acting through a district attorney, county attorney, state's attorney, or attorney general is the plaintiff and the person charged with the crime is the defendant. The cases are usually styled as *The State of Minnesota versus* (often written as *"v."*) (*defendant's last name*).

In almost all criminal cases, juries act as fact-finders and a judge rules on questions of law (ie, motions and objections) and gives instruction to the jury on legal principles that apply to the case. In juvenile court, the decision is called an *order* or *ruling*. In criminal court, the ultimate decision is called a *verdict*.

A PRACTICAL GUIDE TO TESTIFYING IN COURT

Medical professionals become involved in child sexual abuse cases because they treated or diagnosed a child's injuries, illnesses, or conditions. Such situations invariably result in medical professionals being asked to appear in court as expert witnesses.

The testimony of expert witnesses is governed by special rules in a jurisdiction's Rules of Evidence. These rules are generally uniform from one state to another. They provide that a witness qualified by knowledge, skill, experience, training, or education may testify about scientific and medical concepts in the form of an opinion or otherwise. Unlike fact witnesses, who receive a standard witness fee, expert witnesses may receive payment for time spent preparing for and giving testimony. An expert witness is never paid "for her testimony." That would be improper. However, payment for an expert's time is entirely appropriate.

There are a number of rules, both formal and informal, that govern to what an expert witness can testify. These rules additionally dictate how an expert witness, or really any witness, should testify.

FORMAL RULES

A jurisdiction's Rules of Evidence allow experts to testify about what they perceive, what they conclude, and about other opinions and conclusions on which they reasonably and regularly rely in forming opinions, which includes consultations with other experts. Experts can testify about what other experts have told them or what other experts have written if that information helps develop the testifying witness' opinions. Statements made by those outside of the courtroom that are presented by third-party witnesses *in court* for the truth of the matter are generally considered hearsay and thus inadmissible. The Federal Rules of Evidence, specifically Rule 801(c), define hearsay as "a statement, other than one made by the declarant while testifying at the trial or hearing, offered in evidence to prove the truth of the matter asserted"; the states' definitions are similar in this regard.[1]

There are, however, many exceptions to the hearsay rule. For example, if a witness testifies in court that she was told that it rained in Philadelphia last week in order to prove that it did, in fact, rain in Philadelphia last week, the statement is deemed hearsay because the witness is reporting second-hand information. However, if the witness provides that testimony only to offer evidence that a conversation about the weather in Philadelphia last week took place and not to establish the truth of the statement, it would not be considered hearsay. In other words, in the second situation, the testimony does not serve to prove the truth or validity of the content of the conversation—it merely attests to the fact that a conversation did occur, regardless of the accuracy or veracity of the conversation's content.

The exception to the hearsay rule most applicable to medical professionals is related to statements for purposes of medical diagnosis or treatment. This exception to the hearsay rule, of which a version is found in every jurisdiction, states:

803(4). Statements for the purpose of medical diagnosis or treatment. Statements made for the purpose of medical diagnosis or treatment and describing medical history, or past or present symptoms, pain, or sensations, or the inception or general character of the cause or external source thereof insofar as reasonably pertinent to diagnosis or treatment.[2]

Thus, statements made to a medical professional by a child seen for purposes of diagnosis or treatment may be testified to in court as proof of the veracity of what the child said. Statements by children could include information about the abusers' identities. Identification of a child's abuser is essential to the treatment of that child because it is imperative that there is no further contact between the abuser and the child.

Another exception to the hearsay rule is important in some cases: that is, statements made outside of court conveying present sense impressions, containing excited utterances, or about then-existing mental, emotional, or physical conditions. These statements are not excluded by the hearsay rule, and are often witnessed by other officials who are not medical professionals per se (eg, police officers, 911 operators). Of course, when a rule of evidence is involved in the case of a medical professional, that professional should consult with the lawyer who is calling that professional as a witness, prior to providing any testimony, about the application of the rule. There are other elements relating to the formal rules of evidence that might affect the testimonies of medical professionals: namely, the testimony's relevance, the weight of the evidence (ie, its prejudicial versus probative value), and business records and learned treatises. It is not the responsibility of medical professionals to seek training in the law so that they can be effective witnesses. The lawyer calling medical professionals as witnesses should be thoroughly versed in the formal rules and other conditions of testifying. The lawyer should be the one to advise witnesses about the rules that will apply to their testimony.

It is important for medical professionals being called as witnesses to communicate quickly and directly with the lawyer calling them as witnesses. Medical professionals should anticipate that the lawyer will explain the nature of the case, the times at which and places where the professional will testify, and any special circumstances or legal issues affecting the testimony. If this information is not provided in a timely manner, it is well within protocol for the medical professional to diplomatically demand it from the lawyer. The better the communication between the medical professional and the lawyer, the more effective and useful the testimony will be.

Medical professionals who treat children should be sensitive to the social dynamics of cultural and ethnic diversity. In some cultures, for example, making eye contact with a stranger or an elder is considered rude and disrespectful. In other cultures, failure to make eye contact is indicative of deception or fear. Medical professionals who treat children from different cultural, religious, and ethnic backgrounds should actively learn about cultural differences so they can more meaningfully care for their patients. Of particular importance to medical professionals who treat children from sovereign tribes is the Indian Child Welfare Act of 1978 (ICWA).[3] This federal law governs all children who are enrolled or eligible to be enrolled in a recognized Native American nation and has particular relevance in child neglect, dependency, and abuse cases. The ICWA also raises the standard of proof in certain child welfare cases from "clear and convincing" to "beyond a reasonable doubt." The medical professional and the lawyer have a heightened need to communicate thoroughly when handling cases involving children of diverse cultural, religious, or ethnic backgrounds.

INFORMAL RULES

Besides the formal rules of testifying, there are many important informal rules to know on *how* to be an effective witness. **Table 16-1** provides specific suggestions for witnesses, which helps them prepare and understand what is expected of them.

Table 16-1. Informal Rules of Testifying

BEFORE THE TRIAL

— Be prepared, and know the case before the trial.

— Review and be familiar with notes and reports and any medical articles relied upon to inform opinions.

— Meet with the lawyer before the hearing and trial—you should call the lawyer to arrange the meeting.

— Review the reports of other experts who are involved in the case and ensure that the attorney is aware of your own research in scholarly journals that pertains to the subject matter of your testimony.

— Assist the attorney with difficult words, phrasing, and concepts so that he or she can be sure to substitute them with simpler terminology at the trial.

DURING QUESTIONING

— First listen to a query in its entirety; then take a moment to think about the answer second; and, finally, answer the question.

— Do not begin thinking about your answer until the question has been fully stated.

— A question's answer does, and probably should not, take more than 1 or 2 seconds.

— Easy questions require no thinking (eg, "What is your name?"; "What is your job?").

— Answer the question asked, which is a corollary to listening to the full question.

— Do not volunteer unrequested information.

— Always be truthful, regardless of the anticipated outcome of the testimony.

— Do not anticipate where the questioning is leading. If you are anticipating where the questioning is leading, you are not concentrating on listening to the questions.

— Bear in mind that it does not matter what you think about the direction of the questions.

— Be a vessel of truth and information.

— Realize that it is extremely rare that the answer to any one question changes the outcome of the proceeding or trial.

— If you either misunderstand or did not hear a question, you can ask for it to be repeated. However, do not ask for a question to be repeated because you do not understand its purpose.

— Remember that it is acceptable to say "I do not know" if you do not know the answer to a question.

— You are also permitted to say "I do not remember" if you are uncertain of the facts relevant to a question; however, this answer should be used sparingly to preserve your credibility.

— Use common sense when you answer. For instance, if the question is, "Did this incident occur on Thursday or Friday?" and your memory is that it occurred on Wednesday, Thursday, or Friday, but you are unsure which day, you should answer "I am not sure which day, but it was Wednesday, Thursday, or Friday." The answer should not be simply "no."

(continued)

Table 16-1. *(continued)*

DURING QUESTIONING

— When in court, address your answers to the fact-finder—that is, either the jury or the judge.

— Give answers naturally, not theatrically or flamboyantly.

— Avoid using highly technical words and phrases, as it is critical that the fact-finder understand your testimony.

— Do not read from notes unless absolutely necessary.

— During cross-examination, if you are asked about an article, book, or study, you should ask to see it and read it before answering questions about it.

— Avoid overreaching in your offered opinions; that is, do not profess to have knowledge in topics outside your area of expertise. If you are asked a question that pertains to matters outside your area of expertise, you should briefly state so, then remain quiet.

— When an objection is made, stop talking until the judge rules.

— Be stoic. Do not attempt to argue with, fence, debate, outguess, trick, engage in wordplay with, deceive, charm, or flirt with opposing counsel during cross-examination.

— Do not let the questioning become a contest between you and the lawyer.

— In formulating your answers, focus on the words in the question, not the tone of the lawyer.

— Do not think of answers as either helping or hurting the opposing lawyer; instead, think of them as assisting the fact-finder.

— You should shun jokes and wisecracks, because the general rule is that only the judge, not the lawyers or witnesses, is allowed to make jokes.

There are also unwritten rules about what medical professionals can and cannot say substantively when testifying. They are permitted to testify about what information a child provided to them at the time of diagnosis or treatment of the child. This does not mean that they should conduct a forensic interview of the child for the planned purpose of acting as a conduit for the child's testimony. In a recent US Supreme Court case, *Crawford v. Washington*,[4] the court considered the question of whether an out-of-court statement sought to be introduced at trial was "testimonial" or "nontestimonial." The Supreme Court held that if the out-of-court statement is testimonial (ie, elicited with a purpose to develop testimony for trial), it is inadmissible because it violates the Confrontation Clause of the Sixth Amendment, which guarantees a defendant the right to be confronted with those providing testimony against him, unless the witness is available to be cross-examined at trial. Since *Crawford*, many courts have applied the *Crawford* ruling to various types of out-of-court statements. Of particular interest to medical professionals is whether statements made by a patient for purposes of medical diagnosis or treatment are now inadmissible under *Crawford*. Almost all courts considering the issue have concluded that statements made for purposes of diagnosis and treatment are nontestimonial and therefore still admissible. Medical professionals are well advised, however, to be certain that the interviews with children they see are solely for purposes of diagnosis and treatment. Medical professionals should not conduct investigation-like forensic interviews with children as a way of seeking to elicit more information than is necessary for diagnosis and treatment.

Medical professionals are allowed to testify that an evaluation of a child is consistent with sexual abuse. Medical professionals may say they cannot rule out sexual abuse and can even say that it is their professional opinion that a child has been sexually abused.

However, medical professionals can neither testify that a particular person sexually abused a child, nor can they testify that a child or other witness is telling the truth or is believable. Experts generally cannot testify about the profile of a sexual abuser of children and its similarity to the defendant's profile.

Ultimately, when medical professionals testify in court as expert witnesses, their purpose is to tell the truth and inform the fact-finder about information related to their area of expertise. An expert's role in this setting is not as an advocate for the child or a particular position. Rather, advocacy in this situation is the responsibility of the lawyer. When called as an expert witness, it is especially incumbent upon the medical professional to speak truthfully and objectively. If the medical professional is prepared and informed, the experience of testifying in court can be effective and rewarding.

REFERENCES

1. Myers JEB. *Myers on evidence in child, domestic and elder abuse cases.* New York, NY: Aspen Publishers; 2005.

2. Utah R. Evid. 803(4) (2008).

3. Indian Child Welfare Act of 1978, 25 USC § 1901.

4. *Crawford v Washington*, 541 US 36 (2004).

Chapter 17

CHILD SEXUAL EXPLOITATION

Sharon W. Cooper, MD, FAAP
Dan D. Broughton, MD

Child sexual exploitation encompasses several types of sexually based crimes. Each has significant impact on the victim. Often, children and youth are victims of more than a single type of exploitation at one time. The most important fact to remember regarding sexual exploitation of children is that it is rooted in child sexual abuse. A child who is sexually abused may be further traumatized by exposure to others, either visually or physically. The child may develop psychological problems associated with such maltreatment in addition to any psychological problems originating from the original abuse.

The vulnerability of children is clear and ties into sexual abuse and exploitation in tragic proportions. Two thirds of convicted rapists victimized children under 18 years of age, with 40% victimizing children under 12 years of age. However, it often is surprising that, in some ways, adolescents may be even more at risk than younger children. Those aged 12 to 17 years are victimized at twice the rate of the general population, with the incidence of violent crimes being 3 times as high.

A discussion of child sexual abuse can no longer take place without rethinking the entire aspect of child exploitation in the 21st century. Most homes in the United States have at least one computer, and many have several. The advent of the Internet has brought great advances in communication and information retrieval and exchange. Unfortunately, there are aspects of this information and communication technology that have been commonly used as tools for the exploitation of children and youths.

There are 5 types of sexual exploitation perpetrated against children and teenagers: child pornography, cyber-enticement for sexual purposes, prostitution and commercial sexual exploitation, child sex tourism, and human trafficking. Each of these forms of sexual exploitation has sexual abuse as the primary basis of victimology.[1] A thorough understanding of this broadening definition of sexual abuse can assist multidisciplinary teams in addressing the needs of exploited children in a more empathic and effective manner.

Child pornography is often referred to as child sexual abuse images, child abuse images, digital crimes of sexual abuse, and violence against children in cyberspace. Realization that pictures depicted on the Internet are actual children and not virtual morphed images takes time, and members of child abuse multidisciplinary teams are working hard to catch up with the technology of abuse.

Cyber-enticement is a form of sexual exploitation that often entails child pornography victimization. This form of abuse may present in many ways. A youth may go online and meet an adult pretending to be another youth desiring a casual date or may blog onto the page of an adult who is looking for an adventurous teenager on a social networking site. Cyber-enticement can also present as a lure to upload self-made erotic and pornographic images as a form of grooming of youths who may have excellent computer expertise but marginal cyber awareness skills.

Prostitution is the most underreported type of child sexual abuse. Controversy exists regarding the terms *prostitution, commercial sexual exploitation*, and *human trafficking*. Many consider these terms to be synonymous. Others purport that they are 3 distinct forms of sexual abuse and prostitution is the common thread. The term *commercial sexual exploitation* is sometimes used to refer to extrafamilial prostitution. Human trafficking involves the movement of victims from one place to another (eg, from one city to another or one country to another). Prostitution as an intrafamilial form of child sexual abuse has been highly unrecognized in the past. The role of the Internet in the marketing of children and youth as well as an increasing social acceptance of prostitution culture and terms have increased awareness of exploitation. Terms such as *pimps, hos, tricks, players, the game*, and *bling* have become so mainstream that communities have finally begun to recognize that sexual exploitation through prostitution and sexual slavery is a huge concern around the world.

The nexus of pornography production and prostitution is most apparent in ***child sex tourism*** cases, which usually involve sex offenders traveling from one country to another to have sex with children. The offender may take a child from his or her country of origin to a destination that has weak proactive and reactive laws against the sexual abuse of children. At times, children are marketed online for tourists who are often registered sex offenders in their own country. This form of sexual exploitation is highly associated with the production of child pornography as a keepsake or souvenir. Often, the prey in this form of abuse are very young children who are indigent and who may be victims of intrafamilial prostitution.

Human trafficking may be either domestic or international. Sex trafficking is a subset of this form of exploitation, with other aspects including illegal labor, forced marriages, and civil rights violations. Youths may be trafficked for prostitution, where mobility is somewhat available, or for sexual slavery, where victims are kept imprisoned with locks or guards and must perform dozens of sexual acts per day. International human trafficking often involves child abductions or tricking indigent families into believing that they are sending their children to a destination that will provide more prosperity and the possibility of income to be sent home.

With the accessibility and anonymity offered by the Internet and advancing mobile phone technology, each of these forms of abuse has grown significantly and requires new information and understanding by all who deal with abused and exploited children as well as enhanced investigative skills for those investigating these crimes.[2] With the exception of cyber-enticement, child sexual exploitation can and often does occur without computer facilitation. However, typically Internet or mobile phone technology is used in the commission of these kinds of crimes against children. In response to this realization, most states in the US have established individual law enforcement teams who are specially trained to understand and investigate computer-facilitated or -initiated crimes involving the sexual abuse of children. These teams are commonly referred to as Internet Crimes Against Children (ICAC) Task Forces.

CHILD PORNOGRAPHY

Sexual exploitation occurs in several ways (see **Table 17-1**). Each can have a negative impact upon the child.

Although adult pornography is clearly legal in most instances and a completely different issue than child pornography, it still plays a significant role in child sexual exploitation.

> ## Table 17-1. Pornographic Exploitation through Information and Communication Technology.
>
> — Exposure to adult pornography
>
> — Children who are abused through prostitution online for sexual abuse offline
>
> — Children who are abused through prostitution with the use of the Internet and mobile phone technology to contact the abusers
>
> — Adults or youths who engage in written cybersex with children online
>
> — Youths who post pornographic images of other youths or younger children online
>
> — Children living in the home of a parent or guardian who is downloading or distributing child pornography
>
> — Children and youths who download child pornography
>
> — Children who are groomed online with the use of pornography for sexual abuse offline
>
> — Children who are sold online for Webcam–facilitated live sexual abuse online
>
> — Children who are the subjects of child pornography that would include the following scenarios:
>
> > — Offenders who show child pornography to children to normalize the act of sex between an adult and a child
> >
> > — Children who are made to view their own images of pornography, which serves the purpose of intimidation and extortion into silence
> >
> > — Children who are made to be recruiters for friends and acquaintances for the purpose of child sexual abuse and child pornography production
> >
> > — Children who are encouraged to offend against other children for child pornography production purposes, either with the offender or at the direction of the offender
> >
> > — Children who are encouraged to place images of themselves online
>
> — Youths who become compliant victims and use live Webcam–facilitated means of posting autoerotic images online

Often, exposure to pornography is used by an offender in grooming potential victims. To this end, children who are shown adult pornography are introduced to the continuum of offender behaviors. Adult pornography is readily available on the Internet, rendering prior impediments to access passé.

It takes little effort to find pornographic images on the Internet. Most search engines will lead to a display of thousands of pornographic sites with a few clicks of a mouse. Some studies have found that nearly 1 in 4 youths has been exposed to unwanted pornography.[3] Other studies indicate that the number is closer to 1 in 3 despite efforts to make pornography less accessible and to educate families on how to protect children on the Internet. These numbers do not take into account those who seek pornography.

Chronic exposure to pornography may lead to desensitization to viewing sexual encounters, an expectation that sex is often linked with violence, and the belief that a relationship is based upon an expectation of unhealthy sexual interactions.

Analyses of child sexual abuse cases have revealed that offenders will initially introduce children to adult pornography in chat rooms with the intent to subsequently introduce child sexual abuse images as the next phase of grooming. Grooming the child in this manner has 2 purposes: to encourage the youth to believe that having sexual relations with an adult is normal and to feed the fantasy of the groomer who gains sexual gratification from sharing the images. Another purpose of adult pornography is to educate a child on the preferred types of sexual interactions depicted in the images. Even in cases where parents are not involved in the sexual exploitation, the fact that a child is able to view adult pornography for significant periods of time brings up the question of appropriate supervision. In many jurisdictions, exposure of a minor to adult pornography is often a misdemeanor offense.

In contrast to adult pornography, child pornography is always illegal and is never acceptable. In its 1973 decision upholding child pornography statutes, the US Supreme Court stated that "...the use of children as subjects of pornographic materials is harmful to the physiological, emotional, and mental health of the child, easily passes muster under the First Amendment."[4] This effectively removed child pornography from the general debate over pornography and obscenity and all of its controversy. Unfortunately, even with such firm wording from the Supreme Court, child pornography remains a major problem.

There is a direct link between the possession of child pornography and child sexual victimization. In one study of child pornography offenders, 56% had a prior criminal record, 24% had prior contact sexual offenses, and 15% had prior child pornography offenses.[5] Also, approximately 40% of arrested offenders who met or attempted to meet children online also possessed child pornography.

During a personal interview in March 2007, Michelle Collins reported that the Child Victim Identification Program (CVIP) of the National Center for Missing and Exploited Children (NCMEC) has reviewed 7 million pornographic images of children on the Internet through March 2007. Although there are no firm data, it is clear that there is a trend toward younger victims, often depicted in a domestic environment. Images of infants as young as 2 months of age have been documented. Older print versions of child pornography that appeared in magazines rarely showed preschool-aged children. Likewise, younger children were identified infrequently in the Internet images reviewed when the CVIP analysts began processing contraband. However, of the more than 1100 victims who have been identified, 6% are infants or toddlers and 58% are prepubescent. It is important to note that often older teenagers who are still minors may not be included in the victim database because of the evident advanced degree of sexual maturation. Research in the US reveals that the majority of Caucasian, African-American, and Hispanic girls reach sexual maturation by 14 to 16 years of age. Boys are typically indistinguishable from a mature adult male within the parameters of sexual maturation at 15 to 16 years of age.[6]

Victims of this form of exploitation are faced with a lifetime of anxiety because of the perceived and often real threat that others will have access to images of their sexual abuse and that it will never completely go away. Aversion to the use of a computer has been described by victims and therapists when it is known that images have been traded in cyberspace. In addition, these images of young children serve as a means of freezing them at a moment in time, potentially preventing them visually, and therefore psychologically, from being able to move on from these abusive events. Such concerns complicate the long-term effects of sexual abuse. Research is needed to better characterize the impact this type of abuse has on these victims and to define the best practices in the psychological support and legal management of cases involving such children. The best interest of the child should be the guiding tenet in these types of cases, and careful discussion with nonoffending parents and caregivers is necessary to decide the extent of case information that should be provided to the child.

A large number of child pornography users trade images without attempting to produce their own, while an even larger group of adults participate in downloading images of sexually abused children and youths, generally for a fee.[7] Child pornography has become a billion-dollar industry. Many of those involved fail to recognize that downloading images objectifies child victims and promotes a cycle of further abuse by increasing demand for the images.

Children who live in the home of an adult who is downloading or distributing child pornography present a special problem. There is a relationship between downloading images, trading, and ultimately producing images. Some offenders sexually abuse children directly and document the experience with photographs or videography. As is the case in child sexual abuse, family members are often involved with the production of child pornography. Among cases identified by the NCMEC, photographs were produced by parents in 38% of the cases and, in another 10% of cases, by other family members. It is not known whether these relatives were sexually abusing the children and became involved in child pornography subsequently or whether they became involved with viewing such images and then began to abuse and photograph their own children.

The body of knowledge regarding those who possess child pornography is growing. An analysis of those arrested for Internet-related child pornography possession between July 2000 and June 2001 revealed that almost all were male, 95% were Caucasian, more than 85% were over the age of 25, and only 5% were under the age of 18. The majority of offenders (55%) were or had been married. Nearly half of the offenders were from urban/suburban areas and 11% were from rural areas. A total of 95% had graduated from high school and at least 20% had college or higher degrees. Nearly 80% were employed full-time.[8] Research has revealed that a person in possession of child pornography may have a higher risk of an ultimate diagnosis of the paraphilia pedophilia than an actual contact sex offender.[9]

ROLE OF THE HEALTH CARE PROVIDER

The role of the health care provider in child pornography often entails image analysis for legal purposes. A faulty belief that the majority of images on the Internet are virtual and not real children has existed; however, thousands of investigations have proven that real children are being abused and more and more new images continue to appear in cyberspace. Knowledge of the growth, development, and sexual maturation of children is essential to provide a reasonable estimate of the age of victims depicted in sexual abuse images. Medical providers need to be able to assess whether images are consistent with children under 18 years of age, under 12 years of age, or consistent with children who may have a developmental disability. This task is accomplished through knowledge of motor milestones in toddlers, dentition and body habitus in early school-aged children, and sexual maturation ratings in "tweens," preteens, and teenagers. Many in the field now analyze child pornography using more universal age matches for sexual maturation rating instead of the original Tanner stages of puberty.[10] The key point in an analysis of this type is to determine whether a law has been broken. Consequently, discerning the age of a child within the 2 important age ranges of legal prepubescence (age 12 years or under) or legal adolescence (age 18 years or under) is a task for pediatricians, family medicine practitioners, and forensic and sexual assault nurse examiners. Knowledge that the onset of puberty for girls in the US is between 9 and 10 years of age and that puberty is essentially completed by 14 to 15 years of age is essential for recognizing that images of children with incomplete sexual maturation are almost assuredly consistent with an age of less than 18 years. The age ranges for boys are about one year later. Syndromes associated with delayed puberty are uncommon and not likely to be relevant in the circumstance of an offender who has hundreds or thousands of images of children. It is not likely that an offender would find multiple examples of children with abnormal pubertal development.

Because of the increasing number of infant and toddler sexual abuse images, practitioners must become very familiar with motor milestones, because these are the best markers for age in very young children. Normal walking is typically accomplished by 15 months of age, and many toddlers are walking well by 12 months. Often, sexually abused toddlers whose images are online are victims of sadistic abuse either by bondage and beatings or by penetration. These particularly gruesome images result in more severe penalties when in the possession of an offender. Consequently, a health care provider should not only be aware of the age ranges for such victims, but also the degree of depicted sexual depravity.

Specialists who are attempting to identify and locate victims have the leeway of much more speculation regarding the possible age of a child in an image. This latter form of analysis is typically implemented by forensic specialists such as those in the Child Victims of Internet Pornography Unit found at the NCMEC in the United States. These dedicated specialists spend numerous hours analyzing images in order to locate and rescue children whose sexual and emotional abuse is present every day on the Internet as the cycle of abuse continues.

A great deal has been learned about child pornography, and efforts are being made to combat this problem. For example, in 2004, leading US credit card companies and the International Centre for Missing and Exploited Children formed a coalition to stop the flow of money used for the purchase of child pornography on the Internet in an attempt to stop the commercial use of such pornography. In June 2006, a technology coalition of 5 major online companies (Yahoo, America Online, Microsoft, EarthLink, and United Online) and the NCMEC was launched to combine resources to develop and deploy technology solutions to disrupt predators using the Internet to exploit children or to traffic in child pornography.

DISCLOSURE

Delayed disclosure is common in child sexual abuse. This is particularly true when the offender is a family member or an acquaintance. In such circumstances, only 12% of female victims reported to authorities during childhood.[11] In light of this fact, it is not surprising that most children do not disclose sexual abuse in childhood. When they do, however, it is typically due to empowerment from a supportive friend or family member; a desire to see the abuse stop, possibly to protect a younger sibling; or, occasionally, within the context of an angry outburst. When a child is not ready to disclose sexual abuse, but images of the child's victimization have been discovered, defense mechanisms to avoid guilt and self-blame play an important role in the denial of involvement. Children often become arrested in the phase of denial, even when in a therapeutic environment. This realization for counselors and forensic interviewers is key in supporting a victim and avoiding coercing them to lie about their victimization.

There is empirical evidence from investigators, prosecutors, and other members of multi-disciplinary teams that children who have been sexually abused and pornographically photographed are particularly silent regarding the photographic victimization. Many children who have been found to be victims of pornography may disclose sexually abusive acts upon questioning, but often deny the involvement of pictures or videotapes. This phenomenon is referred to as "double silencing" and reflects strong protective defense mechanisms on the part of the child victim.[12]

YOUTH AS OFFENDERS

Children who download child sexual abuse images present a particular concern for those in the fields of juvenile justice and youth welfare. The general consensus is that a significant number of Internet child pornography offenses are committed by minors. These images may have been sent to the child either from an adult offender or from a similar-aged chat room friend who is trying to groom a fellow youth for an ultimate sexual encounter.

Children who download child sexual abuse images are at risk for sexual stimulation and disinhibition, with a resultant faulty belief that children are not harmed by such sexual contact. If a youth offender has access to online adult or child pornography while caring for younger siblings or relatives, there may be a resultant scenario of opportunistic sexual victimization. It is important to ask child victims about the events immediately preceding a sexual assault involving a youth offender. The preceding events may be overlooked by victims unless they are carefully questioned. It is essential to avoid characterizing Internet images in a derogatory manner to a victim of a youth who may have been viewing them before a sexual assault. Negative remarks about the images might deter a victim from disclosing a history of sexual exploitation by the youth through information or communication technology. Images made under these circumstances are almost assuredly for the purpose of extortion into silence. If no pornography was produced but a youth offender was viewing online pornography, such exposure might ultimately provide mitigating circumstances within the context of legal action involving such an offender.

The challenge in dealing with youthful perpetrators in this circumstance is twofold. First, it is likely that they have had access to adult pornography for some period of time. As they become desensitized to the visual images, they (as well as adults) will often begin to seek more graphic and even violent images, which tend to depict younger victims. Thus, the transition from adult to child images may be an inadvertent move on the part of the youth offender.

The second concern, which may have greater psychosexual developmental implications, is that the ease of access and anonymity of downloading child pornography may not reflect an intent for child sexual exploitation, but rather *sexual exploration*. If an image has a file name that indicates the age of the child in the image, and that age is similar to the offender's age, the desire to collect these images is likely an attempt at virtual sexual experimentation. A serious consequence in this circumstance is the potential for mandatory sex offender registration of adolescents who may have a poor understanding of the criminal nature of their behavior.[13]

CYBER-ENTICEMENT

A discussion of sexual exploitation in the 21st century requires a continued under-standing of social trends in adolescent behaviors and emerging technology. It is often difficult to keep abreast of changes in society because of the almost instant receipt of information via the Internet and the behavioral reactions that teenagers so quickly adopt. An example is the emergence of online videogaming. The advent of the ability to play games with thousands of online gamers opened the door to a much broader market of games as well as a need on the part of participants to spend far more time interacting with this type of technology. Reports from other countries reveal that online games constitute 1 of at least 3 types of popular Internet pastimes that are becoming addictive to teenagers to such a degree as to spawn mental health clinics for treatment. Other sources of Web addiction for both teenagers and adults include sex sites, shopping, and online gambling.

Compliant victimization is an important component of Internet activity, and a discussion regarding risks and outcomes is essential to understanding information and communication technology crimes against children. Defined as a pattern of behaviors and beliefs by child sexual exploitation victims that promotes active and passive acceptance of sexual abuse by an adult, compliant victimization reflects a complex response influenced by social trends, grooming, and at times accommodation. Exhibitionism, consumerism, and brain maturation are other factors that influence the acceptance of behaviors and social trends propagated by the Internet. For example, the well-publicized DVDs marketed as *Girls Gone Wild* promote the message that mixing alcohol and group vacationing justifies being filmed in a sexually provocative manner for the reward of a skimpy T-shirt with the *Girls Gone Wild* logo. Several large federal fines have been successfully levied against the owner and producer of this business, primarily due to a failure to document proof of age of the victims of this form of exploitation. Unfortunately for the victims, footage of their exploitation has been found on Internet pornography sites and even on pay-per-view televised pornography channels, such as Playboy, Inc.

At times, youths who network with adults may use Web cameras to show mutual autoerotic images (a form of exhibitionism). Typically, adult offenders expose themselves as a show of trust as well as a strategy to dissolve personal barriers of self-exposure. Victims are frequently rewarded with gifts, money, and online attention when they comply with the wishes of such offenders. Victims have described the seduction as slow and gradual, with each encounter leading to a little more exposure. This was the experience of one victim, Justin Berry, whose case rose to the level of Congressional testimony after the *New York Times* uncovered the incredible degree of victimization that was facilitated by the use of a Webcam.[14] Eventually, with much verbal (via telephone) and online chat encouragement and positive reinforcement, youths mirror the behaviors of the offenders. Sometimes offenders link a reluctant victim with another youth who has already been groomed into compliance so that the former will believe that this is a common and acceptable online behavior among close sexual friends. Once a youth has gone to this degree of self-exposure, it is far easier for an offender to negotiate an offline meeting with the agreement and sometimes even anticipation of the now-compliant victim. The masturbatory behaviors associated with Webcam use may become habitual, both for the sender and the recipient. There are often multiple recipients of these images. Live interactions may escalate from this form of child sexual abuse, resulting in an offender traveling to have contact with the youth or vice versa.

The use of photographs is not the only form of child exploitation found on the Internet. Cybersex (also referred to as "cybering") is a form of written sexually explicit language meant to provide a virtual format for sexual intercourse. It is a form of role play and is often facilitated by the use of Internet emoticons, which are computer keyboard icons popularly used to denote emotions. Also called a smiley, an emoticon is a sequence of ordinary printable American Standard Code for Information Interchange

(ASCII) characters. Emoticons are a form of paralanguage commonly used in e-mail messages, in online bulletin boards, online forums, instant messages, or in chat rooms. Examples include the following:

:-) (used to inflect a sarcastic or joking statement)

;-) (used to denote a wink)

:-* and :-** (used to denote giving a kiss and returning a kiss, respectively)

:9 (used to denote tasty or licking lips)

:-*) (used to denote "I am blushing")

!:-) (used to denote "I have an idea")

Acronyms and abbreviations, in conjunction with emoticons, may be used in cybersex involving youths out of a desire to keep communications a secret, particularly from parents. The secret encrypted nature of such communications is a form of grooming and luring of youths. Common acronyms and abbreviations that are used include the following:

LOL (laughing out loud)

MUSM (miss you so much)

POS (parent over shoulder)

OLL (online love)

WTGP (want to go private?)

LMIRL (let's meet in real life)

Cybersex often entails the use of sexually explicit language and is similar to pornographic magazines that only depict written language. Emoticons are often mixed with simple strings of letters to denote sexual stimulation, excitation, and ultimate gratification. Teen chat rooms are a common place for the initiation of such online dialogue and typically more explicit communication occurs in a personal e-mail or an instant message encounter.

The special and secret nature of this form of exploitation frequently sets the stage for further complicit behaviors, including the use of a Webcam for the transmission of illegal autoerotic images of the youth. Cybersex is often a precursor to an enticement that results in the youth traveling to meet the adult who initiated or participated in this form of sexual exploitation. These meetings almost always result in a sexual encounter.[15] New challenges include the risk for cybersex via mobile phone technology with text messaging and the ability to access the Internet at all times. In addition, offenders may use peer-to-peer communications that bypass the use of an Internet service provider, or 3G technology, which allows transmission of digital images from one mobile phone to another without use of the Internet at all. These methods allow youths access while in school, without them having to place a mobile phone to their ear, and facilitate further covert communication.

Online grooming of children in order to entice them to meet for a sexual encounter is often referred to as "cyber-enticement" or "traveler cases." Recent studies that reviewed offender and victim dynamics in this form of child abuse from 2000 to 2001 revealed that, in the majority of cases, youths voluntarily left their homes to meet this type of predator at least twice before an arrest was made. Although 76% of online encounters occurred in a chat room, 13% originated at a sexually oriented site.[16] This research predated the emergence of social networking sites.

Adult perpetrators are very patient, and often will contact many children in search of a victim. They have often educated themselves in the popular vernacular of teenagers as well as their interests in music, videogames, entertainment stars, and sports activities. They cultivate a relationship over many months and look for children who appear vulnerable and who admit in online blogs that they are lonely or that they are having family problems. Also, if a youth is online very late at night, an offender might assume that the computer is in the youth's bedroom and that the youth is poorly supervised. Approximately 40% of arrested offenders who met or attempted to meet children online possessed child pornography.

Many youths meet predators in teen chat rooms or via instant messaging, but attention is also being focused on social networking sites such as myspace.com, Facebook.com, or Bebo.com. Whereas chat rooms are similar to virtual conferences with several individuals, a social networking site is more like a virtual community. An individual sends out messages to personal friends to join his or her site for the purpose of online communication, sharing of interests, posting pictures, and meeting new people. These personal friends do the same to their friends, thus broadening the network of an online community. In this way, individuals come into contact with people from everywhere the Internet reaches. More and more, different people become interconnected in this way. The problem is that some of these contacts may be quite different from the original person's intended audience and some, including child predators, may be using a false identity.

Social networking sites began to become popular in 2001 with the Circle of Friends, followed in 2003 by a Web site called Friendster. In 2005 one of the largest American sites, myspace.com, became a household term, hosting more than 10 million adolescent users and 110 million total participants. A 2006 Cox Communications and NCMEC study found that 61% of teenagers aged 13 to 17 years had personal files on social networking sites and at least half of these youths had posted pictures of themselves online. The huge financial significance of MySpace is illustrated by its purchase by News Corp for $530 million.

In conjunction with the growing popularity of these sites, reports began to emerge of cyber-enticement cases that resulted from youths on such sites voluntarily leaving their homes to meet child sex offenders.[17] In response, some of the sites began to post new rules to provide a safer environment. For example, in June 2006, myspace.com hired a director of security and introduced a series of measures aimed at protecting their younger clients. Many of these rules restrict older users' access to the sites or information of younger members. However, rules related to age are difficult to enforce as they are dependent on truthful reporting of age by both the younger and the older age groups.

In an effort to alleviate concerns regarding the inability of parents to monitor their children online, MySpace developed the software Zephyr, released in 2007, which allows parents to know what name, age, and location their children use to represent themselves. The program also alerts the youth to the fact that someone is accessing this information.

Bullying has become a major concern for schools, youth groups, youth advocates, and the criminal justice system. Cyber-bullying, enhanced by child pornography production or sexual solicitation or intimidation, can become a tool in the sexual victimization of teenagers by peers (youth offenders). The purpose of the production and transmission of such images may be a prank, but may also represent a desire to humiliate, hurt, or seek revenge on another youth. The use of mobile phone cameras during a gang sexual assault as well as photographs taken surreptitiously in public bathrooms are examples of how sexually explicit images of innocent victims can result in online victimization. Such depictions can be extremely traumatic for victims and difficult to trace. Comparison data indicate that this type of harassment has increased over the past few years from 6% to 9%, and this trend is expected to continue. Another example of this form of sexual exploitation involves a consensual sexual encounter between school classmates who choose to take pictures with mobile phone cameras. If there is an argument or dissolution of the relationship, one partner may share the intimate pictures online with others in the school. In a personal conversation with John Smith of the Ontario Provincial Police, he reported that the female partner is almost always the victim in these cases, and consequences are difficult to gauge because this constitutes the production of child pornography, which could result in a very stiff penalty.

PROSTITUTION OF CHILDREN AND YOUTH

Abuse through prostitution has traditionally been a more hidden form of child sexual abuse, and often children and youths are reluctant to disclose details about this form of victimization because of a history of intimidation or grooming into the belief that they are coconspirators with the offender. Additionally, teenage prostitution is often considered a victimless crime or even the responsibility of the prostituted youth. It is important to note that there is frequently a nexus between pornography and prostitution, both of children and youths, as a later complication of child sexual abuse. Victims of child sexual abuse have a much higher risk (28 times) of arrest for exploitation through prostitution than children who have never been sexually abused.[18]

Children may be victims of prostitution from within their own home and their plight is typically poorly recognized.[19] Children who are prostituted by their families (including exploitation online for sexual abuse offline) are at great risk for all of the traditional complications of prostitution: physical violence; sexual violence; multiple offender sexual abuse; sexually transmitted infections; exposure to alcohol and drugs; and psychological trauma, including posttraumatic stress disorder, depression, dissociation, anxiety, and compulsive disorders. When the Internet is involved in the commission of this type of crime, commercial sexual exploitation is either intrafamilial, where a parent or caregiver is marketing the child with accompanying child pornography teasers, or an offender is using an online classified site such as www.craigslist.org.

The leading causes of death for persons exploited through prostitution are murder and human immunodeficiency virus/acquired immunodeficiency syndrome (HIV/AIDS). When there is a more organized criminal aspect to this form of exploitation, there are often connections with domestic or international human traffickers.

Some youths are victims of commercial sexual exploitation as a form of survival on the streets. This is particularly true when teenagers are struggling with sexual orientation and may have been thrown out of their homes. It is also often the case in internationally trafficked youths. At other times, underage youths are marketed from brothels or from remote locations where they are often kept in sexual slavery.

Child welfare intervention for children in the care of exploitive individuals is indicated under the Child Protective Service's clause for moral turpitude, found in many state statutes. It is incumbent upon the social worker to ensure that no contact offenses have occurred related to the offender's clear preference for children as sexual partners. Some protection is offered for victims trafficked into the US through the Trafficking Victims

Protection Act. Victims are allowed to remain in the US and may be granted a T Visa permitting them to stay for up to 3 years. They may also apply for permanent residency. The federal government is also directed to monitor and combat trafficking under the Office to Monitor and Combat Trafficking in Persons.

When pornography is produced within the context of exploitation through prostitution, sexual abuse and extortion are often involved. The extortion often involves runaways who are duped by offenders as they initially attempt to ingratiate themselves with the youths. Then, with the use of date rape drugs or brute force, they sexually assault the youths and make pornographic photographs or videotapes. The offenders subsequently blackmail the youths into working for them in what may be a lifetime of exploitation.[20]

CHILD SEX TOURISM

Another aspect of childhood sexual exploitation through pornography production is demonstrated in child sex tourism cases. In this particularly deceptive form of abuse, individuals will leave their country of residence to travel to countries whose laws are lax regarding the prostitution of young children and youth for the purpose of finding children who will become their victims.[21] It is also notable that some sex tourists travel to another country with the child whom they will sexually abuse. A pornographic record is generally produced as a keepsake of the trip.

The most common sex tourists are Americans. This form of child sexual exploitation has become popular, in part, in response to required sex offender registration. Often, American perpetrators would rather accept the risk of overseas travel for the purpose of child sexual abuse than be caught abusing an American child with the associated high risk of incarceration and registration. Fortunately, many countries have enacted laws making it a crime in the home country for its citizens to travel to a foreign country for the purpose of sexually abusing a child. In the US, this provision is part of the PROTECT Act passed in 2003. It is only necessary to prove that the abuse took place, not that the perpetrator left with the intent of abusing a child.

HUMAN TRAFFICKING

Professionals who work in inner cities with large immigrant populations or in rural communities with migrant workers must be cognizant of the increased risk for international human trafficking. Women and girls are particularly at risk for illegal labor in massage parlors, sexually oriented businesses, domestic work with sexual abuse as an additional form of exploitation, and other associated civil rights violations. The risk of death is significant, and victims are often indentured. It is common for victims to incur large debts during their transport, which the lenders never intend to be paid off. There are an estimated 18 000 to 20 000 victims in the US, and interaction with the Department of State resources as well as federal investigators is mandatory in providing adequate services.

Children and youths who are trafficked from one city to another for sexual exploitation in prostitution make up nearly 20 times the number of internationally trafficked victims. ECPAT-USA cites the fact that foreign national victims receive many more services than similar victims who are born in the United States. Many cities are beginning to mount task forces to address this issue, particularly as Internet facilitation has made the marketing and movement of persons much more difficult to track. Once state lines are crossed, federal investigators and prosecutors become responsible for these kinds of cases and a great deal of attention is warranted because of the careful manipulation, intimidation, and extortion of victims and witnesses.

OTHER FORMS OF EXPLOITATION

ONLINE LIVE SEXUAL ABUSE

A particularly distressing, albeit rare, form of child sexual exploitation is that of pay-per-view online live sexual abuse of children. This type of case is contrary to the traditionally held concept that child sex rings usually involve an offender who is a trusted adult, not a family member, who abuses children in small groups. In the original descriptions of child sex rings, only syndicated rings involving multiple adults, multiple children, and a wide range of exchange items including child pornography and sexual activities were involved.[22] The reality is that online live sexual abuse is more often perpetrated by family members who belong to a closed network of like-minded parental offenders. The perpetrators voice their requests, live or via e-mail, for the type of sexual acts that they desire at the specified meeting time. The use of live streaming video is the technology of choice for these types of transmissions.[23] Those who participate in this type of child sexual abuse frequently collect large amounts of child pornography and trade with an international group of participants. International cooperation is essential in investigating these crimes. Children who are rescued have often been sadistically sexually abused and typically are very young so they are not able to disclose or provide evidentiary details.

An additional challenge in the field of children and the law focuses on a federal mandate, the Justice for All Act of 2004. The bill has 4 parts that are meant to enhance protection of victims of federal crimes. The section relevant to child sexual exploitation victims is Title I, which requires that victims not be excluded from certain legal proceedings relevant to their victimization. Translated into everyday language, this law mandates that if the identity of a child whose images of exploitation through pornography are involved in a legal proceeding such as a sentencing, et cetera, is known, the child and family have a right to be notified. The problem with this particular type of criminal justice action is that the victim is at risk of knowing that his or her sexual abuse images have been collected and traded over and over via the Internet. This will potentially reinforce the fears and anxiety expressed by school-aged victims that friends and acquaintances will one day find out that their sexual abuse pictures are online and available for anyone to see. In addition, notification continues until the victim reaches the age of 18 years. He or she then has the option to continue the notification or opt out of the mandated plan. Careful consideration and counseling of both victims and their families are necessary to reach the best decision in each case.

THE SEXUALIZATION OF GIRLS

The American Psychological Association released a study that acknowledges that girls are being sexualized as a result of numerous societal influences such as media, advertising, entertainment, music videos, and fashion. The study states that the sexualization of girls occurs when any of the following occur:

— A person's value comes only from her sexual appeal or behavior to the exclusion of other characteristics.

— A person is held to a standard that equates physical attractiveness (narrowly defined) with being sexy.

— A person is sexually objectified—that is, made into a thing for others' sexual use rather than being seen as a person with the capacity for independent action and decision making.

— Sexuality is inappropriately imposed upon a person.

The study notes that much of the evidence evaluated was specific to the third part of the definition (sexual objectification).[24] This concept is central to commercial sexual exploitation of children and youths. When youths are seen as chattel, objects, or forms of barter and exchange, they are not only at great risk of abuse, but also likely to assume the validity of such objectification and become compliant victims.

The sexualization of girls may also result in offenders viewing children as appropriate sexual partners. This only reinforces a well-known cognitive distortion frequently present in child sex offenders who believe that children proactively seduce them into behaviors that they would otherwise not have considered.

PREVENTION

Parents can do a number of things to try to make Internet use safer for their children. First, communication between parents, children, and adolescents is of great importance.

— Discuss Internet concerns with children and teenagers.

— Know children's and teenagers' identifiers, including passwords, screen names, and account information.

— Encourage appropriate behavior (eg, no bullying, sexual communication, or soliciting by youths).

— Enter a safe-computing contract with children and youths or do not let them use the Internet.

— Encourage children and teenagers to tell a trusted adult or law enforcement authorities if they are being sexually abused and images are part of the victimization.

— Parents must learn about computers and the Internet. Children generally have far more savvy than their parents in this area.

— Supervise children's and teenagers' use of the Internet.

— All computers should be in a public part of the home and never in a child's room or where a door can be closed and locked.

— Install monitoring software to identify which sites have been visited by users of the home computer.

— Enable or consider purchasing filtering programs that can restrict what sites can be visited with a computer, especially with younger children.

— Be aware of PDAs and mobile phones that connect to the Internet.

— Recognize that technology exists that allows the transmission of digital pictures from mobile phone cameras without the use of the Internet.

Suggestions for children and teenagers include the following:

— Do not share personal information unless you absolutely know who is on the other end of the connection.

— If uncomfortable with a message, do not respond.

— Talk to parents or a trusted adult if you become concerned about a site or communications you receive.

— Never arrange a meeting with anyone you meet on the Internet unless you will be accompanied by a parent (or a group of trusted friends if an older teenager).

— Never send a photograph of yourself unless you know the person to whom you are sending it.

The following suggestions are good for safety when blogging or using social networking sites:

— Never post personal information.

— Never give out your password.

— Add only people you really know.

— Check privacy settings.

— Be aware that personal photographs may contain inadvertent identifying information.

— Protect your friends and avoid being a bystander.

CONCLUSION

Child sexual abuse and its close link to sexual exploitation are important aspects of child maltreatment that all professionals in the field must understand. The various types of sexual exploitation—pornography, prostitution, cyber-enticement, sex tourism, and human trafficking—are all closely linked to sexual abuse images. These online or offline videos and images are used to educate children for sexual abuse, extort them into prostitution and silence, to commemorate a sexual encounter as is seen in sex tourism cases, to coerce entry into an eventual cyber-enticement episode, and to facilitate domestic and international trafficking of victims for sexual abuse through prostitution. The Internet poses ongoing dilemmas that require careful attention and resolution by cohesive multidisciplinary teams seeking to eradicate child abuse worldwide.

REFERENCES

1. Cooper SW, Estes RJ, Giardino AP, Kellogg ND, Vieth VI, eds. *Medical, Legal, & Social Science Aspects of Child Sexual Exploitation: A Comprehensive Review of Pornography, Prostitution, and Internet Crimes.* Vol 1-2. St. Louis, MO: G.W. Medical Publishing, Inc; 2005.

2. Muir D; ECPAT. Violence Against Children in Cyberspace: A Contribution to the United Nations Study on Violence Against Children. http://www.ecpat.net/EI/Publications/ICT/Cyberspace_ENG.pdf. Published 2005. Accessed March 16, 2010.

3. Finkelhor D, Mitchell KJ, Wolak J. Online Victimization: A Report on the Nation's Youth. National Center for Missing and Exploited Children. 2000.

4. *Miller v California*, 413 US 15 (1973).

5. MC Seto, Eke AW. The criminal histories and later offending of child pornography offenders. *Sex Abuse: J Res Treatment.* 2005;17(2):201-210.

6. Sun SS, Schubert CM, Chumlea WC, et al. National estimates of the timing of sexual maturation and racial differences among US children. *Pediatrics.* 2002;110(5):911-919.

7. Taylor M. IXth ISPCAN European Conference on Child Abuse and Neglect: Promoting Interdisciplinary Approaches to Child Protection. August 29-30, 2003; Warsaw, Poland.

8. Mitchell KJ, Finkelhor D, Wolak J. The Internet and family and acquaintance sexual abuse. *Child Maltreat.* 2005;10:49-60.

9. Seto MC, Cantor J, Blanchard R. Child pornography offenses are a valid diagnostic indicator of pedophilia. *J Abnorm Psychol.* 2006;115(3):610-615.

10. Rosenbloom A, Tanner JM. Misuse of Tanner puberty stages to estimate chronologic age. *Pediatrics.* 1998;102(6):1494.

11. Hanson RF, Resnick HS, Saunders BE, Kilpatrick DG, Best C. Factors related to the reporting of childhood rape. *Child Abuse Negl.* 1999;23(6):559-569.

12. Proceedings from Expert Working Group on Children and Young Persons with Abusive and Violent Experiences Connected to Cyberspace; Sweden, 2006.

13. The Adam Walsh Child Protection and Safety Act of 2006.

14. Eichenwald K. Through his webcam, a boy joins a sordid online world. December 19, 2005. *New York Times.* http://www.nytimes.com/2005/12/19/national/19kids.ready.html. Accessed March 16, 2010.

15. O'Connell RA. Typology of Child Cybersexploitation and Online Grooming Practices. Paper presented at: Society, Safety and the Internet; July 2003; New Zealand.

16. Wolak J, Finkelhor D, Mitchell K. Internet-initiated sex crimes against minors: Implications for prevention based on findings from a national study. *J Adolesc Health.* 2004;35(5):424.e11-424e20.

17. Hunter G, Pardo S. MySpace teen put on tether. The *Detroit News.* May 12, 2006. Available at: http://en.wikipedia.org/wiki/Emoticon. Accessed June 16, 2006.

18. Widom C. Victims of childhood sexual abuse—Later criminal consequences. National Institute of Justice Research in Brief; Victims of Childhood Sexual Abuse; March 1995.

19. Estes R, Weiner N. The commercial sexual exploitation of children in U.S., Canada, and Mexico. Available at: http://www.sp2.upenn.edu/~restes/CSEC_Files/Exec_Sum_020220.pdf. Accessed March 16, 2010.

20. Arenberg GS, Bartimole CR, Bartimole JE. *Preventing Missing Children: A Parental Guide to Child Security.* New York, NY: Avon Books; 1984. 35-37.

21. US Department of State. The Facts About Child Sex Tourism. US Department of State; 2005. Available at: http://www.state.gov/documents/organization/51459.pdf. Accessed June 16, 2006.

22. Burgess AW, Grant CA. *Children Traumatized in Sex Rings.* National Center for Missing & Exploited Children. Alexandria, VA; 1988.

23. Sherman M. US charges 27 in online child porn ring. ABC News and The Associated Press; Chicago, IL; March 15, 2006. Available at: http://www.abcnews.go.com/US/wireStory?id=1729069&page=1. Accessed June 16, 2006.

24. American Psychological Association, Task Force on the Sexualization of Girls. Report of the APA Task Force on the Sexualization of Girls. Washington, DC: American Psychological Association; 2007.

Chapter 18

Child Sexual Abuse: An International Perspective

Marcellina Mian, MDCM, FRCPC, FAAP

Child sexual abuse is a crime, and each abused child represents a betrayal of childhood by society. Commercial sexual exploitation reaches a level of crime and betrayal that many practitioners working to prevent child maltreatment in developed countries would find difficult to comprehend. Yet it is critical that all of society have a better understanding of the kind of entrapment and misery that some children—too many children—endure on a daily basis.

The nature of commercial sexual exploitation of children (CSEC) in its many forms is described in this chapter. How widespread is CSEC and how does it unfold? What renders children vulnerable and what can be done to prevent it? In what ways can society intervene to protect the children who are already in its clutches, without contributing further to their suffering?

What is known about the types of female genital mutilation (FGM) is also reviewed. Why is it done? Where is it done? When a cultural tradition harms children, what can be done to eliminate its practice?

There are many actors on the global stage, including the United Nations and other international organizations, governmental and nongovernmental agencies, and those involved in grass roots projects, whose aim is to protect children. Each sees and contributes to addressing the problem and collecting data to learn more about what can be done to achieve a safer childhood for all children in the world.

COMMERCIAL SEXUAL EXPLOITATION OF CHILDREN

DEFINITIONS

A *child* is defined by the Convention on the Rights of the Child (CRC) in Article 1 as "every human being below the age of eighteen years."[1] The CRC came into force in September 1990 and has been ratified by all states in the world except for Somalia and the United States of America.[1] It is the primary instrument to articulate the right of children to grow up free from harm and provides common ground on which governments and communities can base their work of child protection.

Child labor is a more restricted category than working children since it excludes all children working legally in accordance with International Labour Organization (ILO) Conventions 138 and 182.[2]

Unconditional worst forms of child labor are defined in ILO Convention 182: Convention Concerning the Prohibition and Immediate Action for the Elimination of the Worst Forms of Child Labour, Article 3, as comprising[3]:

(a) all forms of slavery or practices similar to slavery, such as the sale and trafficking of children, debt bondage and serfdom and forced or compulsory labour, including forced or compulsory recruitment, of children for use in armed conflict;

(b) the use, procuring or offering of a child for prostitution, for the production of pornography or for pornographic performances.

Conversely, "slavery is a crime against humanity that includes forced labour, serfdom (forced labour on another's land), debt bondage (undertaking by a debtor for his personal service or service of a person under his control as security for or in payment of a debt, if the terms of the debt payment are not defined and limited), trafficking, forced prostitution, sexual slavery, forced marriage, the sale of wives and child servitude."[4]

In 1999, the World Health Organization (WHO) stated, "Commercial or other exploitation of a child refers to use of the child in work or other activities for the benefit of others. This includes, but is not limited to, child labour and child prostitution. These activities are to the detriment of the child's physical or mental health, education, or spiritual, moral or social-emotional development."[5]

CSEC is now more broadly defined as "criminal practices that demean, degrade and threaten the physical and psychosocial integrity of children. There are 3 primary and interrelated forms of commercial sexual exploitation of children: prostitution, pornography and trafficking for sexual purposes. Other forms of CSEC include child sex tourism, child marriages and forced marriages."[6]

ECPAT (the network to End Child Prostitution, Child Pornography, and Trafficking of Children for Sexual Purposes) clarifies the full scope of the term CSEC.[7] The word *commercial* does not mean that the commercial gain must be obvious and require the exchange of money. In some situations, such as child marriage, the exploitation involves contractual or commercial exchange, gain of prestige, land transfer, or other services. The use of the word *children* may take the focus off the adult perpetrators and facilitators of the activity, among whom are parents, other family members, teachers, friends, and peers, besides procurers, pimps, traffickers and those who engage in sex with a child. It is necessary to keep in mind that CSEC is abuse, that there is a clear link between prior non-commercial sexual abuse of a child and that child's increased vulnerability to commercial sexual abuse and that the exploitation is characterized by violence.

The key element to CSEC as compared to other forms of child sexual abuse is that it involves a commercial transaction, or exchange, in which one or more parties make a gain. The beneficiaries of these transactions are the adults immediately involved in them, as well as the larger circle of facilitators. The child may benefit from some transactions, sometimes monetarily, but usually much less than the adults, and the benefits may be no more than what should be the child's by right. This includes services such as protection, shelter, or food. The child may agree to sexual favors in exchange for these benefits, but this does not in any way imply true consent.

Child sex tourism (CST) "involves people who travel from their own country to another and engage in commercial sex acts with children."[8]

Child trafficking is "the recruitment, transportation, transfer, harbouring or receipt of a child for the purpose of exploitation."[9]

Article 2 of the Optional Protocol to the Convention on the Rights of the Child on the sale of children, child prostitution, and child pornography states[10]:

(a) Sale of children means any act or transaction whereby a child is transferred by any person or group of persons to another for remuneration or any other consideration;

(b) Child prostitution means the use of a child in sexual activities for remuneration or any other form of consideration;

(c) Child pornography means any representation, by whatever means, of a child engaged in real or simulated explicit sexual activities or any representation of the sexual parts of a child for primarily sexual purposes.

The exploitation of children under 18 in prostitution, in child and adolescent pornography or sex shows, constitutes prima facie violence against them.[11]

Child soldiers are "any person under 18 years of age who is part of any kind of regular or irregular armed force or armed group in any capacity, including but not limited to cooks, porters, messengers and anyone accompanying such groups, other than family members. The definition includes girls recruited for sexual purposes and for forced marriage. It does not, therefore, only refer to a child who is carrying or has carried arms."[12]

These definitions are important because they help create a common language for the study and prevention of CSEC at a global level.

SCALE OF THE PROBLEM

One of the conclusions of the Second World Congress against Commercial Sexual Exploitation of Children was that "CSEC mutates and intensifies."[13] Because of limitations in data collection, including variable definitions, problems with study design or feasibility, and the concealment of CSEC, the number of children who are involved in CSEC in its various manifestations is difficult to quantify. With these limitations in mind, the following estimates have been derived.

Between 1995 and 2003 the proportion of women aged 20 to 24 years who were married prior to age 15 years varied between a low of approximately 0.4% in South Africa and a high of almost 30% in Niger. These figures are based on demographic and health surveys of nationally representative households in parts of Africa, South America, South East Asia, and the Pacific.[14] These figures represent a trend toward increasing age at time of marriage in most states, including Niger and South Africa, where the proportion of women older than 40 years of age at the time of the survey, who had married by the age of 15 years, was about 50% and 3%, respectively.

Early marriage is also associated with unions in which the man has more than one wife. As the rate of child marriages decreased, so did the proportion of young women who were married by age 18 years and in polygamous relationships. In Cameroon and Zimbabwe, for example, 55% and 34% of women, respectively, who were in monogamous marriages entered into those relationships by age 18, compared to 75% and 56%, respectively, for women who were in polygamous marriages. This association did not always hold true, however. In 5 countries, women who entered into marriage before age 18 years were more likely to make a monogamous, rather than polygamous, union.[14]

Young women aged 20 to 24 years were more likely to have more children if they married before age 18 years.[14] In South Africa, 2% of women with no children were married by age 18 years, 11% of women with 1 or 2 children were married by age 18 years, and 43% of women with 3 or 4 children were married by age 18 years.[14] However, the data cannot be considered definitive as women in that age group (20 to 24 years) are still having children, so the final tally may show less difference.

Child labor in the 5- to 17-year age group declined globally from 246 to 218 million children between 2000 and 2004, representing a decline of more than 11% in incidence rate to roughly 1 in 7 children.[2] In 2000, 5.7 million children were estimated to be in forced and bonded labor. Close to 97% of these children were concentrated in the Asia-Pacific region. It is estimated that there were 1.2 million trafficked children and 1.8 million children in prostitution and pornography worldwide.[15] Another estimate is that minors represent 10% to 30% of all trafficked prostitutes.[16] The US Department of State, however, reported that children constitute up to 50% of the 600 000 to 800 000 people trafficked across international borders each year, including 14 500 to 17 500 into the United States, mostly for commercial sexual exploitation.[8]

The UN Secretary General's Study on Violence Against Children states that, in 2002, 150 million girls and 73 million boys under the age of 18 years suffered forced sexual intercourse or other forms of sexual violence.[11] Most discouragingly, it suggests that CSEC is increasing, with greater criminal activities related to child trafficking, sex tourism, pornography, and Internet crimes. There has been a decline in some exploitative cultural practices, such as giving girls to temples; however, trafficking within nations and regions, and also across nations, regions, and continents, is on the rise.[13] Millions of child domestic workers live in the homes of others and suffer various forms of maltreatment.[11] As an example, 80% of children employed as domestics in Fiji reported sexual abuse.

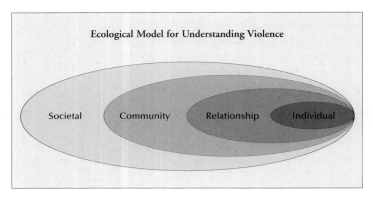

Ecological Model for Understanding Violence

Societal — Community — Relationship — Individual

Figure 18-1.
The ecological model for understanding violence.

CONTRIBUTING FACTORS

The World Report on Violence and Health applied an ecological model to explain susceptibility to violence.[17]

In **Figure 18-1**, risk factors pertaining to the individual nest within those related to the family and other relationships, which in turn nest within those of the community, which lie within those that exist in society. The factors contributing to violence at each level influence those at all other levels and determine the level of risk related to violence.

In CSEC, the contributing factors are at all levels of the ecological model. The root causes of CSEC have been defined multifarious, and include "poverty, inequality, illiteracy, discrimination, persecution, violence, armed conflicts, HIV/AIDS, dysfunctioning families, the demand factor, criminality, negative traditional practices, and violations of the rights of the child."[13]

Globally, the stage for the commercial sexual exploitation of a child may be set at birth. Article 7 of the CRC states, "The child shall be registered immediately after birth and shall have the right from birth to a name, the right to acquire a nationality and, as far as possible, the right to know and be cared for by his or her parents."[1]

Notwithstanding this obligation, a 2002 report stated that the births of only 59% of the world's children were registered.[2] The total number of children worldwide whose births are unregistered is reported to be around 50 million.[18,19] In 2004, the lowest rate of registration was in Afghanistan, Tanzania, and Uganda (under 7%) in contrast to almost 100% in the Occupied Palestinian Territory and the Democratic People's Republic of Korea.[19] **Figure 18-2** gives regional rates for birth registration in the developing world.[19]

A child who has a birth certificate has an identity that is registered in law, which entitles the bearer to access certain rights of personhood or citizenship. These include the right

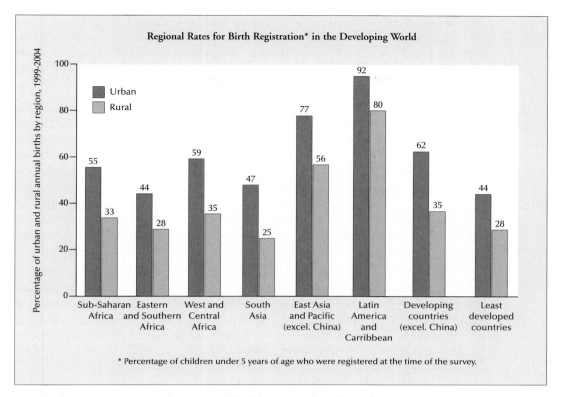

Regional Rates for Birth Registration* in the Developing World

* Percentage of children under 5 years of age who were registered at the time of the survey.

to a family environment, to education and health, to state benefits and participation in society, to protection against exploitation and abuse, and access to juvenile justice.[18]

In some countries (Cameroon, Lesotho, and the Maldives), a birth certificate is required to go to school, while in others it allows progress beyond a primary or secondary education (Turkey and Tanzania). At times local authorities demand a birth certificate before enrolling a child in school, even though no legal requirement exists. Beyond school, a birth certificate is usually required to obtain a marriage license, secure employment, access a pension or other benefits, have a bank account, or inherit property.

A birth certificate is also necessary to obtain a passport or to access the democratic benefits of civil society, such as the ability to vote or to stand for elective office. In most states, national citizenship is conferred by the birth of a child within their jurisdiction, while some confer it on the basis of the parents' nationality, and many have a combination of the two. In other states the system is more complex. In Myanmar, for example, there are 3 classes of citizens: full, associate, and naturalized. Full citizenship is granted only to those who can trace Myanmar ancestry back to 1824 and only they can train to be doctors or engineers, stand for election, or work for a foreign company. Palestinian children who are born in Israel are subject to restrictive procedures so that they may be denied an Israeli birth certificate. In Yemen, a mother cannot transmit her nationality to her child if she is married to a foreigner.

Not having a birth certificate may deny a child to any of the above rights and render the child more vulnerable. Where laws exist against child labor and child marriages, the absence of a birth certificate allows employers and families to work and marry children more easily. For example, in India, where the law states that children less than 14 years of age cannot be employed in hazardous industries, widespread abuses persist and children less than 14 years of age labor in glass, fireworks, or other risky factories. Lack

Figure 18-2.
Regional rates for birth registration.

of registration and nationality are considered significant factors for child trafficking and exploitation, since these children are more easily hidden or passed off as young adults. A female child can be hired ostensibly as a young adult domestic worker and then made to work in the sex trade. Where the law recognizes the special status of young offenders, not having a birth certificate exposes the youth to prosecution as an adult, incarceration with hardened criminals, and potentially to harsh penalties, including death.

Thus, the absence of the birth certificate facilitates illegal adoptions and trafficking of children across national borders, many of whom are intended for commercial sexual exploitation.

Gender and age are risk factors that determine the type of abuse to which children will be more vulnerable. Sexual violence affects girls more than boys, and particularly adolescents.[20] Boys are more likely to be trafficked for forced labor on commercial farms, in the drug trade, or in petty crime. Girls are more likely to be trafficked for commercial sexual exploitation and domestic service. Most child domestic workers are girls between 12 and 17 years of age, but surveys identified children as young as age 5 years.[21] As a group, girls work longer hours than boys.[22]

The absence of protective families predisposes children to maltreatment, leaving them vulnerable to the predatory behavior of others. As an example, 25% of child domestic workers in Togo, West Africa, were orphans.[22] A prior history of violence predisposes individuals to encounter violence again; children who are abused physically, sexually, or emotionally within their families are more likely to be revictimized.[11,23] Families may be the actual intermediaries who introduce the children to the world of commercial exploitation.

Poverty

Poverty is the first among a number of factors cited as contributing to child labor in general, CSEC, and child marriages. It should be noted, however, that CSEC takes place not just in poor, but also in affluent countries and that not all poor countries take part in CSEC.[13] According to the United Nations Population Fund, "Human trafficking is a global phenomenon that is driven by demand and fuelled by poverty and unemployment."[4] Affluent countries contribute by the demand they create for children as sex objects, either by seeking child pornography or sex with children. This usually falls in the category of sex tourism, wherein individuals who might be too inhibited or frightened of legal consequences to engage in sex with children in their own community, travel to other communities, countries, or continents in order to indulge their pleasure.

Child marriage is most common among the poorest 40% of the general population compared to the richest 40%.[14] When subsistence becomes a critical issue for families, the need for all members to contribute to the family's economic survival comes to weigh on even its youngest members. Options for gainful employment may be quite limited in the economically disadvantaged countries, thus making the less desirable alternatives more compelling. When families have to borrow, they may give a child in exchange or use the child to discharge an outstanding debt. The child does not receive any pay, and the length of the servitude may be indeterminate.[21]

The choices made by families to have their children go to work as domestics, to be given as security for a debt, or to be married young are not invariably fueled by greed on the part of the family. The family may be putting the well-being of the children first. They may believe that their children will be living in more affluent surroundings and may view their choice as one of giving their children an opportunity they will not have if they remain with their families.[11]

The poorest 20% of the population of the countries studied had the highest rate of childbirth in those less than age 18 years compared to the richest 20%.[24] The birthrate was highest in Niger (72% in the poorest 20% versus 39% in the richest) and lowest in Turkey (19% versus 8%). Based on data from 56 countries, women between 15 and 19 years of age from the poorest groups were 3 times more likely than their richer peers to give birth in adolescence, and have twice as many children.

Economics may interact with other factors, such as education, to explain the likelihood of child marriages. Women 20 to 24 years of age who had attended primary school, or primary and secondary school, were less likely to be married by age 18 years than those who had not. The husbands tended to be better educated than their young mates.[14] Among couples resulting from child marriages in Egypt, there was no education gap between husband and wife in 22% of marriages, although in 38% the husband had more education. Further, more than 1 in 4 married girls had a husband who was 5 to 9 years older than she was. In Burkina Faso, 65% of the girls who were married had a husband who was more than 15 years older. An older, better-educated man is or may be seen to be more likely to be able to look after his wife and family, or he may simply be in a better position to procure a young wife.

The setting of the child's employment may also contribute to abuse, violence, and exploitation of children. Violence is "rife against children in closed workplaces, such as domestic laborers employed in private households."[11] In some countries, domestic work is designated one of the worst forms of child labor. Children live and work in an environment completely controlled by the people who have power and authority over them. They work hard and long 16-hour days; they may be physically, sexually, and emotionally abused, and deprived of food. This has the dual disadvantage of depriving them of any schooling and making them more vulnerable to further abuse. It is very distressing to the children to be constantly treated as inferior, insulted, belittled, and deprived of peer relations. In some communities, their status as domestics is considered to be tantamount to being sex workers. If they displease their employer, they may be arbitrarily transferred to another home. All of these factors expose them to additional privation and suffering, including illiteracy, ignorance, social ostracism, psychological trauma, and unwanted motherhood.[21] In turn, these further predispose them and their progeny to disadvantage and violence.

Natural disasters increase the opportunities for the abuse and trafficking of children. On December 26, 2004, a tsunami struck the countries bordering the Indian Ocean, causing the greatest destruction in Indonesia, Sri Lanka, India, and Thailand. Within days, CBS News reported the following story[25]:

On a pilgrimage to a temple, the 18-year-old and her family stopped for a picnic by the beach. That's when the tsunami struck. Flailing in the water, the teenager heard a voice. "He told me to grab his hand, that he will save me," she said. She and the stranger were swept into a muddy river. When they reached a bank, he pushed her into a bed of brambles and raped her.

In response to reports on the vulnerability of orphaned children to exploitation by criminal elements, governments and nongovernmental organizations made the prevention of human trafficking, particularly child trafficking, an integral component of disaster-relief planning.[8]

Armed Conflict

Armed conflicts, and the disruption, displacement, and disorientation they provoke lead to further violence even in noncombatants. Rape may be used as a means of terrorizing civilians in a factional conflict. Refugees are subjected to violence and rape, particularly if they go outside the camp perimeter to collect firewood, water, or other resources, or if the latrines are positioned close to the camp's perimeter.[4] Gangs attack the camps to recruit or abduct children as combatants and girls as sexual slaves, cooks, and cleaners. Adult male refugees who are unemployed and stressed become more aggressive, particularly toward adolescents and young women. Unfortunately, even some who are involved in the humanitarian response use physical and sexual violence against the refugees, demanding sex in exchange for staples and services.[26,27] In Mozambique, for example, after the signing of the peace treaty in 1992, girls aged 12 to 18 years were recruited into prostitution by soldiers of the United Nations peacekeeping force.[28]

Human Immunodeficiency Virus/Acquired Immunodeficiency Syndrome

Another source of devastation for children that leaves them orphaned, homeless, and without protection is human immunodeficiency virus/acquired immunodeficiency syndrome (HIV/AIDS). The Joint United Nations Programme on HIV/AIDS (UNAIDS) reports that 15 million children have lost at least one parent to AIDS and 75% of these children are in Sub-Saharan Africa.[29] In South Africa, where there are 10 000 to 12 000 children who are without caregivers or homes because of HIV/AIDS, there are an estimated 28 000 children being sexually exploited. In Cape Town, 25% of prostitutes are children.[11] The prevalence of HIV/AIDS may be as high as 60% in child prostitutes.[11] In addition, the myth of virgins having the power to cleanse men of their HIV/AIDS may be the reason that South Africa has seen an increase in the rape of infants less than 1 year of age.[30]

Cultural Factors

Cultural practices and myths contribute to the sexual exploitation of children. In India and Ghana, girls are given to priests as ritual forms of slavery.[11] The priests then sell their services, including sexual ones. In a study in India, 28% of prostitutes entered into their profession through this ritual.[31] In contrast to other sex trade workers, they were about 6 years younger when they became prostitutes (average age 15.7 years), and they were more likely to be illiterate.

Legal and cultural factors affect what is considered appropriate or acceptable in terms of the treatment of children. Customs or religious doctrines that condone child marriage and female genital mutilation are juxtaposed against the adequacy of legislation against these forms of maltreatment and the ability to enforce that legislation to influence the existence of the abusive practices.[14] Similarly, child trafficking is more likely to flourish if parents and other relatives, friends, peers, and teachers are complicit in allowing, encouraging, or benefiting from it. Negligent authorities and a systemic failure to respond are also contributing to the problem.[13]

Community mores influence the treatment of domestic workers and the maltreatment of children, including child sexual exploitation. Minimally, the community at large does not place sufficient moral sanctions on such behavior. They may view some behaviors as harmless (eg, "It's just looking at pictures."). They may feel the child deserved the maltreatment or that it is none of their business. They also may have become inured to the harshness of their circumstances, as may happen in refugee camps or among sex trade workers and their children. This is in part due to the stigmatization of exploited children, wherein the community does not consider them worthy of any attention, let alone positive intervention.

LOGISTICS

How do children enter into the world of commercial sexual exploitation? For the reasons given previously, a family may be ready to send a child out to work, or adolescents may wish to seek employment or opportunities to improve their education. The family or youth may then respond to advertisements for babysitting, modeling, domestic work, or marriage as a mail order bride.[4] Conversely, recruiters, who are sometimes family members or other girls involved in CSEC, may actively search for and enlist children and adolescents who are ready and willing to go for the promise of a better life. Finally, children may be abducted from their homes and communities.

A child's entry into CSEC may be swift if the initial encounter is with someone whose direct intention is to sell their sexual services or traffic them for that reason. For others their descent into that world may be slower as they pass through other forms of child labor that expose them to maltreatment, unwanted pregnancy, eviction from their employer's home, homelessness, and stigmatization.

Once the children are in the clutches of the people whose intention is to exploit them, they are in a very difficult position. They are confined and their documents and whatever resources they had are taken from them; they may be drugged and are often raped and beaten into subjugation.[4] They are often sold then resold and trafficked again to other destinations.

The biggest suppliers of trafficked people are Southeast and South Asia. These people are trafficked within the region, just as Western Europe receives people mostly from Eastern Europe.[4] Other sources are the former Soviet Union countries, Latin America, and Africa. Some countries are also transit zones. The destination countries are Australia, the United States and Western Europe, as well as India, Pakistan, Thailand, Turkey, and the Middle East. Some countries, such as Thailand, serve as source and destination countries, as well as transit hubs for other countries.

The greatest demand for child sex tourism comes from the developed countries. Tourists, who may hold positions of trust in their own countries, seek the anonymity of foreign countries to engage in sex with children. They come from all socioeconomic backgrounds and travel to developing countries because of the availability of children as prostitutes together with weak law enforcement and corruption.[8]

ECONOMICS

The 2 top-grossing illicit industries are arms and drug trafficking; the third is human trafficking. For first-time transactions this is reportedly a $7 to $12 billion per year business.[4] An additional $32 billion a year is generated in the destination countries, through resale and the avails of the trade generated by the sex trade workers. Reportedly, one third is generated in Asia and one half in industrialized countries.

Child pornography is said to be a multibillion dollar commercial enterprise and among the fastest-growing businesses on the Internet, enabled by easy access and facilitated by credit cards and other payment methods.[32] The Financial Coalition Against Child Pornography has been formed to "disrupt the economics of this despicable business."[32] The coalition includes leading banks, credit card companies, third-party payment companies, and Internet services companies.

A global average indicates that for every additional year of schooling, wages increase by 11% of future earnings per year.[33] An IPEC study estimated the cost and gains involved in replacing child labor with education. It was based on the hypothetical application of an action plan and the study of the economic impact of each element of the program. The net benefit of replacing child labor with education as a percentage of gross national product would be 22%, with the greatest increase in Sub-Saharan Africa (over 54%), Asia (27%), North Africa and the Middle East (23%), and 5% in transitional countries, that are changing from a centrally planned economy to a free market. From 2001 to 2020, the total global cost would be $760 billion, while the accrued benefit would be over $5 trillion. This represents an internal rate of return of about 44%, with benefits exceeding costs by a ratio of 6.7 to 1. The benefit cost ratio is highest in North Africa and the Middle East at 8.4:1 and lowest in Sub-Saharan Africa (5.2:1). The cost of the program exceeds its return for approximately 15 years and then turns dramatically positive. After 2020 there are no more costs, only benefits. The average annual cost of the program would be $55 billion the first decade and $136 billion in the second. This represents 11% and 28%, respectively, of the annual global spending for the military ($493 billion) and 5.5% and 14% of debt service ($1 trillion).

These figures indicate that, even without considering the considerable benefits in human and social terms, economically, the cost of CSEC is higher than the cost of eliminating it. The difficulty is that different people stand to benefit from the continuation or elimination of CSEC. Further, CSEC results in fairly immediate profits, while reaping the benefits of an investment in prevention takes a period of time that often exceeds the term of an elected official's or government's term in office.

CONSEQUENCES OF CSEC

There are a multitude of potential lifetime physical and mental health consequences for children who have suffered sexual violence, including children who have been involved in CSEC. What is more notable about CSEC victims is the scale of their suffering because of the quantity of children involved, the harshness of the conditions, and the limited resources available to many of them.

Two major consequences are pregnancy and HIV/AIDS. Children are particularly vulnerable to both in terms of size, nutritional status, and limited or no access to health care resources. The violence with which they are assaulted creates easier access for HIV infection. Once they are infected, access to health care is problematic and if they have an infected infant, the problem becomes multiplied. In addition, being infected makes them objects of derision and rejection beyond what they were before. Even if they are not infected, they may be AIDS orphans—which frequently subjects them to discrimination. Health, education, and other necessary services are more difficult for orphans to access, especially if they are living in child-headed households or on their own on the streets.

One-quarter to one-half of girls in developing countries become mothers while they are still children, as defined by the CRC.[24] Reported births per 1000 population in the 15- to 19-year age group numbered 53 worldwide, 25 in the most developed regions, 57 in the less developed regions, and 67 in the least developed regions.[4] Mothers less than 20 years of age account for almost 1 in 5 births (14 million) and 1 in 4 abortions (20 million) in the least developed countries.[34] Pregnancy, whether it results in an unsafe abortion or a complicated term birth, is a leading cause of death for teenaged women. Abortions account for nearly 70 000 deaths each year worldwide. Women 15 to 19 years of age and those less than 15 years of age are 2 and 5 times as likely to die in childbirth, respectively, as women in their twenties.[34] The main cause of death is obstructed labor, which is especially common in young women who are not yet physically mature. In the survivors, sequelae include anorectal fistulae that makes them incontinent and, as a result, social pariahs.

Even assuming that victims of CSEC can be liberated from their exploiters, reunification with their families may not be possible.[28] In the course of their trafficking, and without a birth certificate or other official documents, the children, especially those taken from their families at a young age, may lose any clear concept of their original identity or place of residence. Locating their families may be difficult, especially if they have no resources with which to accomplish the task.

In the case of children who were child soldiers or were otherwise exploited during times of conflict or disaster, reunification may be impossible because the families may no longer be alive, or they may have been displaced and relocated. In the case of sex workers, the families may not be prepared to take them back because of the shame they would bring to their families.[11] Child brides are expected to stay in their new home and family. Having had children may make return of an exploited child to a childhood home particularly difficult, because the new generation is evidence of a shameful experience.

Child workers have very low self-esteem associated with the treatment they have received from their employers and other members of the community. Added to this is the limited range of functional social skills they may have due to the lack of schooling and dehumanizing experiences they have suffered. Some child soldiers are forced to commit acts of atrocity, which interferes with their ability to return to normal society.[28] They may be feared or be targets of revenge for members of the community who fought on opposite sides. The double burden of social ostracism and limited social skills makes these children's reentry into normal society difficult.

INTERVENTIONS

Since the ratification of the CRC in 1990, and especially during the last decade of the 20th century, the activity of UN agencies and other international nongovernmental organizations has proliferated in the interest of preventing violence in general and violence against children in particular. The WHO entered into the efforts directed at violence prevention with their publication of the World Report on Violence and Health in 2002.[35] Although pediatricians had recognized the problem of child abuse since 1962, violence had been considered at the international level to be simply a social and legal problem.[36,37] The WHO has gone on to publish a number of evidence-based guidelines and frameworks on what can be done to advance the campaign against violence.

Three world congresses have been held on the issue of CSEC; the first in 1996 in Stockholm, the second in 2001 in Yokohama, and the third in Rio de Janeiro in 2008.[38,39] Networks and coalitions, such as ECPAT and the Coalition to Stop the Use of Child Soldiers (CSC), have been formed to help address the issue in a coordinated fashion.

International protocols have been signed and ratified by a majority of nations.[3,9,10,40] Two special reports on children were completed for the UN Secretary General.[11,28] The many agencies working on the prevention of child exploitation have produced a number of publications to provide information on the progress being made against CSEC in its many forms and to recommend next steps.

Improving education contributes to improved economic well-being, later marriages, fewer children, and better protection of children in general.[41] Children who go to school are more likely to learn how to stay healthy and to protect themselves from HIV infection. They are less likely to be trafficked, exploited, or to suffer abuse or violence.[2,19,41] The education of girls is especially beneficial since it also benefits the next generation.[41] Educated girls are more likely to have healthier children who are better nourished. Extensive evidence from the developing countries shows that for each extra year of maternal education, the rate of mortality for children under the age of 5 years decreases by 5% to 10%.

A study by the International Programme on the Elimination of Child Labour proposed 3 elements in the program it devised to replace child labor through education.[33] One is increasing the availability of education by expanding school capacity and upgrading school quality. The second is income for transfers, which means providing funds to families to defray the costs of transferring children from work to school. The third is non-school interventions, such as the program of interventions for the urgent elimination of the worst forms of child labor.[2]

Violence against children, especially the worst forms of child labor, requires integrated interventions including practical programs, advocacy, and data collection.[11] Depending on the community, its resources, the size of the problem in that community, and the agency that is intervening, different responses may be set in motion. Emergency responses, such as the immediate rescue of children requiring shelter, may involve a small-scale project, while international agencies will have more complete and extensive programs that may include components aimed at preventing children from being abused in the first place.

There is some evidence of the positive impact of ILO conventions, with resulting effective action.[2] Of the more than 200 reports made by governments since 1999 in response to these conventions, over 50% stated they had plans of action to eliminate child labor in its worst forms, with 38% reporting prohibition of hazardous work, 35% and 29% enacting legislation to prohibit trafficking and prostitution, respectively, and 23% having programs for withdrawal of children from the labor force and their rehabilitation. Monitoring of the situation and preventive measures were reported by approximately 20% of reporting nations.

Among the measures to reduce CSEC has been the attempt to reduce demand by focusing on prosecution of offenders beyond the national boundaries of their home states.[10] At least 32 countries have provisions for extraterritorial prosecution of child sex tourists, so the offender who commits such a crime abroad is prosecuted at home, thereby losing the protection previously afforded by anonymity, weak law enforcement, and corruption.[8] In the United States there have been more than 20 indictments and more than a dozen convictions of child sex tourists since legislation was passed in 2003. These laws provide for penalties of up to 30 years' imprisonment. Sentences in other countries include the death penalty in China for traffickers who force girls under age 14 years into prostitution. In Singapore, slavery is punishable by up to 10 years in prison, a fine, and caning.

Also helpful in this regard are the efforts of the tourist industry to eliminate sex tourism, which began in the early 1990s. The global Code of Conduct for the Protection of Children from Sexual Exploitation in Travel and Tourism is an initiative developed in collaboration with ECPAT International, funded by UNICEF and supported by the World Tourism Organization.[42] As of May 2009, 984 travel companies from 54 countries have signed the code.[43] The code requires signatories[42]:

1. To establish an ethical policy regarding CSEC

2. To train their personnel in the country of origin and at travel destinations

3. To introduce a clause in contracts with suppliers stating the common repudiation of CSEC

4. To provide information to travelers by means of catalogues, brochures, in-flight films, ticket slips, Web sites, etc.

5. To provide information to key local persons at the destinations

6. To report annually. The reporting is to the Code Steering Committee and to the national ECPAT partners, on the way they are implementing the Code of Conduct.[44]

National law enforcement agencies in the countries of origin or destination of trafficked children or pornographic images, such as the Federal Bureau of Investigation (FBI) in the United States, are continually honing their skills at identifying and locating victims of abuse in order to release them from bondage.[45]

Once exploited children have been identified and located, contact needs to be made with them to remove them to safety. Possible means to this end are hotlines and peer-to-peer contact in public places, such as churches, parks, or shops where the child workers go when they are off duty.[11] The removal of the children from exploitative situations requires skilled intervention so the child is not further traumatized. In an emergency, this may require rescue operations; in more stable situations, there may be time for more considered action. For child soldiers, any peace agreements must acknowledge their involvement in the war so that there can be effective plans for them on a national scale.[28]

The rehabilitation of children must include attention to their physical and mental health needs.[11] Programs must help children establish lives based on their individual capabilities and experiences. Because exploitation interferes with children's normal physical, emotional, and intellectual development, they need to be provided with an environment that fosters dignity and self-respect.[11,28] Good relations with a supportive family are beneficial, but some families may be too stressed themselves to take the returning youth back, or may not be prepared to accept them. Conversely, the youth may not wish to return home and should not be forced to do so.[11] Settings that provide peer group living and are integrated into communities are viable alternatives to institutions.

One of the changes in monitoring intervention efforts in the child labor movement has been the shift in focus from the industry to the child.[2,11] This shift aims to ensure that children removed from work are provided with satisfactory alternatives with which to reenter mainstream society. Coordinated efforts involve the identification, referral, verification, and tracking of children. This approach focuses on monitoring long-term changes in all types of child labor within specific geographical areas and includes all aid agencies and organizations working within a given geographical area. With these data a better understanding of children's experiences with physical and psychological violence can be garnered, which will improve future prevention strategies.

FEMALE GENITAL MUTILATION

Female genital mutilation is not a form of CSEC, but is included in this chapter because it is a practice that affects the sexual apparatus and sexuality of girls in many parts of the world, and it affects individuals immigrating to countries where it was previously unknown.

Female genital mutilation is also known as female genital cutting or female circumcision. The WHO states it "comprises all procedures involving partial or total removal of the external female genitalia or other injury to the female genital organs whether for cultural, religious or other non-therapeutic reasons."[46] Although there are variations in how it is practiced, there are 4 main types. These are summarized in **Table 18-1**.

The global prevalence of women and girls who have been subjected to FGM is estimated to be between 100 and 140 million.[47] Each year, about 3 million girls are at risk of undergoing FGM. This practice takes place in 28 African countries, in the area extending across the middle part of the continent and up the Nile valley. It also takes place in Yemen and Southern Asia. The prevalence of this practice in various African countries between 1995 and 2001 varied from a high of almost 99% in Guinea to a low of 4.5% in Niger. Self-reporting of FGM has been found to under-report the extent of the procedure undergone by women.[48] The extent or type of FGM varies from country

Table 18-1. Types of Female Genital Mutilation.

TYPE	DESCRIPTION
Type I	Involves excision of the clitoral hood, and may include part or all of the clitoris.
Type II	Involves excision of the clitoris with partial or total excision of the labia minora. This type accounts for approximately 80% of FGM.
Type III	Involves excision of part or all of the external genitalia and stitching/narrowing of the vaginal opening (infibulation). This type accounts for approximately 15% of FGM.
Type IV	Pricking, piercing, incision, or stretching of the clitoris and/or labia; cauterization by burning of the clitoris and surrounding tissue; scraping of tissue around the vaginal orifice; cutting of the vagina; or introduction of corrosive substances or herbs into the vagina for the purpose of tightening or narrowing it.

to country. Nations commonly performing Type III procedures are Chad (eastern part), Djibouti, Egypt (southern part), Eritrea, Ethiopia (eastern part), Gambia, Ghana, Guinea, Kenya, Mali (southern areas), Nigeria (more in northern states), Senegal, Somalia, Sudan, and Yemen (practiced by a small East African immigrant community).[49] In Djibouti, Nigeria, Somalia, and Sudan, Type III is widely practiced.

As emigration from practicing countries has increased, so has the spread of this practice to Europe, North and South America, Australia, and New Zealand.[4] In 1990, it was estimated that 168 000 girls and women in the United States had been or were at risk of undergoing FGM, presumably because they were of an age and culture in which FGM is practiced.[50] This creates the need for training of health professionals to be able to manage the gynecologic and obstetric needs of these girls and women.

Female genital mutilation is performed for many reasons. Some are sexual, related to eliminating or reducing a woman's sexual feeling and desire in order to maintain her chastity before marriage and fidelity after marriage. Some are sociological and tied to cultural tradition to make girls eligible for marriage. Others are due to hygiene, as external female genitals are considered dirty and ugly. Finally, some communities believe FGM is a requirement of Islam, although the Quran does not require it and the practice is not only used by followers of Islam.[46] In Chad, for example, FGM is practiced not only by Muslims, but also by Christians and Animists, while in Ethiopia, it is also practiced by Jews (Falashas).[51]

Where it is practiced, the procedure is performed increasingly by medical personnel as compared to traditional practitioners, who use razorblades, knives, cut glass, sharpened rocks, scissors, burning, and fingernails. The reasons for this are reduction of pain, hemorrhage, infection, and other health complications. However, even under these circumstances, the practice is not to be condoned.[46]

There are many deleterious effects of FGM. Immediate complications include severe pain, severe blood loss and shock, urinary retention, and infections, including HIV/AIDS.[46] Hemorrhage and infection can be fatal. Physical long-term consequences include damage to the urethra and resulting incontinence, sexual dysfunction, and difficult childbirths. Mental health problems include depression and anxiety. Complications can extend into the next generation, with increased neonatal morbidity and mortality. The relative risk of perinatal death or an infant requiring resuscitation at delivery is significantly higher for mothers with FGM Type II and FGM Type III than for those without FGM.[52]

Female genital mutilation is a dual attack on women in that it infringes their rights and compromises their health. This has resulted in UN agencies uniting to try to eliminate the practice. Indications are that attitudes against it are rising and national policy strategies against FGM have been implemented.[46] Several best practice initiatives have been undertaken, such as community empowerment in Senegal and alternative rites of passage in Kenya, and health professionals have received training on FGM-related issues. Overall, communities appear to be more active in this regard than governments, but both the level of activity, the official response, and reductions in the practice are variable.[53] Between 1995 and 2001, rates in FGM were compared in several countries for women 20 to 24 years of age compared to those 40 to 44 years of age.[46] Rates in Guinea and Eritrea remained essentially unchanged, but in Nigeria the rate dropped by almost 50% and in other areas the rate decreased by 5% to 30%.

The death of a 12-year-old girl who underwent the procedure in June 2007 in Egypt prompted several actions against the procedure.[51] A decree was issued by Egypt's Health and Population Minister fully criminalizing FGM and closing a previous loophole involving health professionals conducting the practice. Al-Azhar Supreme Council of Islamic Research, the country's highest Muslim authority, stated that FGM and cutting have no basis in core Islamic law and should not be practiced. Suzanne Mubarak, Egypt's first lady, launched a national campaign to raise awareness about the practice and to accelerate efforts to ensure it is eliminated, including by amending existing child laws.

CONCLUSION

Globally, much has been learned and accomplished in the field of child sexual abuse prevention to try to eliminate any expression of this violence, especially CSEC. Much more still needs to be done through collaborative efforts, careful data gathering and analysis, and monitoring of any interventions taken to ensure that efforts, especially in areas where resources are scarce, represent the most effective ways to protect children.

REFERENCES

1. Office of the United Nations High Commissioner for Human Rights (OHCHR). Convention on the Rights of the Child. http://www2.ohchr.org/english/law/crc.htm. Published 1990. Accessed August 7, 2009.

2. International Labour Organization The End of Child Labour: within reach. http://www.un.org/aroundworld/unics/english/ilo_childlabor_2006.pdf. Published 2006. Accessed August 17, 2009.

3. International Labour Organization. ILO Convention 182: convention concerning the prohibition and immediate action for the elimination of the worst forms of child labour. http://www.ilo.org/public/english/standards/ipec/ratification/convention/text.htm. Published 1999. Accessed August 18, 2009.

4. United Nations Population Fund. State of World Population 2006: a passage to hope: women and international migration. http://www.unfpa.org/upload/lib_pub_file/650_filename_sowp06-en.pdf. Published 2006. Accessed August 7, 2009.

5. World Health Organization. Report of the Consultation on Child Abuse Prevention. http://whqlibdoc.who.int/hq/1999/aaa00302.pdf. Published March 1999. Accessed August 7, 2009.

6. ECPAT-USA. Commercial Sexual Exploitation of Children Overview. http://www.ecpatusa.org/. Accessed August 15, 2009.

7. ECPAT International. CSEC terminology. http://ecpat.net/Ei/Csec_definition.asp. Accessed August 7, 2009.

8. United States Department of State. 2005 Trafficking in Persons Report. http://www.state.gov/documents/organization/47255.pdf. Published June 2005. Accessed August 7, 2009.

9. United Nations. UN Protocol to Prevent, Suppress and Punish Trafficking In Persons, Especially Women and Children, Supplementing the United Nations Convention against Transnational Organized Crime. http://www.uncjin.org/Documents/Conventions/dcatoc/final_documents_2/convention_%20traff_eng.pdf. Published 2000. Accessed August 7, 2009.

10. Office of the United Nations High Commissioner for Human Rights. Optional Protocol to the Convention on the Rights of the Child on the Sale of Children, Child Prostitution and Child Pornography. http://www2.ohchr.org/english/law/crc-sale.htm. Published May 2002. Accessed August 7, 2009.

11. United Nations. UN Secretary General's Study on Violence Against Children. http://www.violencestudy.org/r25. Published 2006. Accessed August 7, 2009.

12. United Nations International Children's Emergency Fund. Cape Town Principles and Best Practices on the Recruitment of Children into the Armed Forces and on Demobilization and Social Reintegration of Child Soldiers in Africa. http://www.unicef.org/emerg/files/Cape_Town_Principles(1).pdf. Published April 1997. Accessed August 7, 2009.

13. Muntarbhorn V. General Rapporteur's Report of the 2nd World Congress Against CSEC. http://csecworldcongress.org/PDF/en/Yokohama/Congress_Reports/General%20Rapporteur's%20report,%20Yokohama.pdf. Published December 20, 2001. Accessed August 15, 2009.

14. United Nations International Children's Emergency Fund. Early Marriage: a harmful traditional practice. http://www.unicef.org/publications/files/Early_Marriage_12.lo.pdf. Published 2005. Accessed August 7, 2009.

15. International Labour Organization. Every Child Counts: New Global Estimates on Child Labour. http://www.ilo.org/public/english/standards/ipec/simpoc/others/globalest.pdf. Published 2002. Accessed April 11, 2007.

16. Tautz S, Bähr A, Wölte S. Commercial sexual exploitation of children and young people. In: Razum O, Zeeb H, Laaser U, eds. *Globalisierung—Gerechtigkeit—Gesundheit*. Einführung in International Public Health. Verlag Hans Huber. Bern; 2006:245-258. Available at: https://www.gtz.de/de/dokumente/en-CSEC-article-2006.pdf. Accessed August 7, 2009.

17. Krug EG, Dahlberg LL, Mercy JA, Zwi AB, Lozano RE. *World Report on Violence and Health*. Geneva: World Health Organization. 2002:1-21. Available at: http://www.who.int/violence_injury_prevention/violence/world_report/en/index.html. Accessed August 7, 2009.

18. United Nations International Children's Emergency Fund Birth Registration: right from the start. http://www.unicef-icdc.org/publications/pdf/digest9e.pdf. Published March 2002. Accessed August 7, 2009.

19. United Nations International Children's Emergency Fund. The State of the World's Children 2007: women and children: the double dividend of gender equality. http://www.unicef.org/publications/index_36587.html. Published December 2006. Accessed August 7, 2009.

20. Krug EG, Dahlberg LL, Mercy JA, Zwi AB, Lozano RE. *World Report on Violence and Health*. Geneva: World Health Organization. 2002:57-86.

21. International Programme on the Elimination of Child Labour. Helping Hands and Shackled Lives: understanding child domestic labour and responses to it. http://www.ilo.org/public/english/standards/ipec/publ/download/cdl_2004_helpinghands_en.pdf. Published 1998. Accessed April 16, 2007.

22. International Labour Organization. International Labour Conference 86th Session 1998—Report VI (1) Child Labour: targeting the intolerable. http://www.ilo.org/public/libdoc/ilo/1996/96B09_344_engl.pdf. Published 1998. Accessed August 7, 2009.

23. Classen CC, Palesh OG, Aggarwal R. Sexual Revictimization: a review of the empirical literature. *Trauma Violence Abuse*. 2005;6:103-129.

24. United Nations Population Fund. State of World Population 2005: the promise of equality: gender equity, reproductive health and the millennium development goals. http://www.unfpa.org/upload/lib_pub_file/493_filename_en_swp05.pdf. Published 2005. Accessed August 7, 2009.

25. Cosgrove-Mather B. Tsunami survivor raped by rescuer. *CBS News*. January 7, 2005. http://www.cbsnews.com/stories/2005/01/07/world/main665533.shtml. Accessed August 19, 2009.

26. UNCHR. Note for Implementing and Operational Partners by UNHCR and Save the Children–UK on Sexual Violence & Exploitation: the experience of refugee children in Guinea, Liberia and Sierra Leone. http://www.unhcr.org/cgi-bin/texis/vtx/search?page=search&docid=3c7cf89a4&query=Sexual%20violence%20&%20exploitation:%20the%20experience%20of%20refugee%20children%20in%20Guinea. Published February 2002. Accessed August 7, 2009.

27. United States General Accounting Office. Humanitarian Assistance: protecting refugee women and girls remains a significant challenge. http://www.gao.gov/new.items/d03663.pdf. Published May 2003. Accessed August 7, 2009.

28. United Nations. Impact of Armed Conflict on Children. http://www.unicef.org/graca/. Published August 1996. Accessed August 7, 2009.

29. Joint United Nations Programme on HIV/AIDS. http://www.unaids.org/en/Issues/Affected_communities/orphans.asp. Published 2007. Accessed April 20, 2007.

30. Pitcher GJ. Infant rape in South Africa. *Lancet*. 2002;359: 274-275.

31. Blanchard JF, O'Neil J, Ramesh BM, et al. Understanding the social and cultural contexts of female sex workers in Karnataka, India: implications for prevention of HIV infection. *J Infect Dis*. 2005;191:S139–S146.

32. National Centre for Missing & Exploited Children. The Financial Coalition Against Child Pornography Adds Four Financial Services Leaders to Its Roster. http://www.missingkids.com/missingkids/servlet/NewsEventServlet?LanguageCountry=en_US&PageId=2851. Published November 2006. Accessed August 7, 2009.

33. International Programme on the Elimination of Child Labour. Investing in Every Child: an economic study of the costs and benefits of eliminating child labour. http://www.ilo.org/public/english/standards/ipec/publ/download/2003_12_investingchild.pdf. Published 2003. Accessed April 20, 2007.

34. United Nations Population Fund. State of World Population 2004: the Cairo consensus at ten: population, reproductive health and the global effort to end poverty. http://www.unfpa.org/upload/lib_pub_file/327_filename_en_swp04.pdf. Published 2004. Accessed August 7, 2009.

35. Krug EG, Dahlberg LL, Mercy JA, Zwi AB, Lozano RE. *World Report on Violence and Health*. Geneva: World Health Organization. 2002.

36. Kempe CH. The battered child syndrome. *JAMA*. 1962;181:17–24.

37. Mian M. World report on violence and health: what it means for children and pediatricians. *J Pediatr*. 2004;145:14-19.

38. ECPAT. World Congress III Against the Sexual Exploitation of Children and Adolescents. http://www.ecpat.net/worldcongressIII/overview2.php#stockholm. Published 2008. Accessed August 7, 2009.

39. World Congress III Against the Sexual Exploitation of Children and Adolescents. Rio Declaration and Call for Action. http://www.iiicongressomundial.net/index.php?pg=docs&inicial=2&id_pg=79&sid=1fc0a0d316fa2820ba1d8d5b4ec3 9934&id_sistema=2&id_idioma=2. Published 2008. Accessed August 7, 2009.

40. Office of the United Nations High Commissioner for Human Rights. Optional Protocol to the Convention on the Rights of the Child on the Involvement of Children in Armed Conflict. http://www2.ohchr.org/english/law/crc-conflict.htm. Published May 2000. Accessed August 7, 2009.

41. United Nations International Children's Emergency Fund. The State of the World's Children 2004: girls, education and development. http://www.unicef.org/publications/index_18108.html. Published December 2003. Accessed August 7, 2009.

42. Code of Conduct. Code of conduct for the protection of children from sexual exploitation in travel and tourism. http://www.thecode.org/. Accessed August 7, 2009.

43. Code of Conduct. The Code Partners: code signatories-may-2009-by region. http://www.thecode.org/index.php?page=6_3. Published 2009. Accessed August 7, 2009.

44. Code of Conduct. The Reporting Process. http://www.thecode.org/index.php?page=4_1. Accessed August 7, 2009.

45. Federal Bureau of Investigation. Innocent Images National Initiative. http://www.fbi.gov/publications/innocent.htm. Published 2006. Accessed August 7, 2009.

46. World Health Organization Regional Office for Africa (AFRO). Elimination of female genital mutilation in the African region. The African Health Monitor. http://www.afro.who.int/press/periodicals/healthmonitor/janjun2004.pdf. Published June 2004. Accessed August 7, 2009.

47. World Health Organization. Female Genital Mutilation: key facts. http://www.who.int/mediacentre/factsheets/fs241/en/. Updated May 2008. Accessed August 7, 2009.

48. Elmusharaf S, Elhadi N, Almroth L. Reliability of self reported form of female genital mutilation and WHO classification: cross sectional study. *BMJ*. 2006; 333(7559):124.

49. United States Department of State. Female Genital Mutilation (FGM) or Female Genital Cutting (FGC): individual country reports. http://www.state.gov/documents/organization/10222.pdf. Published 2001. Accessed August 7, 2009.

50. Kelly E, Hillard PJ. Female genital mutilation. *Curr Opin Obstet Gynecol*. 2005; 17:490–494.

51. UN News Centre. UNICEF hails moves by Egypt to eliminate female genital mutilation. http://www.un.org/apps/news/story.asp?NewsID=23125&Cr=unicef&Cr1=. Published July 2007. Accessed August 7, 2009.

52. World Health Organization. Female genital mutilation and obstetric outcome: WHO collaborative prospective study in six African countries. *Lancet* 2006; 367:1835-1841.

53. Wakabi W. Africa battles to make female genital mutilation history. *Lancet* 2007; 369:1069–1070.

Chapter 19

THERAPY FOR THE CHILD SEXUAL ABUSE VICTIM

Laura K. Murray, PhD
Judith A. Cohen, MD
Anthony P. Mannarino, PhD

Child sexual abuse (CSA) is an all-too-common occurrence that transcends ethnicity, socioeconomic status, and gender.[1] There are multiple variables within a child sexual abuse case that complicate psychological treatment. First, the definition of CSA encompasses a wide range of activities such as intercourse, oral-genital contact, fondling, exposing children to sexual behavior, or the use of a child for prostitution. Second, outcomes of abuse are affected by multiple characteristics such as the age and gender of the child, when the abuse occurred or began to occur; the age and gender of the perpetrator; the relationship between the perpetrator and the victim; the frequency, duration, and severity of the abuse; and the amount of threat. Third, the effects of CSA vary depending on a youth's vulnerability and resilience, preabuse functioning, risk and protective factors, and emotional support. Treatment should address each client's needs and take advantage of their strengths and resources.

This chapter will begin by giving a brief overview of some psychological symptoms commonly seen in children who have been sexually abused, within a framework that is helpful for maximizing treatment approaches. Next, this chapter will outline the importance of early treatment, engagement, and the need for treatments that have demonstrated efficacy and/or effectiveness in well-designed studies. Finally, a treatment that has been considered well researched and efficacious will be briefly described.

SEQUELAE OF CSA

CSA is a devastating experience that may cause negative short- and long-term consequences in the psychological and physical well-being of the victim; however, not all sexually abused children have serious ongoing psychological sequelae.[2] Research shows that approximately 70% of asymptomatic children remain symptom-free over time, and approximately 30% go on to develop symptoms later.[3,4] Mannarino et al[4] have documented evidence of "sleeper effects," with serious symptoms not manifesting until a year after disclosure. For asymptomatic children, treatment focuses on prevention of further abuse incidences, safety planning, normalizing feelings, and psychoeducation for both the child and caregivers.

Unfortunately, the majority of sexually abused children do show psychological symptoms at some point. Research from both clinical and community samples continually demonstrates that sexually abused children exhibit more mental health symptoms than nonabused comparison children.[3,5,6] However, no one symptom manifests in these children. In fact, the effects of CSA commonly span both externalizing and internalizing symptoms and can vary significantly across developmental stages. These may include anxiety; inappropriate sexual behavior and preoccupation[8-10]; anger, guilt, shame, and depression; and other emotional and behavioral difficulties.[7,11-15] Current research demonstrates that a significant proportion of sexually abused children also suffer from posttraumatic stress disorder (PTSD).[9,16-19] For example, McLeer et al[19] report that 48.4% of their sample of sexually abused children aged 3 through 16 years met full diagnostic criteria for PTSD based on the DSM IIIR, with many more displaying partial criteria. A diagnosis of PTSD is also associated with high suicide risk.[20] A history of childhood abuse or trauma more than doubles the likelihood of developing a major depressive episode[21] and conveys a markedly increased risk for suicide and suicidal behavior later in life.[22-26] In fact, even after controlling for other family problems such as parental mental disorder, sexual abuse is found to account for almost 20% of the population-attributable risk for suicide attempts in young people.[23,24]

There is also now a substantial body of research literature that affirms the increased risk child abuse victims have for various mental health disorders and problems in their future, as well as the factors that tend to mediate these risks.[3,13,26-32] For example, one common consequence seen in individuals with CSA histories is adolescent or adult substance use.[33-35]

With regard to the treatment of sexually abused children who have these complex, myriad symptoms, it is often helpful to think in terms of 3 categories of symptoms—cognitive, emotional, and behavioral—rather than only in terms of diagnoses. This allows a clinician or referring practitioner to better tailor treatment to the specific needs and strengths of each youth.

COGNITIVE SYMPTOMS
Many sexually abused youth present with cognitive distortions or "unhelpful thoughts" that may lead to extreme distrust of others, feelings of self-blame, a negative view of the world…etc.).[36] A perceived lack of self-confidence and effective communication skills are also frequently found in abused youths.[37-38] Sexually abused youth also demonstrate unhelpful thoughts of low self-esteem and self-blame.[39-40] For example, youth may display dysfunctional ideas about relationships and difficulty with accurate judgment, which can interfere with their ability to assess risk and lead to poor decision-making, problem-solving, and sense of reality.[37,41] In addition, many children who have been sexually abused report difficulty concentrating in school or a significant drop in school performance, or both.[42]

EMOTIONAL SYMPTOMS
Emotional difficulties concomitant with CSA can include anxiety, sadness, anger, or guilt.[7,11] Deficits in emotion regulation are also consistently recorded in sexually abused children.[43,44] In addition, shame and fear of rejection have been shown to be prominent in sexually abused children and are considered easily triggered emotional states.[37,45,46] Depression symptoms are also highly correlated with child sexual abuse.[24,47-49]

BEHAVIORAL SYMPTOMS
A wide variety of behavioral problems have been associated with CSA in general.[50] Numerous studies have found that sexually abused children exhibit sexualized behaviors more frequently than children in comparison groups.[8,51-53] Other behavioral problems may include aggression, violence, or impulsivity.[54-57] Donenberg et al[58] demonstrated that sexual behavior among adolescent psychiatric patients who were sexually abused was impulsive and spontaneous, rather than a result of sound decision-making. Youths who have experienced CSA are also more likely to show maladaptive behavior patterns such as alcohol or drug abuse[59] and higher numbers of sexual partners.[60]

Even with examining these clusters of symptomatology to help guide appropriate intervention, the typical clinical picture varies widely within and across cases and is often very complex and severe. This can leave clinicians and referring professionals confused regarding where to start with treatment. The first step is for therapists and families to understand the need for and importance of early treatment and then to engage families in therapy from the first contact with any professional.

ENGAGEMENT OF FAMILIES IN THERAPY

It is well documented in the United States that mental health services rarely reach those most in need.[61-65] Among families who do receive and attend treatment, 20% to 60% terminate treatment prematurely.[66-67] Traumatized populations are some of the most difficult to engage and maintain in treatment because of the common existence of avoidance symptoms, as well as parental stress and depression and severity of child dysfunction.[68,69] Moreover, many CSA survivors and their families will go to significant lengths to try to "simply forget," "leave the past behind," or "just deal with it." In the treatment of CSA, engagement needs to be at the forefront of delivery of services, whether that care is rendered by a clinician or any other professional.

Research in the area of engagement has advanced since the late 1990s and has identified numerous barriers that prevent children and families from receiving the care they need.[70] For example, Nock and Kazdin[71] found that parent expectancies were predictive of subsequent barriers to treatment participation and of premature termination from therapy. Family perceptions of the therapeutic relationship and the degree to which they are involved in service planning have also emerged as important issues in the continuation of treatment and in better outcomes.[72-74] McKay et al[75] have also shown that parental attitudes about mental health services, parental discipline effectiveness, family stress, and the presence of or encouragement from a social support network are significantly related to keeping a first appointment within an outpatient mental health program and to longer lengths of stay in services for urban youths and their families.

More recently, there have been impressive strides in engagement strategies that address these barriers and significantly improve service usage for youths and their families, including reminders of appointments and discussions, during the initial telephone contact, of overcoming potential barriers.[63,64,76,77] These strategies have resulted in an approximately 30% increase in attendance at an initial clinic appointment, a significant increase in the number of child mental health sessions, and fewer dropouts.[63] Thus, treatment should include engagement during any and all contact with the child and adult caregiver. Particularly with families that have experienced trauma and carry the distrust, guilt, and shame, it is critical to begin addressing barriers and encouraging treatment immediately.

RESPONSIBILITIES OF REFERRING PRACTITIONERS AND FAMILIES

The engagement of families, encouragement of treatment, and proper referral are intimately connected to knowledge about the treatment options for CSA victims. Often when people are faced with a health-related problem or procedure, someone involved is asking a number of important questions such as what the procedure is, what the risks and benefits are, how long recovery is, how much pain is involved, if the doctor is qualified and experienced, and the number of successful outcomes. Referring professionals and even family members should begin to ask these same questions to mental health care providers. Professionals involved in the care of sexually abused children can effectively advocate for these children by referring them to programs or practitioners with the highest demonstrable treatment effectiveness.

RESPONSIBILITIES OF MENTAL HEALTH PRACTITIONERS

Likewise, mental health care practitioners have a responsibility to choose and deliver the treatments that are most appropriate for their patients. Ours is a generation of "evidence-based" treatments[78-80]; furthermore, these kinds of treatment strategies are not just encouraged, they are quickly becoming mandated by many federal and state funders and agencies. Notably, many of the challenges of connecting science with real-world practice and policy have yet to be ironed out.[81-82] As such, it becomes even more important for practitioners themselves to be intimately familiar with the treatments available for particular populations and to be able to turn a critical eye toward the research behind them.

CLINICAL AND EMPIRICAL LITERATURE ON THE TREATMENT OF CSA

Since the mid-1980s, the mental health treatment of child victims of sexual abuse has been examined by both the clinical and research communities. Theories have been developed that give direction to specific approaches for clinical intervention.[83-85] A large and rich body of clinical treatment literature has resulted, with descriptions of interventions that appear to be theoretically sound and have good clinical utility.[86-89] Most importantly, there now is a growing corpus of research literature detailing efficacy tests of mental health interventions in populations of sexually abused children.[2,90-96] Efficacy research is understood as laboratory-based studies that control for most variables such as child and family diagnoses and characteristics, highly trained therapists, standardized assessments, strict adherence to a manual, and intensive supervision (see Chambless and Hollon[78] or Kazdin and Weisz[97]).

Recent reviews describe certain treatment protocols for the treatment of sexually abused children that have yielded empirical data.[79,91] Cognitive behavioral therapy (CBT) treatment is considered to be one of the most efficacious and well-supported interventions for sexual abuse. This is not to say that other treatments are not effective; rather that CBT has the greatest empirical support whereas other techniques have not been well evaluated. CBT for trauma consists of many well-established components initially developed for the treatment of fear and anxiety in adults[98-99] and commonly used with adult rape victims.[100,101] CBT has been adapted and applied to many problems in children and adolescents such as depression and anxiety.[102-104] The shared components across disorders make sense given the myriad symptoms that a sexually abused child might exhibit. Many cognitive behavioral treatment manuals for a particular disorder or symptom cluster are similar, and thus clinicians are often familiar with many of the components. However, in each evidence-based treatment, there is a particular theoretical basis, system, and flow to the order and application of the components. Most often, one component is designed to build on the next. In this way, it is important to understand that the efficacy of each treatment modality is based on a certain amount of fidelity to the model.

In addition to efficacy trials, some of these empirically supported treatments have benefited from effectiveness research; shared, direct practice experience; and feedback from thousands of clinicians providing these services, all of which created intervention models that were more flexible and applicable to the "real world" (see Schoenwald and Hoagwood[105] for a review of effectiveness and dissemination research). Effectiveness research is important in that it tests the performance of treatments under highly naturalistic conditions.[106] Still, researchers are finding that treatments validated by efficacy trials are not commonly offered in routine mental health practice settings.[107]

EMPIRICAL REVIEWS OF EFFICACIOUS TREATMENTS FOR SEXUAL ABUSE

In recent reviews of treatments for abused children, only one model—trauma-focused cognitive behavioral therapy (TF-CBT)—was found to have enough empirical evidence to be deemed "well-supported and efficacious" by two independent groups.[108,109] The developers, Drs. Cohen, Mannarino, and Deblinger, began testing TF-CBT in the 1990s and contributed to more than 10 randomized controlled trials (RCTs) on this one model. In 1996, Deblinger et al[94] compared TF-CBT across 4 conditions: child only, parents only, both child and parent, and standard community care. The two conditions where children received treatment resulted in the greatest improvement of symptoms, with all TF-CBT conditions performing better than the standard community care. In the same year, Cohen and Mannarino[110] demonstrated that TF-CBT was superior to nondirective supportive therapy (NST) in reducing PTSD, internalizing, externalizing, and sexualized behavior symptoms in preschool children and their caregivers. An additional study by Cohen and Mannarino[93] found that TF-CBT was effective in improving depression and social competence in sexually abused children aged 8 to 14 years. A reduction in PTSD and dissociation symptoms was found in this population at a 1-year follow-up.[111] A more recent multisite RCT with 229 sexually abused children found that TF-CBT was superior to child-centered supportive therapy in improving PTSD, depressive, anxiety, shame, and behavioral symptoms in children.[55] This study also demonstrated decreased depressive symptomatology and an increase in parental support and positive parenting practices in the parents of sexually abused children. A study by an independent researcher (ie, someone who was not a developer of TF-CBT) showed that TF-CBT is superior to a wait-list control group in improving PTSD and depressive symptoms in sexually abused children.[112] Clinically, it is important to note that many of these studies included multiply traumatized children and children with complex PTSD. In summary, several randomized controlled treatment trials and review studies have supported the efficacy of TF-CBT in treating the myriad symptomatology commonly seen in sexually abused children.

TF-CBT has also been used in transportability, dissemination studies, and effectiveness studies that demonstrate its applicability and sustained effectiveness when used in a "real-world" setting. Through the efforts of the National Child Traumatic Stress Network (http://www.nctsn.org; Medical University of South Carolina, http://tfcbt.musc.edu/), TF-CBT is now being extensively disseminated and implemented across the United States, resulting in ongoing effectiveness studies with culturally diverse children who have experienced varied types of traumatic life events. It was also used in the Child and Adolescent Trauma Treatments and Services (CATS) Consortium, which is the largest youth trauma evaluation and treatment project associated with the September 11 attacks.[113] TF-CBT has been adapted and used with several populations including Hispanics,[114] Australians,[112] and refugees of African descent (Center for Multicultural Human Services, http://www.nctsn.org).[115] Recent evidence suggests that TF-CBT maintains its effectiveness with adaptation.[116] In addition, it has demonstrated broad applicability and acceptability among ethnically diverse therapists with varied backgrounds and among children and parents.[117]

TREATMENT DESCRIPTION OF TF-CBT AND ITS EIGHT COMPONENTS

TF-CBT is a hybrid model that integrates elements of cognitive behavioral, affective, humanistic, attachment, family, and empowerment therapies into a treatment designed to address the unique needs of children with problems related to traumatic life experiences such as sexual abuse.[118] This treatment model includes primary treatment components for children aged 5 to 18 years and for their nonoffending parents or

---

Table 19-1. Difficulties Addressed and Core Values by TF-CBT.

DIFFICULTIES ADDRESSED:	CORE VALUES:
Cognitive problems	**C**omponents-based
Relationship problems	**R**espectful of cultural values
Affective problems	**A**daptable and flexible
Family Problems	**F**amily-focused
Traumatic behavior problems	**T**herapeutic relationship is central
Somatic problems	**S**elf-efficacy is emphasized

Table 19-2. Primary Components of TF-CBT.

EIGHT COMPONENTS:

Psychoeducation and parenting skills

Relaxation

Affective modulation

Cognitive processing

Trauma narrative

In vivo desensitization

Conjoint parent-child sessions

Enhancing future development

---

primary caregivers. The mnemonic term *CRAFTS* spells out both the core values and the difficulties addressed by TF-CBT (see **Table 19-1**). These are helpful in understanding the foundation of TF-CBT and in balancing fidelity and flexibility when using this treatment.

There are 8 primary components of TF-CBT: **p**sychoeducation and parenting skills, **r**elaxation, **a**ffective modulation, **c**ognitive processing, **t**rauma narrative, **in** vivo desensitization, **c**onjoint parent-child sessions, and **e**nhancing future development. These 8 elements spell out *PRACTICE* (**Table 19-2**). Many of these are common components found in many cognitive behavioral treatments for children and adolescents.

Each of these components has specific goals that should be achieved in order to maintain fidelity to the model. The flexibility comes in how a therapist actually achieves some of these goals. The remainder of this chapter contains brief summaries of both goals and possible applications for each of the treatment components to give readers a basic understanding of an evidence-based cognitive behavioral treatment plan for sexually abused children. For a more complete understanding of TF-CBT, readers are strongly encouraged to visit the free online training in TF-CBT at the Medical University of South Carolina's Web site (http://tfcbt.musc.edu/) and to obtain a treatment manual available through Sage Publications.[118]

Psychoeducation and Parenting Skills
Goals of Psychoeducation

— To normalize the child's and parent's (or parents') reactions to severe stress

— To provide information about psychological and physiologic reactions to stress

— To instill hope for child and family recovery

— To educate the family about the benefits of and need for early treatment, as well as to present a plan (eg, how long treatment will last)

— To discuss safety planning for the future (if needed)

Application of Psychoeducation

Psychoeducation is a component that can be performed by anyone and should ideally begin with the patient's or caregiver's first encounter with any professional. The information provided to children and their families can take many forms and should vary with respect to the family and the child's developmental level. Some methods commonly used by practitioners include simply talking to the child and caregiver to give them information, asking them to read a book about how stress affects people, using the Internet to research the topic with the patient or caregiver, or handing out written materials to parents. A clinician or referring practitioner talking about the many children they have seen with similar experiences and problems can provide information as well as normalize reactions to stress. Every clinician and referring practitioner should provide families with information on the research behind the treatment choice, because doing so also achieves the goals of providing information, instilling hope, and educating the family about the need for early treatment. Psychoeducation may also include some information about what treatment will look like—for example, what the schedule is and how long it will last. Describing a plan and a time line can help you to assure families, take away any fear of the unknown, and promote attendance.

Goals of Parenting Skills

— To explain the rationale for parent inclusion in treatment

— To begin to establish the parent as the person the child turns to for help in times of trouble

— To emphasize positive parenting skills and maximize effective parenting

Application of Parenting Skills

TF-CBT and CBT treatments in general view parents or caregivers as central therapeutic agents of change and include them in treatment because they can be the child's strongest source of healing.[83,92,94,110,118] Clinicians should convey that "a parent is the expert on their child." This component also includes working as needed on some parenting skills such as praise, selective attention, time-out, reward programs, and other behavior management techniques. These behavioral techniques are applied as needed in the family and are incorporated into the treatment by working on small goals throughout rather than spending multiple full sessions on parenting skills alone.

Relaxation, or Stress Management

Goals

— To explain the body's responses to stress

— To reduce the physiological manifestations of stress

Application

The key to application of relaxation is to make sure that the method taught is personally effective for each individual. Some of the most common relaxation techniques taught include progressive muscle relaxation, deep breathing, and positive self-talk; however, people relax using all types of methods. Other skills include exercise, yoga, meditation, guided imagery, gardening, spending time with pets or those close to the individual, dancing, and so on. Culturally relevant activities should be actively integrated into this component.

Affective Modulation
Goals
— To accurately identify and describe a variety of emotions

— To understand the patient's (or caregiver's) vocabulary of affect

— To gain another way to talk about feelings (eg, as colors, objects)

— To understand the physical/concrete manifestation of emotions (eg, body, facial expressions)

— To comprehend different situations that correspond to the emotions

— To gain a sense of the strength/intensity of different feelings

These goals might also be necessary:

— To teach control over thoughts that are negatively affecting emotions or functioning (eg, traumatic reminders, or flashbacks)

— To increase positive emotions through positive self-talk

Application
This component can be achieved through a number of different techniques and can be altered depending on characteristics such as developmental age and culture. These may include board games or activities such as "color my person," which entails drawing a person and listing each emotion the child can come up with, asking which color "looks like" that feeling to them, drawing where in the body they feel it, and asking about a situation when they may have felt that way. Thought-stopping techniques may be used when a child is having difficulty functioning because of traumatic reminders; such strategies might include visualizing a stop sign as a reminder to stop the intrusive thought and replace it with a more positive one.

A clinician may also teach positive self-talk. A child can learn to repeat a particular phrase such as "I am good at many things" or "Many people like me" to help regulate some of the negative emotions. This is also a very useful tool for parents. Parents of sexually abused children often feel great amounts of shame or guilt and may say things such as "I am a terrible parent." Incorporating positive self-talk with caregivers—eg, "I'm helping my child in many ways"—can help them become more emotionally available to their children.

Cognitive Processing, or the Cognitive Triad
Goals
— To help children and parents understand the cognitive triad: connections among thoughts, feelings, and behaviors, as they relate to everyday events

— To help children distinguish among thoughts, feelings, and behaviors

— To help children and parents view events in more accurate and helpful ways

— To encourage parents to assist children in cognitive processing of upsetting situations and to use this in their own everyday lives for affective modulation

Application
To teach the connections among thoughts, feelings, and behaviors, the cognitive triad is often used (**Figure 19-1**).

First, a clinician guides the child or parent to imagine a familiar situation that is not inherently emotional. For example, a social situation where a child walks into the lunch room and a group of friends are laughing could be used. On the contrary, a heated argument between a mother and a teenager who have a stressed relationship could still be very "raw" and may be more difficult to use in the initial teachings of the triangle.

The clinician walks them through the triangle, asking what they were thinking during the situation, what they were feeling, and what their behaviors were, then pointing out the connections among them. A number of different scenarios are used so that the child or adolescent becomes aware of the interrelatedness of thoughts, feelings, and behaviors.

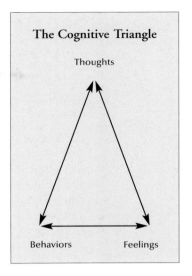

Trauma Narrative, or Exposure
Goals
— To gain mastery over trauma reminders

— To resolve avoidance symptoms

— To correct distorted cognitions

— To model adaptive coping

— To identify and prepare for trauma/loss reminders

Figure 19-1.
A number of different scenarios are used so that the child or adolescent becomes aware of the interrelatedness of thoughts, feelings, and behaviors.

NOTE: The exposure component of processing a trauma is the component most often avoided in the treatment of CSA for a variety of reasons including child discomfort, parent discomfort, and, most commonly, therapist discomfort. There is extensive literature to suggest that exposure treatment has demonstrated its effectiveness in the treatment of a variety of anxiety-related illnesses.[100,101,119]

Application
This component is most often implemented in the form of a book that the child or adolescent creates; however, this so-called narrative can also be in the form of a poem, song, computer presentation, or interview. The trauma narrative often begins with designing a title page; in addition, for those children who are multiply traumatized, the creation of a table of contents or time line in which to lay out the periods of abuse or number of incidences may be used. The first chapter includes innocuous information about the child such as their name, age, school, or hobbies. The child is encouraged to give more and more details of the traumatic event during subsequent sessions. As the child talks about the sexual abuse, the clinician continually walks them around the cognitive triad, asking them what they were thinking at the time, what they were feeling, and what they were doing. The clinician returns to some of these thoughts that may be inaccurate or unhelpful (eg, "I should have known that would happen," "It is all my fault") and tries to restructure them to a more accurate or helpful cognition. The book is re-read during every session to gradually desensitize the child to the event over time. The last chapter of the trauma narrative is about what the child has learned through this treatment or what the child wants other kids to know, or both.

Sharing the Trauma Narrative with the Parent
Ideally, the narrative is shared with the parent after each session, of course after gaining permission from the child or adolescent to do so. Sharing the narrative with the parent moves toward the goals of desensitizing the parent to the trauma and having them understand the child's thoughts and feelings. In this way, the parent or caregiver is being established as the one the child turns to when in need. The parent is most often willing to do this and appreciative that he or she is able to hear the details of the child's experience with the therapist first and gradually over time.

In Vivo Desensitization

Goals

— To desensitize a child to innocuous trauma reminders

— To resolve remaining avoidance symptoms

NOTE: This component of in vivo desensitization as a whole may not be needed in all trauma cases.

Application

Once the specific feared situation or place is identified, there is a plan to have the child gradually remain in the situation or place for longer and longer time periods. Behavioral reinforcement techniques are frequently added to help encourage and maintain the plan. For example, there should be praise for success, statements that the child can do this, and rewards once the child has succeeded. Each plan is highly individualized depending on the avoided reminder and the child or adolescent.

Conjoint Parent-Child Sessions

Goals

— To share the child's trauma narrative

— To correct cognitive distortions (held by the child, the parent[s], or both)

— To encourage optimal parent-child communication and a question-and-answer situation between child and parent about trauma and other topics

— To prepare for future traumatic reminders and to suggest how the child and parent can optimally cope with these

— To model appropriate child support and redirection

— To praise for progress made

Application

This component includes the clinician preparing the parent and child to share the trauma narrative together. A list of questions is developed with both the child and caregiver, and the questions are reviewed in the joint session to help encourage open communication between the child and the caregiver. The clinician then meets with the parent and child and has the child read the book with the parent. The child reads the words and also describes the pictures or color scribbles that represent the thoughts, feelings, and behaviors discussed throughout. Questions are also exchanged between the parent and child.

Enhancing Future Development

Goal

— To prepare plans for dealing with future trauma reminders or safety situations

Application

This component focuses on any remaining safety issues that may exist. Now that the sexual abuse has been openly discussed, different safety plans for a variety of situations can be organized and agreed upon.

CONCLUSION

Child sexual abuse is a highly variable event that can have widely devastating and long-term effects in a range of areas. The resulting symptoms are equally diverse, making the treatment of CSA challenging at best. Throughout the 1990s and 2000s, extensive research has resulted in a number of identified treatments that show efficacy in RCTs. Current efforts are focused on extending these empirically sound treatments into the mainstream and testing their ability to perform under more naturalistic conditions. The available research suggests that CBT is the most efficacious in treating sexually abused children and their complex, myriad symptoms. It is important for both clinicians and other involved professionals to familiarize themselves with the most efficacious treatments now available for addressing the needs of sexual abuse victims.

TF-CBT is currently considered one of the most efficacious and well-supported treatments for sexually abused children. However, it is also clear that effective psychotherapeutic treatment consists of more than a clinician executing the components of a manual for a particular disorder. In fact, treatment is an interdisciplinary effort to weave together engagement, therapeutic alliance, the retention of families, an understanding of development, and the theory and practice of a treatment. In this way, it is becoming increasingly important for all professionals involved in sexual abuse cases to become familiar with the sound treatments available, the research behind them, and of what the treatments themselves consist. Practitioners and researchers will have to collaborate in order to deliver optimal services to sexually abused youth and their families.

REFERENCES

1. Finkelhor D. Epidemiological factors in the clinical identification of child sexual abuse. *Child Abuse Negl.* 1993;17:67-70.

2. Finkelhor D, Berliner L. Research on the treatment of sexually abused children: a review and recommendations. *J Am Acad Child Adolesc Psychiatry.* 1995;34:1408-1423.

3. Kendall-Tackett KA, Williams LM, Finkelhor D. Impact of sexual abuse on children: a review and synthesis of recent empirical studies. *Psychol Bull.* 1993;113:164-180.

4. Mannarino A, Cohen J, Smith J, Moore-Motily, S. Six and twelve month follow-up of sexually abused girls. *J Interpersonal Viol.* 1991;6:494-511.

5. Browne A, Finkelhor D. Impact of child sexual abuse: a review of the research. *Psychol Bull.* 1986;99:66-77.

6. Mannarino AP, Cohen JA, Gregor M. Emotional and behavioral difficulties in sexually abused girls. *J Interpersonal Viol.* 1989;4:437-451.

7. Cohen JA, Mannarino AP. Psychological symptoms in sexually abused girls. *Child Abuse Negl.* 1988;12:571-577.

8. Cosentino CE, Meyer-Bahlburg HF, Alpert JL, Weinberg SL, Gaines R. Sexual behavior problems and psychopathology symptoms in sexually abused girls. *J Am Acad Child Adolesc Psychiatry.* 1995;34:1033-1042.

9. Deblinger E, McLeer SV, Atkins MS, Ralphe D, Foa E. Post-traumatic stress in sexually abused, physically abused, and nonabused children. *Child Abuse Negl.* 1989;13:403-408.

10. Friedrich WN, Grambasch P, Damon L, Hewitt SK, Koverola C, Lang R, et al. The Child Sexual Behavior Inventory: normative and clinical comparisons. *Psychol Assess.* 1992;4:303-311.

11. Koverola C, Pound J, Heger A, Lytle C. Relationship of child sexual abuse to depression. *Child Abuse Negl.* 1993;17:393-400.

12. Wozencraft T, Wagner W, Pellegrin A. Depression and suicidal ideation in sexually abused children. *Child Abuse Negl.* 1991;15:505-511.

13. Briere JN, Elliott DM. Immediate and long-term impacts of child sexual abuse. *Future Child.* 1994;4:54-69.

14. Conte JR, Schuerman JR. Factors associated with an increased impact of child sexual abuse. *Child Abuse Negl.* 1987;11:201-211.

15. Einbender AJ, Friedrich WN. Psychological functioning and behavior of sexually abused girls. *J Consult Clin Psychol.* 1989;57:155-157.

16. Cohen JA, Mannarino AP. Factors that mediate treatment outcome of sexually abused preschool children: six- and 12-month follow-up. *J Am Acad Child Adolesc Psychiatry.* 1998a;37:44-51.

17. McLeer SV, Deblinger E, Henry D, Orvaschel H. Sexually abused children at high risk for post-traumatic stress disorder. *J Am Acad Child Adolesc Psychiatry.* 1992;31:875-879.

18. McLeer SV, Callaghan M, Henry D, Wallen J. Psychiatric disorders in sexually abused children. *J Am Acad Child Adolesc Psychiatry.* 1994;33:313-319.

19. McLeer SV, Deblinger E, Atkins MS, Foa EB, Ralphe DL. Post-traumatic stress disorder in sexually abused children. *J Am Acad Child Adolesc Psychiatry.* 1988;27:650-654.

20. Oquendo M, Brent DA, Birmaher B, Greenhill L, Kolko D, Stanley B, et al. Posttraumatic stress disorder comorbid with major depression: factors mediating the association with suicidal behavior. *Am J Psychiatry.* 2005;162:560-566.

21. MacMillan HL, Fleming JE, Streiner DL, Lin E, Boyle MH, Jamieson E, et al. Childhood abuse and lifetime psychopathology in a community sample. *Am J Psychiatry.* 2001;158:1878-1883.

22. Brent DA, Baugher M, Bridge J, Chen T, Chiappetta L. Age- and sex-related risk factors for adolescent suicide. *J Am Acad Child Adolesc Psychiatry.* 1999;38:1497-1505.

23. Brown J, Cohen P, Johnson JG, Smailes EM. Childhood abuse and neglect: specificity of effects on adolescent and young adult depression and suicidality. *J Am Acad Child Adolesc Psychiatry.* 1999;38:1490-1496.

24. Fergusson D, Horwood L, Lynskey M. Childhood sexual abuse and psychiatric disorder in young adulthood: II. Psychiatric outcomes of childhood sexual abuse. *J Am Acad Child Adolesc Psychiatry.* 1996;35:1365-1374.

25. Kaplan SJ, Pelcovitz D, Salzinger S, Mandel F, Weiner M. Adolescent physical abuse and suicide attempts. *J Am Acad Child Adolesc Psychiatry.* 1997;36:799-808.

26. Mullen PE, Martin JL, Anderson JC, Romans SE, Herbison GP. The long-term impact of the physical, emotional, and sexual abuse of children: a community study. *Child Abuse Negl.* 1996;20:7-21.

27. Beitchman JH, Zucker KJ, Hood JE, daCosta GA, Akman D, Cassavia E. A review of the long-term effects of child sexual abuse. *Child Abuse Negl.* 1992;16:101-118.

28. Duncan RD, Saunders BE, Kilpatrick DG, Hanson RF, Resnick HS. Childhood physical assault as a risk factor for PTSD, depression, and substance abuse: findings from a national survey [published correction appears in *Am J Orthopsychiatry*. 1997 Jan;67(1):161]. *Am J Orthopsychiatry*. 1996;66:437-448.

29. Felitti VJ, Anda RF, Nordenberg D, Williamson DF, Spitz AM, Edwards V, et al. Relationship of childhood abuse and household dysfunction to many of the leading causes of death in adults. The Adverse Childhood Experiences (ACE) Study. *Am J Prev Med*. 1998;14:245-258.

30. Polusny M, Follette V. Long term correlates of child sexual abuse: theory and review of the empirical literature. *Appl Prev Psychol*. 1995;4:143-166.

31. Saunders BE, Kilpatrick DG, Hansen RF, Resnick HS, Walker ME. Prevalence, case characteristics, and long-term psychological correlates of child rape among women: a national survey. *Child Maltreat*. 1999;4:187-200

32. Widom CS. Posttraumatic stress disorder in abused and neglected children grown up. *Am J Psychiatry*. 1999;56:1223-1229.

33. Luster T, Small SA. Sexual abuse history and number of sex partners among female adolescents. *Fam Plann Perspect*. 1997;29:204-211.

34. Miller BA, Downs WR, Testa M. Interrelationships between victimization experiences and women's alcohol use. *J Stud Alcohol Suppl*. 1993;11:109-117.

35. Saunders BE, Berliner L, Hanson RF. *Child Physical and Sexual Abuse: Guidelines for Treatment*. Charleston, SC: National Crime Victims Research and Treatment Center, US Department of Justice; 2003.

36. Finkelhor D, Hotaling GT, Lewis IA, Smith C. Sexual abuse and its relationship to later sexual satisfaction, marital status, religion, and attitudes. *J Interpers Viol*. 1989;4:379-399.

37. Brown LK, Kessel SM, Lourie KJ, Ford HH, Lipsitt LP. Influence of sexual abuse on HIV-related attitudes and behaviors in adolescent psychiatric inpatients. *J Am Acad Child Adolesc Psychiatry*. 1997;36:316-322.

38. Carey MP, Carey KB, Kalichman SC. Risk for human immunodeficiency virus (HIV) infection among persons with severe mental illnesses. *Clin Psychol Rev*. 1997;17:271-291.

39. Jehu D. *Beyond Sexual Abuse: Therapy with Women Who Were Childhood Victims*. Chichester, UK: John Wiley; 1988.

40. Jehu D, Gazan M, Klassen C. Common therapeutic targets among women who were sexually abused in childhood. *J Soc Work Hum Sex*. 1984;3:25-45.

41. Brown LK, Danovsky MB, Lourie KJ, DiClemente RJ, Ponton LE. Adolescents with psychiatric disorders and the risk of HIV. *J Am Acad Child Adolesc Psychiatry*. 1997;36:1609-1617.

42. De Bellis MD, Keshavan MS, Clark DB, Casey BJ, Giedd JN, Boring AM, et al. Developmental traumatology. Part II: brain development. *Biol Psychiatry*. 1999;45:1271-1284.

43. Catanzaro SJ. Mood regulation and suicidal behavior. In: Joiner TE, Rudd MD, eds. *Suicide Science: Expanding the Boundaries*. Boston: Kluwer Academic Publishers; 2000:81-103.

44. Eisenberg N, Cumberland A, Spinrad TL, Fabes RA, Shepard SA, Reiser M, et al. The relations of regulation and emotionality to children's externalizing and internalizing problem behavior. *Child Dev.* 2001;72:1112-1134.

45. Cohen JA, Mannarino AP. Addressing attributions in treating abused children. *Child Maltreat.* 2002;7:82-86.

46. Feiring C, Taska L, Lewis M. A process model for understanding adaptation to sexual abuse: The role of shame in defining stigmatization. *Child Abuse Negl.* 1996;20:767-782.

47. Beitchman JH, Zucker KJ, Hood JE, daCosta GA, Akman D. A review of the short-term effects of child sexual abuse. *Child Abuse Negl.* 1991;15:537-556.

48. Brand EF, King CA, Olson E, Ghaziuddin N, Naylor M. Depressed adolescents with a history of sexual abuse: diagnostic comorbidity and suicidality. *J Am Acad Child Adolesc Psychiatry.* 1996;35:34-41.

49. Hotte J, Rafman S. The specific effects of incest on prepubertal girls from dysfunctional families. *Child Abuse Negl.* 1992;16:273-283.

50. Nagy S, Adcock AG, Nagy MC. A comparison of risky health behaviors of sexually active, sexually abused, and abstaining adolescents. *Pediatrics.* 1994;93:570-575.

51. Friedrich WN, Fisher JL, Dittner CA, Acton R, Berliner L, Butler J, et al. Child sexual behavior inventory: normative, psychiatric, and sexual abuse comparisons. *Child Maltreat.* 2001;6:37-49.

52. McClellan J, McCurry C, Ronnei M, Adams J, Eisner A, Storck M. Age of onset of sexual abuse: relationship to sexually inappropriate behaviors. *J Am Acad Child Adolesc Psychiatry.* 1996;34:1375-1383.

53. Paolucci EO, Genuis ML, Violato C. A meta-analysis of the published research on the effects of child sexual abuse. *J Psychol.* 2001;135:17-36.

54. Brodsky BS, Oquendo M, Ellis SP, Haas GL, Malone KM, Mann JJ. The relationship of childhood abuse to impulsivity and suicidal behavior in adults with major depression. *Am J Psychiatry.* 2001;158:1871-1877.

55. Cohen JA, Deblinger E, Mannarino AP, Steer RA. A multisite, randomized controlled trial for children with sexual abuse–related PTSD symptoms. *J Am Acad Child Adolesc Psychiatry.* 2004;43:393-402.

56. Finkelhor D, Kendall-Tackett K. A developmental perspective on the childhood impact of crime, abuse, and violent victimization. In: Toth S, ed. *Developmental perspectives on trauma: theory, research, and intervention.* Rochester, NY: University of Rochester Press; 1997.

57. Rosenfeld S, Lewis D. The hidden effect of childhood sexual abuse on adolescent and young adult HIV prevention: rethinking AIDS education, program development, and policy. *AIDS Public Policy J.* 1993;8:181-186.

58. Donenberg GR, Schwartz RM, Emerson E, Wilson HW, Bryant FB, Coleman G. Applying a cognitive-behavioral model of HIV risk to youths in psychiatric care. *AIDS Educ Prev.* 2005;17:200-216.

59. Hussey DL, Singer M. Psychological distress, problem behaviors, and family functioning of sexually abused adolescent inpatients. *J Am Acad Child Adolesc Psychiatry.* 1993;32:954-961.

60. Rotheram-Borus MJ, Mahler KA, Koopman C, Langabeer K. Sexual abuse history and associated multiple risk behavior in adolescent runaways. *Am J Orthopsychiatry*. 1996;66(3):390-400.

61. Wang PS, Lane M, Olfson M, et al. Twelve-month use of mental health services in the United States: results from the National Comorbidity Survey Replication. *Arch Gen Psych*. 2005;62:629-640.

62. Burns BJ, Costello EJ, Angold A, et al. Children's mental health service use across service sectors. *Health Aff (Millwood)*. 1995;14:147-159.

63. McKay M, McCadam K, Gonzales JJ. Addressing the barriers to mental health services for inner city children and their caretakers. *Community Ment Health J*. 1996;32:353-361.

64. McKay M, Stoewe J, McCadam K, et al. Increasing access to child mental health services for urban children and their caregivers. *Health Soc Work*. 1998;23:9-15.

65. Ringel JS, Sturm R. National estimates of mental health utilization and expenditures for children in 1998. *J Behav Health Serv Res*. 2001;28:319-333.

66. Gould MS, Shaffer D, Kaplan D. The characteristics of dropouts from a child psychiatry clinic. *J Am Acad Child Psychiatry*. 1985;24:316-328.

67. Wierzbicki M, Pekarik G. A meta-analysis of outpatient therapy dropout studies. *Professional Psychol: Res Pract*. 1993;24:190-195.

68. Kazdin AE, Mazurick JL, Bass D. Risk for attrition in treatment of antisocial children and families. *J Clin Child Psychol*. 1993;22:2-16.

69. Koverola C, Murtaugh C, Connors KM, et al. Children exposed to intra-familial violence: predictors of attrition and retention in treatment. *J Aggression, Maltreat & Trauma*. 2007;14(4):19-42.

70. Kazdin AE, Wassell G. Predictors of barriers to treatment and therapeutic change in outpatient therapy for antisocial children and their families. *Ment Health Serv Res*. 2000;2:27-40.

71. Nock MK, Kazdin AE. Parent expectancies for child therapy: assessment and relation to participation in treatment. *J Child Fam Stud*. 2001;10:155-180.

72. Garcia JA, Weisz JR. When youth mental health care stops: therapeutic relationship problems and other reasons for ending youth outpatient treatment. *J Consult Clin Psychol*. 2002;70:439-443.

73. Frank JD, Frank JB. *Persuasion & Healing: A Comparative Study of Psychotherapy*. Baltimore, MD: Johns Hopkins University Press; 1991.

74. Garfield SL. Research on client variables in psychotherapy. In: Bergin AE, Garfield SL, eds. *Handbook of Psychotherapy and Behavior Change*. 4th ed. New York: Wiley; 1994:190-228.

75. McKay MM, Pennington J, Lynn CJ, et al. Understanding urban child mental health service use: two studies of child, family, and environmental correlates. *J Behav Health Serv Res*. 2001;28:475-483.

76. Shivack N, Sullivan T. Use of telephone prompts at an inner-city patient clinic. *Hosp Community Psychiatry*. 1991;40:851-853.

77. Szapocznik J, Perez-Vidal A, Brickman AL, et al. Engaging adolescent drug abusers and their families in treatment: a strategic structural systems approach. *J Consult Clin Psychol.*1988;56:552-557.

78. Chambless DL, Hollon SD. Defining empirically supported therapies. *J Consult Clin Psychol.* 1998;66:7-18.

79. Chorpita BF et al. Toward Large-Scale Implementation of Empirically Supported Treatments for Children: A Review and Observations by the Hawaii Empirical Basis to Services Task Force. *Clinical Psychology: Science and Practice.* 2002; 9(2):165-190

80. Weisz JR, Hawley KM, Pilkonis PA, et al. Stressing the (other) three Rs in the search for empirically supported treatments: review procedures, research quality, relevance to practice and the public interest. *Clin Psychol-Sci Pract.* 2000:7:243-258.

81. Kazdin AE. Bridging the enormous gaps of theory with therapy research and practice. *J Clin Child Psychol.* 2001;30:59-66.

82. Weisz JR, Donenberg GR, Han SS, et al. Bridging the gap between laboratory and clinic in child and adolescent psychotherapy. *J Consult Clin Psychol.* 1995;63:688-701.

83. Deblinger E, Heflin AH. *Cognitive Behavioral Interventions for Treating Sexually Abused Children.* Thousand Oaks, CA: Sage Publications; 1996.

84. Friedrich WN. *Therapy for Sexually Abused Children and Their Families.* New York, NY: Norton; 1990.

85. Wolfe DA, McMahon RJ, Peters RD. *Child abuse: new directions in prevention and treatment across the lifespan.* Thousand Oaks, CA: Sage Publications; 1997.

86. Bolton FG, Bolton SR. *Working with Violent Families: A Guide for Clinical and Legal Practitioners.* Thousand Oaks, CA: Sage Publications; 1987.

87. Gil E. *Systemic Treatment of Families Who Abuse.* San Francisco, CA: Jossey-Bass; 1995.

88. Karp CL, Butler TL, Bergstrom SC. *Treatment Strategies for Abused Children: From Victim to Survivor.* Thousand Oaks, CA: Sage Publications; 1997.

89. Maddock JW, Larson NR. *Incestuous Families: An Ecological Approach to Understanding and Treatment.* New York, NY: W.W. Norton; 1995.

90. Berliner L, Saunders B. Results of a controlled two-year follow-up study. *Child Maltreat.* 1996;1:294-309.

91. Cohen JA, Berliner L, March JS. Treatment of children and adolescents. In: Foa EB, Keane TM, Friedman MJ, eds. *Effective Treatments for PTSD: Practice Guidelines from the International Society for Traumatic Stress Studies.* New York, NY: Guilford Press; 2000.

92. Cohen JA, Mannarino AP. A treatment outcome study for sexually abused preschool children: initial findings [published correction appears in *J Am Acad Child Adolesc Psychiatry.* 1996 Jun;35(6):835.]. *J Am Acad Child Adolesc Psychiatry.* 1996;35:42-50.

93. Cohen JA, Mannarino AP. Interventions for sexually abused children: initial treatment findings. *Child Maltreat.* 1998;3:17-26.

94. Deblinger E, Lippman J, Steer R. Sexually abused children suffering from post-traumatic stress symptoms: initial treatment outcome findings. *Child Maltreat.* 1996;1:310-321.

95. Cohen JA, Deblinger E, Mannarino AP, et al. A multi-site, randomized controlled trial for children with sexual abuse–related PTSD symptoms. *J Am Acad Child Adolesc Psychiatry.* 2004;43(4):393-402.

96. Deblinger E, Mannarino AP, Cohen JA, et al. A follow-up study of a multisite, randomized controlled trial for children with sexual abuse–related PTSD symptoms. *J Am Acad Child Adolesc Psychiatry.* 2004;45(12):1474-1484.

97. Kazdin AE, Weisz JR. Identifying and developing empirically supported child and adolescent treatments. *J Consult Clin Psychol.* 1998;66:19-36.

98. Wolpe J. Basic principles and practices of behavior therapy of neuroses. *Am J Psychiatry.* 1969;125:1242-1247.

99. Beck AT. *Cognitive Therapy and the Emotional Disorders.* Oxford: International Universities Press; 1976.

100. Foa EB, Rothbaum BO, Riggs DS, et al. Treatment of posttraumatic stress disorder in rape victims: a comparison between cognitive-behavioral procedures and counseling. *J Consult Clin Psychol.* 1991;59:715-723.

101. Keane TM, Fairbanks JA, Caddell JM, Zimering RT. Implosive (flooding) therapy reduces symptoms of PTSD in Vietnam combat veterans. *Behav Ther.* 1989;20:245-260.

102. Weisz JR, Hawley KM, Doss AJ. Empirically tested psychotherapies for youth internalizing and externalizing problems and disorders. *Child Adolesc Psychiatr Clin N Am.* 2004;13:729-815, v-vi.

103. Kazdin AE, Weisz JR. *Evidence-Based Psychotherapies for Children and Adolescents.* New York, NY: Guilford Press; 2003.

104. Ollendick TH, King NJ. Empirically supported treatments for children and adolescents. In: Kendall PC, ed. *Child and adolescent therapy: cognitive-behavioral procedures.* 2nd ed. New York, NY: Guilford Press; 2000:386-425.

105. Schoenwald SK, Hoagwood K. Effectiveness, transportability, and dissemination of interventions: what matters when? *Psychiatr Serv.* 2001;52:1190-1197.

106. Henggeler SW, Bourduin CM, Schoenwald SK, Rowland MD, Cunningham PB. *Multisystemic therapy for antisocial behavior in children and adolescents.* 2nd ed. New York, NY: Guilford Press; 2009.

107. Torrey WC, Drake, RE, Dixon L, et al. Implementing evidence-based practices for persons with severe mental illnesses. *Psychiatric Serv.* 2001;52(1):45-50.

108. Saunders BE, Berliner L, Hanson RF. *Child Physical and Sexual Abuse: Guidelines for Treatment (Revised Report: April 26, 2004).* Charleston, SC: National Crime Victims Research and Treatment Center, US Department of Justice; 2004.

109. Hensler D, Wilson C, Sadler BL; Kaufman Foundation. Closing the Quality Chasm in Child Abuse Treatment: Identifying and Disseminating Best Practices. The Findings of the Kauffman Best Practices Project to Help Children Heal from Child Abuse. http://www.chadwickcenter.org/Documents/Kaufman% 20Report/ ChildHosp-NCTAbrochure.pdf. Publish March 2004. Accessed January 12, 2010.

110. Cohen JA, Mannarino AP. Factors that mediate treatment outcome of sexually abused preschool children. *J Am Acad Child Adolesc Psychiatry*. 1996;35:1402-1410.

111. Cohen JA, Mannarino AP, Knudsen K. Treating sexually abused children: 1-year follow-up of a randomized controlled trial. *Child Abuse Negl*. 2005;29:135-145.

112. King NJ, Tonge BJ, Mullen P, et al. Treating sexually abused children with posttraumatic stress symptoms: a randomized clinical trial. *J Am Acad Child Adolesc Psychiatry*. 2000;39:1347-1355.

113. CATS Consortium. Implementing CBT for traumatized children and adolescents after September 11: lessons learned from the Child and Adolescent Trauma Treatments and Services (CATS) Project. *J Clin Child Adolesc Psychol*. 2007; 36:581-592.

114. de Arellano MA, Danielson CK. *Culturally-Modified Trauma-Focused Treatment (CM-TFT)*. Unpublished manuscript, Medical University of South Carolina; 2005.

115. Northern Virginia Family Service. http://www.nvfs.org/pages/page.asp?page_id= 91764. Accessed January 18, 2010.

116. de Arellano MA, Danielson CK. Culturally-Modified Trauma-Focused Therapy for Treatment of Hispanic Child Trauma Victims. Workshop at the Annual San Diego Conference on Child and Family Maltreatment; January 2006; San Diego, CA.

117. Kolko DJ, Cohen JA, Mannarino AP, et al. Community Treatment of Child Sexual Abuse: A survey of Practioners in the National Child Traumatic Stress Network. *Adm Policy Ment Health*. 2009;36:37-49.

118. Cohen JA, Mannarino AP, Deblinger E. *Treating trauma and traumatic grief in children and adolescents*. New York, NY: Guilford Press; 2006.

119. Riggs DS, Cahill SP, Foa EB. Prolonged exposure treatment of posttraumatic stress disorder. In: Follette VM, Ruzek JI, eds. *Cognitive-Behavioral Therapies for Trauma*. New York, NY: Guilford Press; 2006:65-95.

Chapter 20

CHILD SEXUAL ABUSE IN CHILDREN WITH DISABILITIES

Roberta A. Hibbard, MD
Sharon W. Cooper, MD, FAAP

Sexual assault can affect any child from any family at any age. Victims may be adults or children, healthy or ill, and able or disabled. Service providers need to be familiar with the special needs and circumstances of disabled victims. This chapter addresses these special considerations in evaluating and treating sexual assault of disabled children and adolescents.

EPIDEMIOLOGY

There is currently no universally accepted definition of what constitutes a disability. The lack of a single uniform definition used by researchers results in variable findings on the incidence, attributes, and experiences of children with disabilities. The Centers for Disease Control (CDC) describes developmental disabilities as a diverse group of severe chronic conditions that are caused by mental and/or physical impairments and result in problems with major life activities such as language, mobility, learning, self-help, and independent living.[1] The Americans with Disabilities Act defines "disability" as a physical or mental impairment that substantially limits one or more of the major life activities of an individual.[2] This definition includes all types of disabilities; including physical disabilities; cognitive or learning disabilities; motor and sensory dysfunctions; mental illness; or any other kind of physical, mental, or emotional impairment.[3] The phrase "children with special health care needs" is less limiting than some other phrases.[4]

Child sexual abuse can be conceptualized as any sexually stimulating activity that is considered inappropriate for the child's age, level of development, or role within the family. It can be any kind of sexual act that is perpetrated on an individual without consent or by force, either psychological or physical. The developmental level of the child is an important factor because it indicates the problem of cognitive delay that may influence the child's ability to consent, even when old enough chronologically to consent by local statutes or typical maturity. Sexually abusive acts may include exposure to sexually explicit materials; not respecting personal privacy in bathing or toileting; exhibitionism; fondling; oral, anal, or vaginal intercourse; incest; and other more extreme forms of perverse sexual acts. It is important to recognize that any kind of disability may influence the child's or adolescent's risk of and response to victimization and determines his or her special needs during the evaluation and treatment phases.

The Children's Bureau reported that an estimated 872 000 children were determined to be victims of abuse or neglect in 2004.[5] More than 60% of child victims experienced neglect, almost 20% were physically abused, and 10% were sexually abused. Of the 36 states that reported on disabilities, child victims who were reported to have a disability accounted for 7.3% of all victims. Children with the following conditions were considered as having a disability: mental retardation, emotional disturbance, visual impairment, learning disability, physical disability, or behavioral problems. It was believed these conditions were underrecognized and underreported, as not every child received a clinical diagnostic assessment when child maltreatment was suspected.

The Child Abuse and Prevention, Adoption, and Family Services Act of 1988 included a mandate to study the incidence of child maltreatment among children with disabilities. The National Center on Child Abuse and Neglect (NCCAN) reported that 14.1% of children whose maltreatment was substantiated by child protection service workers in 35 states had one or more disabilities. Of the children who were abused, 17.2% had disabilities; of those sexually abused, 15.2% had disabilities. Children with disabilities were found to be at greater risk of being victims of abuse and neglect than children without disabilities. Another study found the overall incidence of child maltreatment to be 39% in 150 children with multiple disabilities admitted to a psychiatric hospital. Of those children, 69% had been physically abused, 45% had been neglected, and 36% had been sexually abused; 52% of those children experienced multiple forms of maltreatment.[6]

Sullivan and Knutson reported maltreatment in 9% of non-disabled children and 31% of disabled children in a school setting.[7] In this study of more than 4500 maltreated children, children with disabilities were 3.4 times more likely to be abused and neglected when compared to non-disabled children. The most common form of maltreatment for children with disabilities was neglect, but sexual abuse was found to occur 3.1 times more often in the disabled population. Children with behavioral disorders were found to be at the highest risk of all types of maltreatment. One recent study reported 18.5% of children with autism had been physically abused and 16.6% sexually abused.[8] Cross and colleagues reported in 1993 that the disability itself directly contributed to child abuse in 47% of maltreated children with disabilities. The most common disabilities noted were emotional disabilities, learning disabilities, physical disabilities, and speech or language delay.[9] Sobsey reported that 48.1% of perpetrators of sexual abuse against people with disabilities gained access to their victims through disability services.[10]

RISK FACTORS

Why are children with disabilities at increased risk for child maltreatment in general and sexual assault specifically? There is no single risk factor that places a child at specific risk for abuse or neglect. A child with a disability may be more vulnerable to abuse because of society's beliefs or responses to his or her condition, rather than the condition itself. The interaction of factors seems to be most important. An integrated ecological model based on child development takes into account cultural and environmental factors as well as characteristics of the parent and child and their interactions.[10] Substance abuse on the parents' part is a well-known risk factor for maltreatment of all children. Other identified risk factors placing any child at risk include parents' poor coping skills, psychiatric conditions, financial stressors, poor impulse control, and a history of violence. Parents who lack positive parenting role models and suffer from low self-esteem and depression are more likely to maltreat children.

Additional factors that influence risk of maltreatment in children with disabilities relate to societal attitudes, stress, families, children, and non-familial caregivers. Some individuals may believe that children with disabilities are unlikely to be abused, which results in a lack of awareness and less effort at providing protection. Children with disabilities may be offered less sex education if they are perceived as asexual or unable to understand sex education. This lack of information contributes to placing the children at a higher risk of maltreatment.

Isolating the child from society increases risks by decreasing the child's knowledge and awareness of appropriate behaviors, which lessens the chance that other individuals are aware of maltreatment, while maintaining privacy of contact with the child. The child may be considered unreliable or an untrustworthy source of information. The perception that all caretakers are inherently good results in lack of attention to signs or symptoms of child maltreatment. Caretakers are trusted to provide good care and children are taught to obey authority figures. Many caretakers for children with disabilities provide extensive physical care. Children who have increased dependency on caregivers for their physical needs may be accustomed to having their bodies touched by adults on a regular basis and in private places. Children with some disabilities require assistance in toileting and intimate care. A child may not be aware when the behavior becomes inappropriate, especially if taught to trust the provider to always know what is best. It may be very difficult for the child to comprehend the distinction between appropriate assistance in activities of daily living and behaviors that become intrusive. The child is often dependent on the caretaker to put the nature of the behavior in context; if taught that the behavior or activity is normal or necessary, the child is unlikely to question it, or to report it.

With respect to sexual abuse, infrequent contact between a child with disabilities and other children and adults may enable molestation, because there is decreased opportunity for the child to develop a trusting relationship with an individual to whom he or she may disclose the abuse and decreased opportunity to learn to resist molestation.[3] On the other hand, children with disabilities who require multiple caregivers may have contact with numerous individuals in private, which increases the opportunity for abuse, including sexual abuse. However, an advantage of having a large number of caregivers is both the increased chance of someone's detecting the injuries or signs of abuse, and additional assistance that lessens the amount of stress placed on the primary caregiver. Thus, the presence of multiple providers may heighten or reduce the risk. Risk can be minimized by careful screening and selection of providers, sporadic and unscheduled monitoring of care, and keeping an open mind to recognition that any child may become a victim.

Children with disabilities often have limited access to critical information pertaining to personal safety and sexual abuse prevention. Parents often object to their child being provided with education on human sexuality. They feel that their children will never need it because of their special needs, without recognizing that their child still experiences sexual feelings and needs to know what behavior is acceptable and what is not. Children with disabilities are often unintentionally conditioned to comply with authority, which could result in their failing to recognize abusive behaviors as maltreatment.[11] Children with disabilities are often perceived as easy targets or "good victims" because their intellectual limitations may prevent them from being able to discern the experience as abuse; they may not be able to communicate the experience; or perpetrators think no one would believe the child if he or she does try to tell. The disclosure may be explained away by a perpetrator as the child's misunderstanding of routine care.

Parents and other providers often cannot imagine that their child might become a victim, thus missing opportunities to identify or prevent future abuse. The parent may hesitate to voice concern for fear it may result in dismissal from a program or services, and they might lose all assistance in providing care for a child with special needs. There are also fears of not wanting to accuse someone without proof that inappropriate activity actually took place.

It is important to recognize that disabled victims may be assaulted regardless of their apparent "attractiveness" or lack thereof. Sexual assault is rarely romantically motivated, and the bias to suggest the victim is unattractive to an offender should be addressed to ensure the highest motivation of the investigative process.[12]

Table 20-1. Myths regarding persons with disabilities.
— The dehumanization myth
— The damaged merchandise myth
— The feeling no pain myth
— The disabled menace myth
— The helpless myth

In 1990, Sobsey and Mansell outlined five "cultural myths" that contribute to the erroneous thinking about persons with disabilities (**Table 20-1**).[13] The acceptance of these myths may perpetuate psychological justification that a perpetrator may employ.

The ***dehumanization myth***. Labels such as "vegetative state" suggest that a person with the disability is something less than a full member of society and serves to dehumanize the individual. Perpetrators may rationalize their abusive behavior as not really injuring another person.

The ***damaged merchandise myth***. Similar to dehumanization, this myth asserts that the life of the individual with the disability is "worthless" and that he or she has nothing to lose. Such philosophy can lead to the justification of cessation of minimal support (ie, providing food, water, or medication) to a person who is otherwise relatively functional, especially after a catastrophic event such as a traumatic brain injury. This thinking is aligned with advocates for euthanasia of children with severe disabilities, who rationalize that such killing is in the best interest of the child.

The ***feeling no pain myth***. People with disabilities are thought of as having no feelings or as being immune to pain and suffering. There is no basis for this myth; individuals with disabilities experience the same range of emotions found in any person.

The ***disabled menace myth***. Perceived as different, individuals with disabilities are often considered unpredictable and dangerous, whether or not there is any foundation for the fear. Adherence to this myth may motivate people to prevent community facilities, such as group homes for adults with mental retardation, from being developed in their neighborhoods.

The ***helpless myth***. Beliefs or perceptions that individuals with disabilities are helpless and unable to take care of themselves undermine their self-esteem and ability to make decisions related to daily life. Such thinking makes the individual with a disability more vulnerable to abuse and manipulation.[13]

The prevalence of these myths with respect to the views of disabled children is unknown; however, in-depth case analysis of crimes against disabled children might direct prevention strategies to target these widely held misconceptions.

CLINICAL PRESENTATION OF CHILD SEXUAL ABUSE

There is no typical clinical presentation of sexual abuse for a child with or without disabilities. Physical abuse and sexual abuse often occur together; physical or behavioral indicators of child maltreatment are similar. Indicators of possible child sexual abuse may consist of behaviors, physical symptoms or signs, or a statement by the child. Indicators suggest the possibility of abuse, but do not prove it by themselves. Child sexual abuse is most easily recognized when the child makes a clear, consistent statement about the activity, the activity has been witnessed by others, or there is clear forensic evidence. Unfortunately, these conditions do not always occur. As discussed, the child with a disability may be less capable or incapable of making a clearly credible statement. To compound the difficulties, these events are rarely witnessed and forensic evidence is unlikely to be present by the time sexual abuse is considered. Added diligence and recognition of the possibilities are necessary to identify the suspected child sexual victim who also has a disability. Any parental caregiver or child report of concern about sexual abuse must be carefully explored.

BEHAVIORAL INDICATORS

Behavioral indicators encompass a variety of patterns, all of which may be the child's response to the stress or distress of what he or she is experiencing. Patterns may encompass, but are not limited to, unusual fear of people or places, aggression, withdrawal, regression in behaviors, wariness of physical contact, fear of going to a specific location, and destructive behaviors. Defensive startle behaviors such as covering of the eyes or ears, extreme reluctance to accept assistance, recent onset of sleeping in the fetal position, withdrawal, and self-imposed isolation are some behavior changes that might cause concern. Emotional lability, easy agitation, and fearfulness during bathing or toileting form another group of signs that may be encountered. The difficulty is that these behaviors are nonspecific and simply reflect the child's stress. They do not identify what the underlying stressor is—maltreatment, death in the family, financial problems in the home, marital discord, or otherwise. Behavioral changes, rather than a specific behavior, are usually more concerning; however, if the child has been sexually abused for a long period of time, the behavior may have been evident for a prolonged period of time and is not recognized as a "new" behavior. One must be careful to not automatically attribute behavioral changes to the child's disability. This is sometimes difficult when the child's disability may provide an alternate explanation for the symptoms of abuse. If the child is viewed as unreliable or not trustworthy, behavioral observations may go unheeded. Careful and thoughtful attention to all possibilities is warranted.

PHYSICAL SIGNS AND SYMPTOMS

The physical signs and symptoms may be multivariate or completely absent. Multiple somatic complaints are not unusual in victims of child sexual assault: headaches, chest pain, abdominal pain, fatigue, and a general malaise. More specific symptoms referable to the genitourinary tract or an area of the physical assault may be present. Children may complain of discomfort in the genital area, dysuria, or painful defecation. They may have specific signs such as genital bleeding, vaginitis, or blood in the stool. The child may have bruises, "hickies," or bite marks that may indicate physical trauma coexistent with the sexual assault. It may be the physical findings of bruising, bleeding, or vaginitis in nonverbal children that raise initial concerns of sexual abuse. Changes in signs and symptoms, diapering, and underlying medical problems must be explored. Vigilance is required to refrain from automatically assigning etiologies to the underlying disability without considering sexual abuse. Just as behavioral indicators may have multiple etiologies, so may the physical indicators. They require an appropriate complete medical evaluation considering all possibilities to determine their association with possible child sexual abuse or other unrelated medical conditions.

DISCLOSURE BY THE CHILD

The child's verbal disclosure about the sexual contact, when possible, is typically the most helpful information in ascertaining what has happened to the child and who was involved. The child with a disability that significantly influences communication skills and cognitive functioning may have more difficulty in communicating the activities that occurred or who was involved. Disclosures must be interpreted in the context of the child's cognitive and behavioral ability. Any physical disability (motor, sensory, hearing, or visual) may also influence the timing, context, and content of the disclosure.

In documenting a history of sexual assault or child sexual abuse, a careful understanding of the method and content of disclosure is critical. If a patient has a developmental level within the very early childhood range, the disclosure might be blurted out within the context of toileting or bathing. Often, children who are cognitively less than 5 years old will not have learned the concept of a "secret" and feel comfortable in revealing private information without hesitation. Some examiners may inadvertently discount such a disclosure if it constitutes a simple environmental contamination and seems to have no validity. However, if the patient has not demonstrated sexually reactive behaviors in the past and has not had a habit of verbalizing in a sexually explicit manner, there is no reason to disbelieve the factual nature of the information anymore than one would disbelieve any other statement the child might make.[14]

A child's disclosure may be incomplete because of the poor understanding or interpretation of the specific events that took place; this is a developmental and cognitive function. Although a child with developmental delay may not understand the concept of inappropriate touch, he or she might still be able to describe the incident within the context of its sensation. Identification of sensations and feelings is important to note as they imply the event was experienced. Sensations of wetness, gagging or choking, "gooey," and others are vivid descriptors. If a child with developmental delay has been told a story about sexual contact, it is not likely that he or she would be able to describe the sensation that would accompany that activity. A detailed description of the feelings of touch, taste, sounds, and smell are unlikely to come from only hearing about these activities and probably represent objective history about the event. Such detail in a disclosure significantly enhances its credibility. For example, one child's disclosure was not believed until the alleged perpetrator's wife learned of the child's description of the sounds and ritual behavior that she had observed in her husband for many years. When she heard the child's description, she knew the child had clearly experienced the contact. This detailed information can also be helpful to investigators in the field and at the scene, where they may find items to corroborate the child's disclosure.

At times, disabled children disclose extremely sexually explicit information, such as forced fellatio or anal penetration. Indication of such forms of abuse may be frankly stated or demonstrated by gestures and reenactment. Such descriptions are outside the normal range of psychosexual development and knowledge. It is unlikely these disclosures have been suggested by others. They should be documented verbatim and as descriptively as possible. Some children may have been exploited through exposure to a significant amount of pornography as a method of grooming for future abuse. This may have definite impact on the child's sexual knowledge and influence the interpretation of the disclosure. This form of desensitization by an assailant does not negate the reality of a true sexual assault and is exploitation by itself. It may also explain a delay in the disclosure or a feeling in the victim that his or her sexual behavior constitutes what grown-ups do. This may be offered to the child as justification for the activity by a perpetrator.

There is sometimes a concern that a child has fabricated a story of sexual abuse. Fabrication may occur in children with disabilities just as it may occur in children without disabilities. Research has revealed that disclosures under these circumstances are rare. It is important to consider the basis of concern for sexual assault; for example, one must determine whether it is the actual content of the child's statement or the adult's interpretation of a statement or behavior. A well-intentioned adult may misinterpret a child's cues and behaviors. There often exists a good faith concern on the part of a parent to ensure that nothing has happened to the child. Without investigation, however, no one will have a good understanding of the child's intent. Clinicians who have experience in evaluating children for sexual abuse readily recognize the risk of false disclosure when there has been a threat or coaching of a statement by a parent.

Individuals with disabilities are at risk to behave in a more compliant manner than those who are not disabled in attempts to ensure that they will be liked and included by others. This increases the risk of sexual abuse, but may also increase the risk of making a coached accusation. Learned compliance is often carefully instilled in them by their parents to facilitate their social acceptability. Children may then disclose details that may not be accurate in order to please the adult who is asking the questions. This should not be assumed, as the details may be accurate. It is important to remember that some inconsistencies and inaccuracies are to be expected from any child's statement—inconsistencies must be interpreted in the context of all the available information and the degree of variance. Is the variation minor, major, or is the child talking about multiple different incidents? A coached statement may be too consistent at a level not expected of the child. The consistency of the disclosure, language used, and details can help sort out the veracity of the disclosure.

The same set of guidelines and standards regarding obtaining a history from a child who is not disabled should be used within the limitations of the availability and need for special services that may be required to interview the child. As with any child, the parent or caretaker of a child with a disability may provide background information and the reason for concern. One must be cautious in assuring that the presence of a care provider serving as an interpreter or support person will not influence the child's willingness to disclose. On the other hand, the disabled victim may require reassurance from the presence of a familiar person. Children with disabilities may be traumatized because of an inability to anticipate an attack or difficulty in communicating with the assailant. It is essential to remember that most assailants are known to the victim and may be in a caregiving role.

SPECIFIC IMPAIRMENTS

HEARING IMPAIRMENT

If the care provider is fluent in sign language, it may be possible to obtain a cursory history from the child with a hearing impairment before having access to a certified language interpreter. One must be very cautious in assuring the care provider is not a perpetrator or someone interested in protecting the abuser before asking him or her to interpret. Actual interviewing techniques with the hearing impaired victim should include careful eye contact despite the fact the questions may be interpreted by a sign language expert. The clinician should follow the standard method of interviewing to include rapport building and free-association conversation before embarking on the sexual assault history. Setting the victim at ease is an important part of the medical evaluation because the use of threats by the perpetrator may cause the victim to fear talking about the incident. Review of the behaviors of the hearing impaired victim should be discussed both with a supportive family member or care provider and with the victim. Often care providers are unaware of sleep dysfunction, situational anxiety, specific fearfulness, intrusive thoughts, or other signs and symptoms the child is experiencing. Because of a high association of posttraumatic stress disorder after either a single incident of sexual assault or multiple occurrences, any symptoms should be discussed with the child as well as the care provider.

When using a sign language interpreter, the interviewer should consider reiterating what he or she has heard back to the victim. The sexual vocabulary of many deaf people may be colloquial or idiosyncratic. An interpreter who is deaf may need to work in conjunction with a hearing interpreter to ensure the best communication. The child should be told that the examiner will repeat back what he or she believes the victim said to ensure complete understanding of the history. The child should understand that this effort is to confirm that the interviewer truly understands the details the victim is communicating, and it is not a challenge to what has been disclosed.

VISUAL IMPAIRMENT

The information in a disclosure by a visually impaired child will include mostly nonvisual sensory information. Details such as the time of day or place of the assault should be explained in more depth based on the victim's normal means for making these determinations. Careful questioning in a step-by-step fashion may provide important information, such as unusual smells on the assailant, the sensation of facial hair, or the recognition of an unusual accent in the voice. If a weapon was used, the victim may recall exactly where on the body the instrument was placed when it was used to touch him or her. The examiner might be able to document the presence of the skin reaction.

Children and adolescents who have lost their sight either from birth or very early in life may have early language delay. Expressive language in severely visually impaired children develops later than in sighted children.[15] Lack of visual stimuli may limit verbal responses to the usual visual cues. Victims of sexual assault who are visually impaired are often able to describe auditory and olfactory details, which may have some value in the resultant identification of an assailant. If the perpetrator is known to the victim, questions during the interview might include the reasons that convince the victim of the identity of the assailant.

Children who lose their vision after age 5 years have a higher incidence of independence and better language development. The lack of visual stimuli is a natural incentive for enhanced vocabulary acquisition in these children. One language parameter noted to be problematic is the incorrect use of personal and possessive pronouns, such as confusing *his* and *their*. This may impact the ability of such a victim to clearly convey the history of the sexual assault; therefore, it is wise to screen language concepts in a visually impaired child and ensure that the child is responding reliably, consistently, and with expressive understanding. Identification of body parts might need to be done with tactile reinforcement, so that the examiner will assuredly understand what the victim is trying to communicate. A review of behaviors and feelings should be conducted in a manner similar to that of the hearing impaired victim, with intentional verbal redundancy to ensure that the examiner has a clear understanding of the information being communicated about the assault of the individual.

When visual impairment accompanies other disabilities such as cognitive delay or hearing loss, the victim may demonstrate tactile defense after a sexual assault. This is manifested as combativeness and is another indicator that might lead investigators to believe the sexual assault could have occurred.

MOTOR DELAY

The child with motor disabilities may present other unique challenges. Motor delays may range from the central nervous system to the distant muscle fiber. Depending on the etiology of the motor delay, cognition may be normal or impaired. Cerebral palsy (CP) is a category of static motor dysfunction that is most often present at or shortly after birth. Many children with CP have normal cognitive function, but may have speech delay. The traumatic brain injury victim often has significant gaps in motor, cognitive, and behavioral function. Of individuals with hemiplegia, 85% have both normal intelligence and the capability of complete independent living. Those persons with athetosis also have a higher incidence of near-normal intelligence, although dysarthria may lead to poor speech intelligibility and the impression that the patient is not cognitively intact. Receptive language in such patients is often age-appropriate. Keeping this in mind is important when determining a patient's ability to respond to questions regarding a sexual assault. A family member or other individual who is accustomed to the victim's communication style (and is neither a suspected perpetrator nor someone likely to interfere with the child's disclosure) is invaluable to assist the examiner in understanding what is being communicated.

INTERVIEW TECHNIQUES

Taking the above information into consideration, interview techniques should be adapted to reflect an appropriate level of interaction for the child's cognitive or developmental level and special needs for a visual or hearing impairment. Once rapport has been established, it may be helpful to frame questions within certain topic areas (ie, home, classroom, school, playground). Children and adults with disabilities may have a more difficult time shifting from topic to topic and may need to be assisted in making transitions. If an event occurred outside, asking about weather conditions may help in the corroboration of the event. One can confirm from other reports easily whether the conditions described by the victim were true on that day. Redundancy in questioning for children and adolescents with disabilities increases the chance that the examiner and the victim will be talking consistently about the same thing at the same time. Rephrasing questions allows one to ask the individual in several ways about the same information. One must be careful not to suggest answers to the questions asked. When a victim is unchanged in the response, the examiner can feel more secure there's no confusion regarding the facts. Simple questions are best; complex sentences and sentences that run together in content and meaning can be confusing. The receptive language age equivalent may be far less than the chronologic age, and the examiner must have realistic expectations of the questions asked. A limited time for the interview based on the child's attention span must also be taken into consideration.

It is critical to use language that the child understands. It is best to use the child's terminology once he or she has identified such. The interviewer must also be skilled at helping children describe all aspects of their experience. If the child does not know terminology or who a specific individual is, the examiner must be creative in helping the child convey as much detail is possible. The child may be able to describe the duties of an individual, what they look like, or for what special occasions they encounter that individual.

In some states and jurisdictions, the hearsay exception associated with a medical history must meet the test that the victim understands that he or she is in a medical encounter. It is important for the medical examiner to introduce himself or herself as a physician or other health care provider, and be sure that the individual is aware they are at a medical facility. If the encounter is for medical diagnosis and treatment, establishing that fact that is essential.

When taking a history from a child victim, it is important to consider a gradual approach to seeking information. The questions about daily routines, such as, "What do you do when you get up in the morning?" encourage open conversation in the rapport-building phase of the medical history. They also establish the victim's ability to recall more activities of daily living. Prompts such as, "What happens after that?" are helpful in affording the examiner the opportunity to evaluate spontaneous language content and the ability of the victim to speak in terms of concrete actions versus more abstract feelings. Questions such as, "Do you stay home all day?" can assist the victim in expressing place and person concepts. They may also allow him or her to speak of an alleged perpetrator in an indirect fashion, so that the examiner might learn the terminology used in reference to this person. The examiner should use the same terms as the child. The child's concept of time may not be fully developed; demonstrating concepts of yesterday, today, and tomorrow help a child to establish whether the child has an understanding of time, if that is the case. Relating incidents to special events, holidays, or locations can assist in establishing a time frame.

Because the most common perpetrator of sexual assault and abuse is most likely an acquaintance, the developmentally delayed victim demonstrates the same degree of confusion as seen in young children in trying to sort out and report an experience. Unfortunately, many children with a developmental disability, for example, are taught to be compliant with authority figures and to seek assistance. Consequently, they may not perceive that anyone has hurt them or touched them in a bad way. Questions should not be asked in a "yes-no" format if they can be avoided. "What happened?" or "Tell me more about that," encourages more spontaneous detail and avoids the introduction of interviewer assumptions.

Corroborative information from family members or others who are frequently with the victim should be obtained to better evaluate the victim's credibility. Such corroborative information could include the weather on the day of the assault, who was present in the house or facility, what time the assault may have taken place, and to whom the victim made a statement or comment about what happened.

MEDICAL EVALUATION OF CHILD SEXUAL ABUSE

The medical evaluation of a child who is disabled and a suspected victim of sexual abuse should progress along the same lines as any medical evaluation; that is a history, physical examination, impression and plan. The evaluation and physical examination must be tailored to the individual needs of the patient. Depending upon the child's ability to make a disclosure and provide detail, additional investigation by child protection services and law enforcement may be necessary to get to the truth of the concern.

HISTORY

The purpose of the medical interview is to understand what happened and to ascertain any medical consequences from a possible sexual contact. In some settings, the medical team obtains the information from the child victim. In other settings, forensic interviewers not in the medical environment interview the child regarding the allegation or experiences. The details of the assault may then be shared with the medical providers, to assist in determining the appropriate medical steps. The interview techniques described in the previous section should be applied when obtaining the medical history.

The child often presents to health care either because of verbal disclosure, or behavioral concerns of assault, or because there were suspicious circumstances leading to an evaluation. A victim with a disability may present with evidence of physical bodily harm or genital trauma. The health care provider must provide a concise but detailed account of the history as given by the victim or any other observer. However the concern comes to light, it is important to speak with someone knowledgeable about the child to understand the child's capabilities, and normal behaviors and to identify any physical complaints. A careful behavioral history is important because family members or care providers who know the child well can attest to any changes in normal routines and any concerning new behaviors. It is necessary to understand the child's usual routines in order to help interpret changes in behaviors. A child may not know someone well enough to be able to name them, but may be able to describe them in ways others would recognize them by the activity in which they participate or a specific physical feature. Behaviors and changing behaviors, as well as a complete review of systems, should be obtained as part of the medical history to look for behavioral and physical consequences of sexual contact or evidence of other medical conditions that may be confused with sexual assault.

Behavioral changes may be the primary evidence warranting an initial evaluation for child sexual abuse in a victim with behavioral and cognitive impairment. A care provider familiar with the habits and behaviors of the child may be included in the evaluation to obtain some perspective. Although instruments have been devised to assess sexualized behaviors in normally developing children, no such studies have been devised for children with serious forms of disabling conditions. Non-abused children without disabilities have more sexualized behaviors at younger ages. As they mature, fewer sexualized behaviors are seen. It is the developmental age equivalence of the child that is important in assessing the appropriateness of any behavior. This realization of cognitive age equivalence is also important in determining the approach to the interview. The approach must match the child's abilities for the examiner to obtain some degree of cooperation and hope for meaningful information.

Physical Examination

The physical examination of the child sexual assault victim should be a complete examination—from the top of the head to the tip of the toes, with a detailed genital exam. Special attention should be paid to those parts of the body with signs or symptoms. The skin, mouth, and anogenital area of every victim is important to evaluate to look for evidence of new or old trauma, infection, or clues to underlying medical conditions. Sexual maturity will also influence medical considerations independent of cognition—specifically the possibility of pregnancy.

The approach to the physical examination, like all other aspects of the evaluation for sexual assault, should be geared to the child's developmental and behavioral level and any physical or sensory handicaps. Adaptations for motor impairments may be necessary in considering examining positions. The visually impaired child should be told what is happening and extra care should be taken in letting him or her feel and touch any instruments that might be used, such as a moistened cotton swab. The hearing impaired child should also see and touch any materials to be used. Keeping all children informed of what is happening, no matter their disability, is an important consideration in gaining their trust and cooperation. Just as a normal child should not be coerced into an examination and held down against his or her will, neither should a child with a disability. Coercion, again, depends on the level of cognition; an 18-month-old child may have to be coerced to have the ears examined. Most examinations can be easily performed by examiners experienced in cajoling and adapting the approach to fit the needs of the child. The benefits of an exam (often with no physical findings) must be weighed against the risks of further emotional trauma of coercion. In rare situations, physical signs or symptoms that require immediate medical attention may warrant sedation or an examination under anesthesia.

Violence associated with sexual assault requires close surveillance for head and neck injury, facial trauma or old trauma, and other bodily injuries. While violence is not typical as part of the sexual assault of children, children who are physically abused are more likely than their peers to be sexually abused. If the victim's disabilities include communication problems, the clinicians must be very thorough, as in examining a very young child, to ensure discovery of all injuries. Defensive wounds, which usually occur to the upper extremities when the victim assumes a defensive posture, should be carefully noted. Injuries that result from defending against the assailant's hand or weapon can be seen in the upper outer arms, shoulders, or palms of the hand. Ligature marks about the wrists or ankles may be seen in the child who has been restrained. There may be marks about the neck from strangulation or choking. Injuries may result to the mouth as a result of oral-genital contact, and bruising may occur anywhere, especially the breasts and inner thighs. Depending on the assault, there may evidence anywhere.

In a sexual assault case, there are 2 crime scenes: the victim and the site where the crime occurred. Both scenes deserve meticulous attention to ensure the integrity of results. Evidence collection is extremely important at the crime scene as well as with a child. Forensic collection from the child may be reasonable when the child presents to the health care system within 72 to 96 hours of a sexual assault. Studies have shown the greatest yield for positive forensic evidence of the prepubertal child sexual assault victim is from the clothing gathered and submitted with the rape kit.[16] In a study by Christian, Lavelle, De Jong, and colleagues, the DNA evidence present in this material was found to be more reliable than those fluids found on the victim's body.[16] Realization of this fact requires a careful retrieval of any and all articles of clothing the child was known to have been wearing at the probable time of the crime. From a crime scene perspective, this includes discarded diapers or clothes that might be present at the scene; bed sheets and towels should also be examined.

MULTIDISCIPLINARY TEAM EVALUATION

The evaluation of children for possible child sexual abuse requires a team approach under all circumstances. There is no single profession or provider who has access to all the information necessary to make a determination of what happened, address medical consequences, interview witnesses or suspects, collect and process forensic evidence, and provide victim and family treatment as needed. Child protection services have a responsibility to ensure safety and protection of the child; law enforcement is responsible for determining whether a crime has been committed; the medical provider assesses and treats the physical and mental well-being of the patient and may need to collect evidence on the child's body.

The social worker in the medical setting can be an invaluable source early in gathering background psychosocial information on the child and family. This may include information on domestic violence, previous child protection involvement, criminal histories, and possible confounding factors or additional risk factors (ie, living with a convicted sex offender) in the child's life. The social worker can also assess the level of anxiety and genuine concern for the child in balance with external issues of a parent who has not dealt with his or her own sexual assault in the past or may be using the allegation to seek custody of a child. A history of the child's functional, behavioral, and cognitive abilities can aid medical providers and social and legal investigators in determining the best approach to questions and examination of the child. The social worker can assist in victim advocacy options should other factors such as domestic violence, substance abuse, or homelessness be contributing factors. He or she can also facilitate referrals for mental health treatment for the child and family.

Team decision-making processes are indicated, particularly when a victim has a disability. Many communities have established sexual abuse response teams or child advocacy centers to address the special issues of child victimization. The expertise of specially trained sexual assault investigators (child protection services, law enforcement, and prosecutors) in conjunction with medical providers with advanced training in sexual assault cases is invaluable. In the circumstances of the disabled victim, physical evidence of an acute sexual assault is self-explanatory. In the circumstance of a nonverbal child victim where no forensic evidence has been collected and who may have no physical evidence of a sexual encounter (most victims), team reviews of all the information can be very helpful. Consultation with providers who have expertise in working with children with disabilities can also be helpful. When a team documents that there has been attention to all of the possibilities explaining the presentation and discerns that enough evidence exists to discount other hypotheses, the credibility of the final decision is increased.

Investigation by law enforcement and child protection services is important in determining what is rumor and what observers directly report. When others receive information and pass it along, it is imperative to note the source of the original information. In this way, investigators can identify and confirm the information from the original source. The sexual assault may have been witnessed or the victim may have been discovered very shortly after the event occurred. For example, if a child with cognitive and communication delay is brought from a residential care facility, the provider accompanying the child may not have any direct information. Providers at the facility who have information should be interviewed rather than others who initially deny any knowledge of the assault or concern. This scenario of an uninformed provider accompanying the child recurs with children in facilities as well as children in public schools and homes. It is often not the individual with the most direct knowledge who brings the child to care. In these cases, child protection services must seek out and interview other sources of information.

It is also important for the investigator to go to the scene of any incident to look for evidence of what may have been described, such as possible forensic evidence on bed sheets and towels. The observations of many providers may be helpful in elucidating what actually happened.

Investigators can learn whether there are what appears to be irrational fears of a specific room or area in the home or facility. This behavior is not different from what is noted in children and adolescents who have no developmental problems. This may be useful insight into the possible location of an assault. It is not uncommon that the acute sexual assault victim comes for medical care after the most recent event in a series of recurrent episodes. Concerning behaviors, physical complaints, or other observations may be reported on by other providers.

Team members can also assist in establishing whether the child victim is capable of giving a reasonable history. This is generally feasible if the child's cognitive developmental level is at least 4 years of age. Care providers familiar with the child can provide information on the child's short- and long-term memory, reliability to recover normal facts, and language abilities in comprehension and expression. Although a disabled individual may not be able to read, he or she may be able to consistently recall incidents that had a major impact on his or her memory.

The question of consent must be addressed in the adolescent with a disability. A sexual assault victim who is nonverbal or developmentally delayed may be reported as a consensual sex partner. Consent is not volition alone but includes the victim's ability to understand the nature of the sexual act and its consequences.[17] Developmentally delayed adolescents typically lack an adequate understanding of a consensual sexual relationship. They often have little or no dating experience, and few have had formal sexual education. Without confirmation of an understanding of sex education, these individuals would likely not satisfy the legal criteria for distinguishing between a consensual sex act and sexual abuse.

Just as issues of competence to testify in a legal setting arise for the young child, they arise in the child with cognitive and developmental delay. Establishing that there is an understanding between the truth and a lie rests on information from care providers familiar with the individual. To allow a child's testimony, certain legal criteria may need to be met depending on the jurisdiction. These criteria typically include demonstrating that the child understands the difference between the truth and a lie, knows there is some compulsion to tell the truth, and knows there are consequences for not telling the truth. Children may pretend play, but this normal behavior does not preclude their ability to understand truth and lies, or to be reliable historians. It is inappropriate to identify all children with disabilities as unreliable witnesses.

TREATMENT AND PREVENTION

Children with disabilities have the same types of medical and mental health treatment needs as other children who have been sexually assaulted. Considerations for medical care, pregnancy, and sexually transmitted infection prophylaxis should not be influenced by the child's cognitive ability. Any medical conditions identified needs appropriate care and treatment. Each case of child sexual abuse that is confirmed or strongly suspected should include a multidisciplinary treatment plan, which includes a mental health assessment and treatment component appropriate for the child's cognitive and developmental level. Counseling for the family is a necessary component for their needs and to assist in helping their child victim. This child and family treatment plan should be integrated with other intervention plans that may have already been developed for the child. Children with disabilities also require mental health services that are appropriately adapted to their special needs—be it a developmental adaptation or sign language interpreter.

Children with disabilities can experience the full range of feelings and emotions that are experienced by children without disabilities. It is a tremendous disservice to assume that the child is disabled and therefore does not comprehend the experience or have any effects from it. It must be remembered that many children are identified as victims because of the behavioral manifestations of the assault. The mental health treatment provider should assess how much the child understands the experience and how the child is dealing with any conflicting emotions. While the treatment provider may be faced with many challenges, counseling and therapy must be individualized to meet the needs of the child. Multiple modalities of treatment including behavior modification, art or music therapy, cognitive and educational methods, and psychoanalytic approaches may be considered.[18]

Prevention of child maltreatment, and child sexual abuse specifically, must be addressed to protect our children. The steps to prevention that any parent or professional can follow include the following[19]:

— Learning the risks and understanding facts

— Minimizing opportunities for the child to be molested, talking about prevention and sex education with their children

— Staying alert to the possible indicators of child sexual abuse

— Making a plan on how to respond if abuse is suspected

— Getting involved in community prevention efforts

At a national level, *A Call to Action: Ending Crimes of Violence Against Children and Adults with Disabilities* recommends establishing prevention as a priority, determining the magnitude and scope of the problem, creating a plan of action and implementation, and instituting an evaluation plan.[20]

Society must recognize children with disabilities as equal citizens who have equal rights to services and protections.[21] Attitudes about children and youth with disabilities must change to empower their positions and decrease their vulnerability to abuse. Institutional policies should include screening and monitoring of employees and volunteers, chaperones, and supervisors of field trips and prompt reporting of allegations of sexual abuse. Children need to be given accurate information about sex education and personal safety.[22]

The keys to success will include informing parents about the reality of the problem and making children aware of the possibilities and empowering them all to stop the abuse. Knowledgeable providers with supportive programs will need to continue to provide ongoing education and services in these areas.

FUTURE EFFORTS

Research has demonstrated that there are significant training needs for collaborative responses in the evaluation of children with disabilities who have been maltreated. Orelove studied parents, educators, and investigators about their understanding of the needs in working with children with disabilities and child maltreatment. Respondents had a cursory awareness of some of the issues; a majority of the respondents were interested in training and ranked recognition of maltreatment of children with disabilities as a priority.[23]

Future efforts need to expand the recognition that children with disabilities may be sexually assaulted and improve prevention techniques and awareness. Research and training initiatives need to incorporate a focus on children with disabilities in order to get a better understanding of their unique responses and treatment needs.

CONCLUSION

Sexual abuse occurs at a higher rate among children with disabilities than among children who are not disabled. Disabilities may include mental retardation, emotional disturbance, visual impairment, learning disability, physical disability, behavioral problems, or another medical problem. Disabled children appear to be more vulnerable to abuse because of numerous societal and cultural factors, as well as increased stress on parents and other caregivers. Sexual abuse may occur along with physical abuse, or separately. When evaluating a child with a disability, modifications in communication or examination technique may be needed. Physical and mental health care should be the same as for children who are not disabled. Increased awareness of the issues surrounding abuse of children with disabilities is needed, and society must recognize children with disabilities as equal citizens, having equal rights to services and protections.

REFERENCES

1. Developmental Disabilities: Topic Home. Centers for Disease Control and Prevention Web site. http://www.cdc.gov/ncbddd/dd/default.htm. Accessed August 12, 2009.

2. *Americans with Disabilities Act.* Pub L No. 101-336, 104 Stat 327.

3. Ammerman RT, Baladerian NJ. *Maltreatment of Children with Disabilities.* Chicago, IL: National Committee to Prevent Child Abuse; 1993.

4. van Dyck PC, Kogan MD, McPherson MG, et al. Prevalence and characteristics of children with special health care needs. *Arch Pediatr Adolesc Med.* 2004;158:884-890.

5. US Department of Health and Human Services, Administration on Children, Youths and Families. *Child Maltreatment 2004.* Washington, DC: US Government Printing Office; 2006.

6. Ammerman RT, Van Hasselt VB, Hersen M, et al. Abuse and neglect in psychiatrically hospitalized multi-handicapped children. *Child Abuse Negl.* 1989; 13:335-343.

7. Sullivan PM, Knutson JF. Maltreatment and disabilities: a population-based epidemiological study. *Child Abuse Negl.* 2000;24(10):1257-1273.

8. Mandell DS, Walrath CM, Manteuffel B, et al. The prevalence and correlates of abuse among children with autism served in comprehensive community-based mental health settings. *Child Abuse Negl.* 2005;29:1359-1372.

9. Cross S, Kaye E, Ratnofsky A, et al. *A report on the Maltreatment of Children with Disabilities.* Washington, DC: National Center on Child Abuse and Neglect, US Dept of Health and Human Services; 1993.

10. Sobsey D. *Violence and Abuse in the Lives of People with Disabilities: The End of Silent Acceptance?* Baltimore, MD: Paul H. Brookes; 1994.

11. Sullivan P, Cork PM. *Developmental Disabilities Training Project.* Omaha, NE: Center for Abused Children with Disabilities, Boys Town National Research Hospital, Nebraska Department of Health and Human Services; 1996.

12. Sorensen DD. *The Invisible Victims.* Minneapolis, MN: University of Minnesota, Institute on Community Integration (UAP)/Research and Training Center on Community Living; 1997.

13. Sobsey D, Mansell S. The prevention of sexual abuse of people with developmental disabilities. *Dev Disabilities Bull.* 1990;18:55-56.

14. Gil E, Johnson TC. *Sexualized Children Assessment and Treatment of Sexualized Children Who Molest.* Rockville, MD: Launch Press; 1993.

15. McConachie HR, Moore V. Early expressive language of severely visually impaired children. *Dev Med Child Neurol.* 1994;36(3):230-240.

16. Christian CW, Lavelle JM, De Jong A, et al. Forensic evidence findings in prepubertal victims of sexual assault. *Pediatrics.* 2000;106:100-107.

17. Parker T, Abramson PR. The Law hath not been dead: protecting adults with mental retardation from sexual abuse and violation of their sexual freedom. *Ment Retard.* 1995;33:257-258, 261-262.

18. Allington-Smith P, Ball R, Haytor R. Management of sexually abused children with learning disabilities. *Adv in Psychiatr Treatment.* 2002;8:66-72.

19. Darkness to Light. http://www.darkness2light.org/7steps/7steps.asp. Accessed May 7, 2009.

20. Marge, DK. *A Call to Action: Ending Crimes of Violence Against Children and Adults with Disabilities: A Report to the Nation 2003.* Syracuse, NY: SUNY Upstate Medical University; 2003.

21. Svevo K. Children with disabilities and child maltreatment. *Off Newsl Int Soc Prev Child Abuse Negl.* 2005;14(2):8.

22. Adolescent Medicine Committee, Canadian Pediatric Society. Sexual abuse of adolescents with chronic conditions. *Paediatr Child Health.* 1997;2(3):212-213.

23. Orelove FP, Hollahan DJ, Myles KT. Maltreatment of children with disabilities: training needs for a collaborative response. *Child Abuse Negl.* 2000;24(2):185-194.

Chapter 21

CHILD SEXUAL ABUSE: REFRAMING AND EXPANDING OUR PERSPECTIVE

John Stirling, Jr., MD

Society has worked diligently to identify abused children and has brought considerable resources to bear in protecting them and bringing their abusers to justice. The past few decades have seen the development of an entire discipline of child protection. An impressive body of literature has accumulated, with dedicated journals and texts: a recent keyword search of the PubMed Internet medical library Web site using the phrase "child abuse" turned up more than 27 000 responses. Successful prosecution has been aided by the advent of child advocacy centers (CAC), multidisciplinary endeavors that seek to minimize trauma to the child victim and family while improving the investigation. Child abuse pediatrics has appeared as a recognized subspecialty in pediatrics, with its own board examination and fellowship requirements.

There is evidence to suggest that these efforts have been successful. In the past decade and a half the number of child abuse cases reported and confirmed in the United States has substantially declined. Sexual abuse cases have fallen the most—by nearly 50%—but physical abuse has appeared to decrease as well.[1] Of the 3 most often reported types of abuse (physical, sexual, and neglect) only neglect has continued unchanged. Although many explanations for the change have been suggested, wider awareness, earlier detection, and increasingly successful prosecution are certainly thought to have played a part.[2,3]

These are heartening figures, but public awareness, early detection, and prosecution of acts that have already been committed will not in themselves eliminate child abuse. In 2004, protective service agencies received 3 million reports of child abuse and were able to substantiate nearly 900 000 of them.[4] Moreover, success in raising societal awareness of child abuse has come at a price. As with any successful social initiative, child abuse awareness has spawned a backlash of criticism of, and even skepticism about, society's efforts to protect its children from harm.[5] Media depictions of child protective services (CPS) concentrate on its failures rather than its successes.[6] While there are now a great number of nonprofit, nongovernmental organizations devoted to child abuse care and prevention, fundraising is becoming ever more difficult. With so many stakeholders in the cause of child welfare, the field has often been marked by an atmosphere of competition rather than cooperation.[7]

The "Good" has often been described as the enemy of the "Excellent." As good and successful as recent efforts have been, there are still many areas that need improvement. While one might understandably wish for a powerful new "weapon" in the "war" against child abuse, new discoveries and practices will not result in dramatic changes without similar fundamental changes in the way society regards the problem of child maltreatment. We already know many of the things we need to achieve: preventing most abuse, detecting and prosecuting it when it does occur, and effectively addressing its consequences. Unfortunately, our biases often prevent us from efficiently using what we know. It is the contention, at the heart of this chapter, that further progress in the field of child protection will be made only by changing our perspective on the problems of child abuse and neglect; that is, by seeing abuse, and the community's role in responding to it, in a different way.

Public relations specialists refer to this process as "reframing."[8] A perceptual frame is a set of internalized values and concepts that help us understand our environment and help us make sense of new information by likening it to what is already known. People have a tendency to configure new information to make it conform to a dominant frame. This keeps us from being overwhelmed by new input and makes novelty more comfortable, but valuable information may be lost in the process. The following sections of this chapter argue that the current dominant frames regarding the prevention, management, and treatment of child abuse have come to limit our progress and risk losing hard-won allies among the public. A reframe is suggested for each domain.

REFRAME 1. PREVENTION: CHILD ABUSE AS A SYMPTOM, NOT A DISEASE

It is hard to imagine anything worse than the deliberate abuse of a child by an adult. Such an act is a betrayal of one of our most sacred compacts: the promise to nurture and protect future generations. Child maltreatment is, of course, a criminal offense. When such an act occurs, society must respond quickly to identify and punish the perpetrator. Although this model is valid, it is not sufficient if we are to end abuse.

Evidence indicates that the maltreatment of a child is a complex and multifactoral event, not so much a discrete occurrence as a reflection of an underlying pathologic condition in the family ecology. Child abuse must be viewed as the result of a preexisting situation. If a patient is hospitalized to treat diabetic shock, the doctor does not simply recalibrate the blood sugar and send the patient home; instead, the underlying condition is diagnosed and the patient is counseled regarding its management. Similarly, child abuse must not simply be seen as an injury, but as one issue in a constellation of causes and effects.

For example, it is clear that the abusive event we see is often not the first the child has suffered. It is recommended, for example, that infants and young children with a recognized abusive skeletal injury undergo a thorough radiologic skeletal examination. This well-accepted practice arose because studies show a significant incidence of other unapparent injuries, many of which have already begun healing.[9] Researchers who study children hospitalized for abusive head trauma find that many have experienced an earlier head injury.[10] As to sexual abuse, it is seldom the case that the first incident reported is the first suffered. The vast majority of child sexual and physical abuse is committed by someone known to the child, often in the household,[4] and is not reported until the child feels safe in doing so, months or years later, if ever.[11] Although physicians can hope to be fortunate enough to detect the child's first abusive injury, this is often difficult.

As damaging as physical and sexual abuse are, researchers and clinicians agree that the worst long-term injury to a child's development can result from early emotional abuse and neglect. Sadly, neglect is the most pervasive form of child maltreatment. In 2004, 60% of all reports to CPS nationwide involved neglect. This is 3 times as many reports as for physical abuse and 6 times the number of sexual abuse reports.[4] Neglected children suffer the highest rates of posttraumatic stress disorder (PTSD), depression, and lack of social success, and emotional abuse is a stronger predictor of later psychopathologic conditions than either physical or sexual maltreatment.[12-15] Early emotional and psychological abuse are destructive because they are ongoing, corrosive processes that act to deprive the child of the very tools he or she needs to survive. A discrete episode of physical or sexual victimization might well be considered emotionally traumatic. If that episode existed in isolation, the child's environmental supports and emotional strengths might be expected to promote healing and recovery. In a pervasive atmosphere of neglect and emotional abuse, however, the child is denied the opportunity to develop self-confidence and the ability to regulate his or her emotional responses.[16] Such children often fail to attach securely to adult figures and lack the ability to seek out other sources of support.[17,18] Sadly, these deficiencies often make neglected or emotionally abused children hard to parent or to teach, as unregulated emotion and distrust manifest as explosive responses to authority.[19] Such behaviors, of course, often prompt harsher treatment at home and can increase the child's chances of further victimization.

The resultant feedback cycle can lead to lifelong challenges. Research has demonstrated that physical or sexual abuse and emotional/psychological maltreatment can alter a child's developmental trajectory and correlate with a variety of maladaptive behaviors, self-injurious practices, and even chronic health complaints in adult life. The Adverse Childhood Experiences Study (ACES) results have demonstrated robust correlation between childhood trauma and a host of adverse outcomes ranging from depression and drug abuse to obesity, diabetes, heart disease, and other conditions usually regarded as purely medical conditions.[20]

Indeed, research has shown that it is misleading to speak of physical abuse, sexual abuse, and neglect as if they were separate and discrete clinical entities. In practice, clinicians find that victims of one type of abuse frequently suffer from others.[21,22] Sexual abuse victims are often physically abused as well, and vice versa. Emotional abuse appears as concomitant to, and possibly a precursor of, both forms of injury.[23]

Nor do the various forms of child abuse coexist only with one another. It has become apparent that the abuse of children often occurs against the background of abusive relationships within the family. Though violence against intimate partners is often thought of as an adult problem, there is little debate that children are frequently affected—often severely. It is estimated that between 3.3 and 10 million children witness domestic violence each year.[24,25] Many are injured physically as bystanders to the parental discord, whereas others are assaulted directly. Child sexual abuse and parental intimate partner violence can also occur in the same household. In one recent study of sexually abused children, 58% of the in-home abusers were found to have also physically assaulted their domestic partners, in addition to sexually assaulting the children.[26] Whether or not the children are directly assaulted, most bear some scars from the acute and chronic stresses of violent interactions between the dominant figures in their lives. Long-term consequences of early exposure to parental violence are many and varied, including depression, anxiety, PTSD, self-destructive and risky behavior, and a greater predisposition to enter violent domestic relationships in the future.[27-31] Indeed, violence between parents is one of the adverse experiences studied by the ACES researchers mentioned earlier.[20-22] Research has shown very little difference between the long-term psychological consequences suffered by children who witness domestic violence and the consequences for those who are directly abused physically or sexually.[23]

Again, it is perhaps inaccurate to think of child abuse and intimate partner violence as distinct problems, occurring separately. Figures obtained from CPS reports and from domestic violence researchers show a remarkable overlap of violence against intimate partners with that against children. Researchers report that between 40% and 50% of batterers are physically abusive to their children.[26,32,33] Research on violence against seniors, not surprisingly, confirms that elders are also frequently abused, taken in the context of violence against other family members of all ages.[34,35] Even the family pet is not spared from this culture of family dysfunction.[36] It is a culture characterized by dominance in relationships and by violence as a response to challenge.

Though it is common to speak of child abuse as an "epidemic," an occasion of abuse is not so much analogous to a disease as to a symptom, in this case of an underlying need for change. The abuse of a child does not happen in a vacuum. It is not a discrete, one-time event, but rather what quality improvement experts refer to as a "signal event," an occurrence that signals a need for change; in this case, a change in the child's environment. Sometimes this change takes the form of dramatic action, as when a child victim is removed from the abusive home and placed in a shelter or when the perpetrator is convicted and sent to prison. Often, however, the putative abuse or neglect cannot be charged as criminal or proven in court, and the child remains in the home. In these cases, attempts should be made to reconcile the family and to provide resources as needed to improve the child's chances of a successful future. These attempts are only hindered by the perspective that defines abuse solely as a criminal event.

In a reconsideration of the approach to child abuse, then, in terms of seeking partners and especially in working toward its prevention, professionals would do well to remember that distinctions among types of abuse, and even of child abuse as distinct from intimate partner and other forms of family violence, are in some respects artificial. Though no doubt useful in some ways, such distinctions ultimately keep us from realizing the underlying problem: the child has lived in an environment in which domination and violence have become a way of life. It is a toxic lifestyle in which damage of many types may occur unless proper resources are brought to bear.

Among professional communities, the view of child abuse as a discrete act can lead to fragmentation of our responses and failure to capitalize on our awareness of its true dimensions. These divisions cannot help but impair our ability to prevent future abuse. In seeking to prevent child abuse, children's advocates must learn to work hand in hand with domestic violence advocates. Both must build bridges to the drug and alcohol abuse communities and to mental health providers, to address factors known to destabilize the child's environment.

A misunderstanding of child abuse as a discrete event leads to its being conceptually framed as a criminal act. When the public at large shares this overly simple frame, the result is at best a lack of support for many community-based efforts at child protection; at worst, a backlash in which the public actively opposes those efforts.

REFRAME 2. DETECTION AND PROSECUTION: SOMEBODY ELSE'S PROBLEM

When child abuse is viewed primarily as a criminal act, it becomes easy to forget that it is so much more. Certainly, the simpler frame has much to recommend it: it is easier to understand child abuse as a crime perpetrated by criminals. For most crimes, society's answer is effective apprehension, conviction, and incarceration. The other consideration that makes this view so attractive is that child abuse, when viewed as a single, criminal act, becomes a problem to be solved by agents of CPS and law enforcement.

As many acts of child maltreatment are in fact criminal, this can be an appropriate response, if a partial one. As mentioned earlier, the recent, well-documented decreases in child abuse are felt, at least in part, to be due to an increasingly effective response by the criminal justice system. The problems with this simplistic perspective arise in 2 areas: many cases cannot be addressed effectively by the justice system and increasing difficulties are being encountered in recruiting community support.

Because child maltreatment occurs across a spectrum of severity, many if not most cases will fail to meet standards for criminal prosecution or foster home placement. Misdemeanor cases of physical abuse, sexual assault between underage peers, and abuse of children too young to be good historians, for example, may not pass the threshold for criminal prosecution or civil adjudication. Many cases of neglectful behavior do not imperil the child enough to require foster placement, though they may raise concerns for future safety.

Traditionally, CPS has been charged with providing social services to compromised families, but in recent years greater pressure has been placed on CPS to act more as agents of public safety and less as service brokers. Increasingly, caseworkers serve as investigators who use risk assessment tools according to statewide protocols. Their assessments are subject to ever more careful scrutiny by the media, by other professionals on multidisciplinary teams, and by the courts.[37] Although a high degree of certainty is no doubt desirable, there is danger of raising the bar too high; for example, situations involving needy families can be dismissed as "unsubstantiated" and the family is left without services that might have prevented further abuse or neglect.

Reframing child abuse requires us to view it as the presenting symptom of a more pervasive and destructive condition. These situations in which children "slip through the cracks" can be seen not only as symbolic of failed justice, but also as missed opportunities for preventing future abuse or even fatalities.

The regrettable tendency to see child maltreatment as somebody else's problem exists even among those who work in the various fields involved in child protection, as tightly circumscribed zones of professional responsibility can allow blame for failures to be easily shifted elsewhere. When a case cannot be charged, it leaves the jurisdiction of law enforcement. If abuse occurs outside of the family unit, it is not a legitimate concern of CPS. Even medical providers, who, of all the professionals involved, should hold a global concern for the child's welfare, admit to being uncomfortable with initiating the reporting process and find it difficult to maintain medical contact with the family during the investigation.[38,39] Here again, the clear-cut jurisdictional divisions of responsibility encourage a "silo" mentality. Each group can pass responsibility for dealing with abuse to others, and children may easily fall between jurisdictions. When child maltreatment is allowed to be somebody else's problem, it can easily become nobody's.

If we see abuse only as a criminal act, it follows that acts that are not legally criminal are not, therefore, "real" abuse, even though minor offenses are often precursors to severe or even life-threatening assaults. The simplistic view of child abuse as a criminal act also serves to divide the child protection and domestic violence communities, communities with a great deal of common ground. Recognition of those common interests can be easily lost in arguments over a battered mother's culpability in a child's abuse or neglect, where attention should instead be focused on the child's best likelihood of future safety. Similarly, if we persist in seeing physical abuse as unrelated to sexual abuse or as distinct from neglect, then we will have divided ourselves into camps that may fail to cooperate in addressing the causative factors common to all three.

The criminal frame can also compromise public involvement in protecting children. A vast and successful effort has been undertaken to raise public awareness of maltreatment as a crime against children. Prior to the "rediscovery" of child abuse following medical descriptions of battered child syndrome and shaken/impact syndrome[40-42] in the 1960s and the unmasking of sexual abuse in the decades following,[43] child abuse was widely thought to be a rare phenomenon. The prevalence of both physical and sexual child abuse can now be much more accurately estimated, with as many as 1 child in 12 suffering some form of sexual victimization, and homicide recognized as a major cause of death in early childhood in the United States.[44,45] Major campaigns have been undertaken to inform the public of the dangers, ranging from public service announcements to talk-show appearances to the now-ubiquitous milk cartons depicting missing children. Surveys have shown the public to be increasingly aware of abuse, concerned about its consequences, and concerned that child abuse is widespread.[46]

The consequences of this awareness have been both good and bad. On the positive side, there has been an outpouring of public support for the agencies tasked with fighting this war against child abuse, from the national to the local level. In 1974, Congress passed the Child Abuse Prevention and Treatment Act (CAPTA), which provides states with monetary grants, as long as they have complied with requirements for reporting and responding to suspected abuse. CAPTA has been amended and regularly reauthorized ever since by Congresses eager to show support for ending these crimes. In fiscal year 2008, according to Prevent Child Abuse America, community-based child abuse programs were funded at $41.6 million and CAPTA state grants provided $26.5 million to improve CPS. Prevention programs received $63.3 million through the so-called Promoting Safe and Stable Families (PSSF) discretionary grant. The actual funding for all programs was well below authorized amounts.[47] Though these amounts are relatively small, the federal grants have encouraged all 50 states to change their laws to conform to the act's standards on the reporting and investigation of abuse.[48]

On a regional and local level, the past two decades have seen the widespread promulgation of CACs, most supported by a combination of private and governmental funds. The National Children's Alliance, accrediting body for CACs, lists more than 500 member organizations.[49] These centers bring the various professionals together so as to minimize the trauma to the child occasioned by repeated forensic interviews during the investigation, while improving the chances of successful prosecution by encouraging information flow among the agencies involved. When intake criteria are broad and case management is thorough and comprehensive, the CAC approach helps to narrow the jurisdictional "cracks" and keep child victims from falling through. Unfortunately, even team efforts can fall short of these ideals. CACs often maintain a prosecutorial bias, in that they are funded and/or managed by local prosecutors' offices or even law enforcement. For many, children cannot be considered for services unless referred by law enforcement agencies or protective services. Children whose cases do not meet the criteria for prosecution or foster placement are often left with few alternatives.

Despite significant positive outcomes from this outpouring of support, the negative consequences of the dominant criminal perspective are significant. Though public service agencies have been unquestionably successful in protecting children and prosecuting their abusers, they will occasionally fail. It is often these failures that make news, and news shapes the public's reference frame on the issue. An analysis of print and electronic media depictions of child abuse by Cultural Logic in 2003 described dominant frames in widespread use. The first was the depiction of child abuse as a "horrible, criminal atrocity some monstrous parent has committed," as well as the portrayal of "the horrible suffering of the child(ren) in question."[5] This framing of abuse as a criminal event focuses the responsibility for the abuse on the parents (or on a dangerous stranger), and the responsibility for stopping it falls to agencies that apprehend criminals. The logical role for the community, in this frame, would be to support those agencies.

Unfortunately, the second common news frame is to depict the failures of those very agencies. A child who dies in foster care necessarily will receive more media attention than one who thrives, but such stories do little to raise public confidence. Rather, they resonate with the deeply held belief that the government cannot effectively protect anyone. The public comes to see the problem of child maltreatment as one without a solution. Without a solution, they cannot move from widespread awareness to engagement and policy support. Instead, they may become frightened and turn away. This sense of futility, especially when coupled with the perception of strangers as dangerous, can lead to widespread distrust, and it erodes confidence in the community as a source of help for families in need.

This erosion of confidence strengthens the belief in what public policy analysts call the "family bubble," in reference to the deeply held belief that the birth family is the sole agency responsible for childrearing, and that the community's interventions cannot be trusted.[50] Unfortunately, this hands-off philosophy coexists with an increasing conviction that the family's failure is to blame for the abuse in the first place. The community is asked to both trust the family and blame it for its failure. The family in turn is told that strangers are not trustworthy and that to turn to the community for help is to fail as a parent. The resulting impasse further reinforces the perception that the problem of child maltreatment is a problem without a solution. The more the public perceives the problem as insoluble, the more difficult it becomes for community agencies to gain support.

This rejection of the community becomes more tragic as research continues to show the power of a strong community in preventing abuse and minimizing its consequences for families and victims. Both physical and sexual abuses of children are associated with community factors such as parental employment, socioeconomic status, and social support for good parenting. Abuse also correlates with social isolation and a poor understanding of child development, a dangerous combination.[51] The degree to which a child is involved in personal social relationships within family and community directly relates to increased resilience in the face of stresses and to better long-term outcomes.[51-54] The most promising interventions for prevention of child abuse are multifaceted and community-based, bringing the resources of the community to address the various needs of populations at risk. Home-visiting programs have been shown to reduce risk factors for abuse,[55] and coordinated social service interventions can reduce neglect.[56] Even programs directed specifically against physical abuse (eg, Abusive Head Trauma) are most effective when undertaken in community hospitals.[57]

Though the community offers the best hope of improving outcomes for families, framing abuse as a discrete, criminal act has consequences that separate the two. A more inclusive frame is needed. A view that emphasizes the dangers of neglect and the continuum of violence, and that recognizes the value of involvement with others, would help focus attention on successful interventions and build confidence in the community's ability to successfully intervene. With this awareness, community members may also come to recognize their own responsibility in dealing with the problem of child maltreatment.

REFRAME 3. THERAPY: PSYCHOLOGY VERSUS PHYSIOLOGY

As the community is responsible for the prevention of abuse, it must also respond to the long-term consequences to victims of maltreatment. Here again, currently dominant frames tend to fragment this response.

In the early 20th century, the work of Freud, Jung, and other practitioners introduced the field of psychoanalysis. Trained as neurologists, these pioneers described abnormal behavior systematically, inventing a rich lexicon of metaphor to describe, in decidedly nonphysiologic terms, the working of the mind. In what became known as psychotherapy, they utilized these metaphors in an attempt to understand and correct maladaptive behaviors. "Neuroses" and "psychoses" were the product of abnormal but ultimately predictable reactions of the "conscious" and "unconscious minds" to stress. Over the ensuing decades, nonphysiologic terms such as "ego," "superego," "libido," and "id" took on lives of their own, as they more or less effectively described functioning systems of behavior. Eventually, their metaphorical nature was, for all practical purposes, forgotten. Though these terms clearly did not refer to parts of the brain, they were known to be part of the mind.

By the end of the 20th century, scientific and technological advances had turned the focus of psychiatrists' attention back to neurology, and specifically to the neurophysiology of the brain itself. Computed tomographic scanning with X-rays or magnetic resonance imaging (MRI) enabled scientists and clinicians to visualize areas of damage or unusual growth in living patients. More recent refinements in positron emission tomography and "functional" MRI scanning allow accurate portrayal of the brain's metabolic activity, so observers can better understand which brain areas are involved with particular human thoughts and feelings. New computer analysis techniques extract more useful information from electroencephalographic tracings. At the same time, refinements in materials and microneurosurgical techniques have allowed ever more sophisticated research in animal models, measuring responses down to the level of the individual neuron.

This flowering of information has changed our perception of both the brain and of the mind. Several axioms of the "new" neurobiology are directly relevant to our response to child abuse, as summarized hereafter.

THE BRAIN IS NOT MATURE AT BIRTH

A newborn human's brain gives little indication of the remarkable problem-solving device it will become. Despite rapid growth in the last trimester of pregnancy, the baby's cortex is simple compared to the adult's, with fewer neurons and synaptic connections, the cells packed together without the insulating myelin sheaths that enhance impulse transmission. This immature state makes for a smaller head at birth, reducing somewhat the potential trauma of vaginal delivery. It also guarantees that subsequent growth will be, at least in part, determined by the postnatal environment.

EXPERIENCE DETERMINES THE BRAIN'S ARCHITECTURE

Over the next several months, given proper nutrition and stimulation, the number of nerve cells and the connections among them increase exponentially, with the number of synaptic connections peaking in childhood. Growth of the neural architecture is guided by the stimulation the brain receives from the sense organs of the child's body. Stimulated areas show increased growth of both neurons and their supporting structures and blood supply.[58,59]

The converse is also true: cells that are not used are "pruned" in a process called apoptosis. Beginning in earnest around age 4, this pruning allows the brain to concentrate its efforts where they are most useful, saving energy and enhancing the processing speed of the cortical net.[60] While the brain of the young child, with its plethora of cells and synapses, can be said to be optimized for learning, the older brain becomes faster at using what it has learned.

TIMING CAN BE IMPORTANT

This process of growth and the subsequent pruning is time-dependent, with different areas of the brain reaching their peak connectivity at different times. The auditory and visual cortices, for example, peak in early infancy, at 3 to 4 months of age, whereas the speech centers in the angular gyrus and Broca's area of the temporal lobe, which depend on vision and hearing, have formed most of their synapses by 8 or 9 months. Higher cognitive centers in the prefrontal cortex reach their highest potential at 3 years of age and are gradually pruned over the next decade.[61]

In the sensory cortex, at least, it appears that deficits can result when brain areas do not receive stimulation within the allotted time.[62] Irreversible visual defects, for example, are seen if a child with congenital visual impairment from severe congenital cataracts or strabismus does not receive treatment in the first few years of life.

RELATIONSHIPS ARE CRITICAL TO DEVELOPMENT

The degree to which such sensitive periods play a role in higher cortical function is unknown, but social deprivation in early childhood can certainly result in serious defects in emotional self-regulation and other skills necessary to social functioning, defects that may be remarkably robust.[17,63,64] The ability to control one's strong emotions and to trust other humans are vital skills that provide the child with the security to explore the world and thus are a prerequisite to further intellectual growth. In studies conducted on children reared in Romanian orphanages, victims of severe neglect demonstrate difficulties with emotional outbursts and anxiety and marked difficulties forming normal relationships, even after being removed from their socially impoverished environments.[17]

Secure, nurturing, and predictable early relationships may encourage healthy development on a cellular level by properly stimulating cortical circuits that researchers have termed "mirror neurons."[65-67] Social visual inputs (as of another person performing an action) trigger neural responses in the same motor areas the viewer would use to perform the same action. These resonant responses would be useful in learning, especially in terms of the social and emotional learning so important in infancy and early childhood.[68]

ADVERSE EXPERIENCES ALTER BRAIN PHYSIOLOGY

Our ability to observe the functioning brain in situ and to study function at the level of the single neuron has allowed us to catalog a variety of changes to the brain's structure and function following early abuse or neglect. Some are anatomic: patients with symptoms of PTSD have been shown to have smaller limbic structures, with smaller and less sensitive amygdalae and hippocampi.[69-71] Decreased size and complexity have been noted in the corpus callosum after childhood neglect.[72]

Other changes are functional: alterations have been described after abuse in the metabolism of the cerebellar vermis, a major site of neurotransmitter manufacture.[73] Electroencephalographic analyses show a reversal of the normal left-brain dominance pattern in PTSD sufferers.[74] Behavioral problems in severely neglected orphans correlate with marked impairment of brain metabolic activity when the orphans' functional MRI scans are compared with those of normally raised peers.[75,76]

Still other sequelae of early abuse and neglect involve the endocrine function of the brain's stress hormones. Children who have suffered abuse demonstrate different baseline levels and diurnal variation in levels of cortisol, the hormone responsible for coordinating the body's stress response.[77,78] Accentuated hormonal reactions to stressful stimuli have been measured in abused infants,[77] adolescents,[79] and in adult victims of childhood abuse suffering from PTSD.[80]

While it is true enough, then, that early abuse or neglect affects a child's behavior, there is a middle step: abuse alters physiology, which in turn results in misbehavior. Abuse and neglect result in dramatic chemical responses in the brain, which in turn heighten the child's perception of, and response to, threat. Attending to a myriad of perceived threats can adversely affect learning, when this increased threat response drives disruptive behaviors such as explosive outbursts, or alternatively, causes withdrawal. Such abnormal activation of the brain's threat responses might best be regarded as a normal response to an abnormal environment. A successful adaptation to an abusive home environment may not work in the classroom or foster home.

This physiologic frame is easier to understand than the more abstract concept of "psychological damage." Public relations researchers have found that parents find the physiologic model more compelling than the psychological. Concrete ideas, such as the image of lasting damage to the brain's systems, are taken more seriously than more subjective concepts of bad behavior or character.[81] Rather than focusing on subjective, mental experiences like defiance or willfulness, the new model emphasizes tangible, physiological processes (unusual hormonal responses, neuronal damage). It is easier for the parent or layperson to understand an altered hormonal response to stress, than, for example, "oppositional-defiant disorder."

When maladaptive behavior is seen as the consequence of misdirected physiologic adaptation, it can be treated as a physical incapacity rather than as a character failing. In the middle of the 20th century, understanding of alcohol dependence as a disease rather than a character flaw led to a more rational approach to intervention and treatment. In much the same way, when an abused child's misbehavior is seen to arise from a disordered physiology, the child's actions are removed from the "black box" of psychology. While the child may still require mental health services, the process becomes less mysterious and proprietary.

Concentrating on altered physiology suggests more constructive responses, both for the caregivers and for the child. Foster parents and teachers can be made to understand that the child's heightened response to threats demands a less emotional, more measured response to a transgression than would a normal child's. The child victim can be brought to see the value of learning to control inappropriate alarm, to recognize the abnormal response before acting. Modern mental health interventions, such as trauma-focused cognitive behavioral therapy and dialectic-based therapy, acknowledge the physiologic underpinnings of the client's maladaptive behaviors and attempt to help the client to gain cognitive control over the anxiety and intrusive emotions that are the product of runaway physiology.[82-85] Others, recognizing the primary value of relationships in healthy brain growth, seek to aid in healing by guiding parents in changing their responses to the child.[86] The National Child Traumatic Stress Network, founded in 2000, seeks to bring mental health workers together and disseminate new, evidence-based therapies that derive from an awareness of early trauma's impact.[87,88] Our new appreciation of the brain's response to childhood trauma allows for a more focused, more accessible approach to therapy.

CONCLUSION

Our efforts in recent years to combat the abuse of our children have been very successful, but that very success threatens to keep us from moving to the next level. It has been easy to "sell" the concept of child abuse as a discrete, criminal act that results in psychological damage to its victims. The public has adopted this dominant frame; unfortunately, so have many professionals involved in child welfare. The concept is simple, and it hands off most of the responsibility to government agencies. The problem, however, is that child abuse is almost never a discrete event. It instead is a symptom of family and community dysfunction that characterizes the child's entire life. While often a criminal event, abuse is almost never that alone. Our current dominant frame assigns responsibility for intervening in child maltreatment to the criminal justice system and blame it when it fails, while minimizing the demonstrated value of family and community involvement. Damage from abuse, in the meantime, is regarded as psychological, rendering it abstract and inaccessible to the child's caregivers.

Broader framing, although challenging to implement, better reflects the reality of the problem and can hold the promise of a more effective response and better prevention. When an episode of abuse or neglect is recognized as a sign of ongoing family dysfunction, the entire community is more likely to take responsibility and less likely to lose sight of the child in the process. When the damage done by maltreatment is seen for the physiologic insult that it is, therapists and caregivers will find it easier to respond effectively.

The beauty of reframing is that it requires no new discovery, no technological breakthrough. It just asks a willingness to see things in a more realistic light, to be able to change perspective, and to put into practice what we already know.

REFERENCES

1. Jones LM, Finkelhor D, Kopiec K. Why is sexual abuse declining? A survey of state child protection administrators. *Child Abuse Negl.* 2001;25:1139-1158.

2. Jones LM, Finkelhor D. Putting together evidence on declining trends in sexual abuse: a complex puzzle. *Child Abuse Negl.* 2003;27:133-135.

3. Jones LM, Finkelhor D. Why have child maltreatment and child victimization declined? *J Soc Issues.* 2006;62:685-716.

4. US Department of Health and Human Services, Administration for Children and Families, Children's Bureau. *Child maltreatment 2004: Reports from the states to the National Child Abuse and Neglect Data System*; 2004. Available from: www.acf.hhs.gov/programs/cb/pubs/cm04.htm.

5. Conte JR. Child sexual abuse: awareness and backlash. *Future Child.* 1994;4:224-232.

6. Aubrun A, Grady J, Cultural Logic. How the news frames child maltreatment: unintended consequences [Prevent Child Abuse America Web site]. August 22, 2003. Available at: http://www.preventchildabuse.org/about_us/reframing/downloads/analysis.pdf. Accessed February 25, 2009.

7. Sadler BL, Chadwick DL, Hensler DJ. The summary chapter—the national call to action: moving ahead. *Child Abuse Negl.* 1999;23:1011-1018.

8. FrameWorks Institute, Bales SN. Making the public case for child abuse and neglect prevention: A FrameWorks message memo [Prevent Child Abuse America Web site]. April 2004. Available at: http://www.preventchildabuse.org/about_us/reframing/downloads/memo.pdf. Accessed February 25, 2009.

9. Kleinman PK, Blackbourne BD, Marks SC, Karellas A, Belanger PL. Radiologic contributions to the investigation and prosecution of cases of fatal infant abuse. *N Engl J Med.* 1989;320:507-511.

10. Jenny C, Hymel KP, Ritzen A, Reinert SE, Hay TC. Analysis of missed cases of abusive head trauma [published correction appears in JAMA. 1999 Jul 7;282(1):29]. *JAMA*. 1999;281:621-626.

11. Lanning KV. Criminal investigation of suspected child abuse: Section I: Criminal investigation of sexual victimization of children. In: Briere J, Berliner L, Bulkley JA, Jenny C, Reid T, eds. *The APSAC Handbook on Child Maltreatment*. Thousand Oaks, Calif: Sage Publications; 1996:247-263.

12. Rossman B. Longer term effects of children's exposure to domestic violence. In: Graham-Bermann SA, Edleson J, eds. *Domestic Violence in the Lives of Children: The Future of Research, Intervention, and Social Policy*. Washington, DC: American Psychological Association Books; 2001:35-65.

13. Mirescu C, Gould E. Stress and adult neurogenesis. *Hippocampus*. 2006;16:233-238.

14. Shonkoff J, Phillips D, eds. *From neurons to neighborhoods: The science of early childhood development*. Washington, DC: National Academies Press; 2000.

15. Wodarski J, Kurtz PD, Gaudin JM Jr, Howing PT. Maltreatment and the school-age child: major academic, socioemotional, and adaptive outcomes. *Soc Work*. 1990;35:501-513.

16. Siegel DJ. *The developing mind: toward a neurobiology of interpersonal experience*. New York: The Guilford Press; 1999.

17. Chaffin M, Hanson R, Saunders BE, Nichols T, Barnett D, Zeanah C, et al. Report of the APSAC task force on attachment therapy, reactive attachment disorder, and attachment problems. *Child Maltreat*. 2006;11:76-89.

18. Kobak R, Cassidy J, Lyons-Ruth K, Ziv Y. Attachment, stress, and psychopathology: A developmental pathways model. In: Cicchetti D, Cohen D, eds. *Developmental psychopathology. Volume 1: theory and method*. 2nd ed. New York: Jan Wiley & Sons; 2006:330-369.

19. Lieberman A, Amaya-Jackson L. Reciprocal influences of attachment and trauma: using a dual lens in the assessment and treatment of infants, toddlers, and preschoolers. In: Berlin LJ, Ziv Y, Amaya-Jackson L, Greenberg MT, eds. *Enhancing early attachments: theory, research, intervention, and policy*. New York: Guilford Press; 2005:100-124.

20. Felitti VJ, Anda RF, Nordenberg D, Williamson DF, Spitz AM, Edwards V, et al. Relationship of childhood abuse and household dysfunction to many of the leading causes of death in adults. The Adverse Childhood Experiences (ACE) Study. *Am J Prev Med*. 1998;14:245-258.

21. Edwards VJ, Holden GW, Felitti VJ, Anda RF. Relationship between multiple forms of childhood maltreatment and adult mental health in community respondents: results from the adverse childhood experiences study. *Am J Psychiatry*. 2003;160:1453-1460.

22. Dong M, Anda RF, Felitti VJ, Dube SR, Williamson DF, Thompson TJ, et al. The interrelatedness of multiple forms of childhood abuse, neglect, and household dysfunction. *Child Abuse Negl*. 2004;28:771-784.

23. Teicher MH, Samson JA, Polcari A, McGreenery CE. Sticks, stones, and hurtful words: relative effects of various forms of childhood maltreatment. *Am J Psychiatry*. 2006;163:993-1000.

24. Fantuzzo JW, Mohr WK. Prevalence and effects of child exposure to domestic violence. *Future Child*. 1999;9:21-32.

25. Lawrence S; National Center for Children in Poverty Domestic Violence and Welfare Policy: *Research Findings That Can Inform Policies on Marriage and Child Well-Being*. http://www.researchforum.org/media/DomVio.pdf. Published December 2002. Accessed November 16, 2009.

26. Kellogg ND, Menard SW. Violence among family members of children and adolescents evaluated for sexual abuse. *Child Abuse Negl*. 2003;27:1367-1376.

27. Ehrensaft MK, Cohen P, Brown J, Smailes E, Chen H, Johnson JG. Intergenerational transmission of partner violence: a 20-year prospective study. *J Consult Clin Psychol*. 2003;71:741-753.

28. Bensley L, Van Eenwyk J, Wynkoop Simmons K. Childhood family violence history and women's risk for intimate partner violence and poor health. *Am J Prev Med*. 2003;25:38-44.

29. Yates TM, Dodds MF, Sroufe LA, Egeland B. Exposure to partner violence and child behavior problems: a prospective study controlling for child physical abuse and neglect, child cognitive ability, socioeconomic status, and life stress. *Dev Psychopathol*. 2003;15:199-218.

30. Griffing S, Lewis CS, Chu M, Sage RE, Madry L, Primm BJ. Exposure to interpersonal violence as a predictor of PTSD symptomatology in domestic violence survivors. *J Interpers Violence*. 2006;21:936-954.

31. Bancroft L, Silverman JG. *The batterer as parent: addressing the impact of domestic violence on family dynamics*. Sage series on violence against women. ed. C.M. Renzetti and J.L. Edleson. Thousand Oaks, CA: Sage; 2002.

32. Suh E, Abel EM. The impact of spousal violence on the children of the abused. *J Indep Social Work*. 1990;4:27-34.

33. Straus MA. The national family violence survey In: M. Strauss and R. Gelles, eds. *Physical violence in American families: risk factors and adaptations to violence in 8,145 families* (pp. 3-16). ed. Transaction Publishers: New Brunswick, NJ; 1990.

34. Salib E, Appleton T, Pembleton A. Elder abuse and elderly abusers. *Med Sci Law*. 2002;42:147-148.

35. Rudolph MN, Hughes DH. Emergency assessments of domestic violence, sexual dangerousness, and elder and child abuse. *Psychiatr Serv*. 2001;52:281-282, 306.

36. Arluke A, Levin J, Luke C, Ascione F. The relationship of animal abuse to violence and other forms of antisocial behavior. *Interpersonal Violence*. 1999;14:963-975

37. Weber MW. The assessment of child abuse: a primary function of child protective services. In: Helfer ME, Kempe RS, Krugman RD, eds. *The Battered Child*. Chicago: University of Chicago Press; 1997:120-149

38. Trowbridge MJ, Sege RD, Olson L, O'Connor K, Flaherty E, Spivak H. Intentional injury management and prevention in pediatric practice: results from 1998 and 2003 American Academy of Pediatrics Periodic Surveys. *Pediatrics*. 2005;116:996-1000.

39. Flaherty EG, Sege R. Barriers to physician identification and reporting of child abuse. *Pediatr Ann*. 2005;34:349-356.

40. Kempe CH, Silverman FN, Steele BF, Droegemueller W, Silver HK. The battered-child syndrome. *JAMA*. 1962 Jul7;181:17-24.

41. Guthkelch AN. Infantile subdural haematoma and its relationship to whiplash injuries. *Br Med J*. 1971;2:430-431.

42. Caffey J. The whiplash shaken infant syndrome: manual shaking by the extremities with whiplash-induced intracranial and intraocular bleedings, linked with residual permanent brain damage and mental retardation. *Pediatrics*. 1974;54:396-403.

43. Kempe CH. Sexual abuse, another hidden pediatric problem: the 1977 C. Anderson Aldrich lecture. *Pediatrics*. 1978;62:382-389.

44. Wiese, D. and Daro, D. (2005) *Current Trends in Child Abuse Reporting and Fatalities: The Results of the 2004 Annual Fifty State Survey*. Chicago: National Committee to Prevent Child Abuse: Chicago.

45. Finkelhor D, Ormrod R, Turner H, Hamby SL. The victimization of children and youth: a comprehensive, national survey. [published correction appears in *Child Maltreat*. 2005;10(2):207]. *Child Maltreat*. 2005;10:5-25.

46. Bostrom M, Public Knowledge. Discipline and development: a meta-analysis of public perceptions of parents, parenting, child development and child abuse [FrameWorks Institute Web site]. May 2003. Available at: http://www.frameworks institute.org/assets/files/PDF/pca_americameta.pdf. Accessed February 26, 2009.

47. Prevent Child Abuse America http://www.preventchildabuse.org/advocacy/legislative_priorities.shtml. Accessed November 16, 2009.

48. U.S. Administration for Children and Families. Progress report to Congress: federal child welfare programs. 2006. Available from: http://www.acf.hhs.gov/programs/cb/pubs/cwo05/. Accessed October 25, 2009.

49. National Children's Alliance Web site. Available at: http://www.nationalchild rensalliance.org/index.php?s=6. Accessed October 25, 2009.

50. Aubrun A, Grady J, Cultural Logic. Two cognitive obstacles to preventing child abuse: the "other-mind" mistake and the "family bubble" [Prevent Child Abuse America Web site]. August 4, 2003. Available at: http://www.preventchildabuse.org/about_us/reframing/downloads/interviews.pdf. Accessed February 26, 2009.

51. Donnelly AC. An overview of prevention of physical abuse and neglect In: Helfer ME, Kempe RS, Krugman RD, eds. *The Battered Child*. Chicago: University of Chicago Press; 1997:579-593

52. Zolotor AJ, Runyan DK. Social capital, family violence, and neglect. *Pediatrics*. 2006;117:e1124-1131.

53. Runyan DK, Hunter WM, Socolar RR, Amaya-Jackson L, English D, Landsverk J, et al. Children who prosper in unfavorable environments: the relationship to social capital. *Pediatrics*. 1998;101(1 Pt 1):12-18.

54. Resnick MD, Ireland M, Borowsky I. Youth violence perpetration: What protects? What predicts? Findings from the National Longitudinal Study of Adolescent Health. *J Adolesc Health*. 2004;35:424, e1-10.

55. Olds DL, Kitzman H, Cole R, Robinson J, Sidora K, Luckey DW, et al. Effects of nurse home-visiting on maternal life course and child development: age 6 follow-up results of a randomized trial. *Pediatrics.* 2004;114:1550-1559.

56. DePanfilis D, Dubowitz H. Family connections: a program for preventing child neglect. *Child Maltreat.* 2005;10:108-123.

57. Dias MS, Smith K, DeGuehery K, Mazur P, Li V, Shaffer ML. Preventing abusive head trauma among infants and young children: a hospital-based, parent education program. *Pediatrics.* 2005;115:e470-477.

58. Black J, Isaacs KR, Anderson BJ, Alcantara AA, Greenough WT. Learning causes synaptogenesis, while motor activity causes angiogenesis, in cerebellar cortex of adult rats. *Proc Natl Acad Sci USA.* 1990;87:5568-5572.

59. Isaacs KR, Anderson BJ, Alcantara AA, Black JE, Greenough WT. Exercise and the brain: angiogenesis in the adult rat cerebellum after vigorous physical activity and motor skill learning [published correction appears in *J Cereb Blood Flow Metab.* 1992 May;12(3):533]. *J Cereb Blood Flow Metab.* 1992;12:110-119.

60. Greenough WT, Black JE. Induction of brain structure by experience: substrates for cognitive development. In: Gunnar MR, Nelson CA, eds. *Developmental Behavior Neuroscience: The Minnesota Symposia on Child Psychology.* Hillsdale, NJ: Lawrence Erlbaum Associates; 1992:155-200.

61. Huttenlocher P, Dabholkar A. Regional differences in synaptogenesis in human cerebral cortex. *Journal Comp Neurol.* 1997;387:167-178.

62. LeVay S, Wiesel TN, Hubel DH. The development of ocular dominance columns in normal and visually deprived monkeys. *J Comp Neurol.* 1980;191:1-51.

63. Beeghley M, Cicchetti D. Child maltreatment, attachment, and the self system: Emergence of an internal state in toddlers at high social risk. In: Hertzig M, Farber E, eds. *Annual progress in child psychiatry and child development.* Philadelphia: Brunner/Mazel; 1996:127-166.

64. Sameroff AJ, Fiese BH. Transactional regulation: The developmental ecology of early intervention. In: Shonkoff J, Meisels SJ, eds. *Handbook of Early Childhood Intervention.* New York: Cambridge University Press; 2000:135-159.

65. Ferrari PF, Rozzi S, Fogassi L. Mirror neurons responding to observation of actions made with tools in monkey ventral premotor cortex. *J Cogn Neurosci.* 2005; 17:212-226.

66. Fogassi L, Ferrari PF, Gesierich B, Rozzi S, Chersi F, Rizzolatti G. Parietal lobe: from action organization to intention understanding. *Science.* 2005;308:662-667.

67. Gallese V, Fadiga L, Fogassi L, Rizzolatti G. Action recognition in the premotor cortex. *Brain.* 1996;119(Pt 2):593-609.

68. Oberman LM, Hubbard EM, McCleery JP, Altschuler EL, Ramachandran VS, Pineda JA. EEG evidence for mirror neuron dysfunction in autism spectrum disorders. *Brain Res Cogn Brain Res.* 2005;24:190-198.

69. De Bellis MD, Keshavan MS, Clark DB, Casey BJ, Giedd JN, Boring AM, et al. Developmental traumatology. Part II: Brain development. *Biol Psychiatry.* 1999;45:1271-1284.

70. Teicher MH, Andersen SL, Polcari A, Anderson CM, Navalta CP. Developmental neurobiology of childhood stress and trauma. *Psychiatr Clin North Am.* 2002;25:397-426, vii-viii.

71. Andersen SL, Teicher MH. Delayed effects of early stress on hippocampal development. *Neuropsychopharmacology.* 2004;29:1988-1993.

72. Teicher MH, Dumont NL, Ito Y, Vaituzis C, Giedd JN, Andersen SL. Childhood neglect is associated with reduced corpus callosum area. *Biol Psychiatry.* 2004;56:80-85.

73. Anderson CM, Teicher MH, Polcari A, Renshaw PF. Abnormal T2 relaxation time in the cerebellar vermis of adults sexually abused in childhood: potential role of the vermis in stress-enhanced risk for drug abuse. *Psychoneuroendocrinology.* 2002;27:231-244.

74. Teicher MH. Wounds that time won't heal: the neurobiology of child abuse. *Cerebrum.* 2000;4:50-67.

75. Eluvathingal TJ, Chugani HT, Behen ME, Juhász C, Muzik O, Maqbool M, et al. Abnormal brain connectivity in children after early severe socioemotional deprivation: a diffusion tensor imaging study. *Pediatrics.* 2006;117:2093-2100.

76. Chugani HT, Behen ME, Muzik O, Juhász C, Nagy F, Chugani DC. Local brain functional activity following early deprivation: a study of postinstitutionalized Romanian orphans. *Neuroimage.* 2001;14:1290-1301.

77. Bugental DB, Martorell GA, Barraza V. The hormonal costs of subtle forms of infant maltreatment. *Horm Behav.* 2003;43:237-244.

78. Cicchetti D, Rogosch FA. The impact of child maltreatment and psychopathology on neuroendocrine functioning. *Dev Psychopathol.* 2001;13:783-804.

79. Duval F, Crocq MA, Guillon MS, Mokrani MC, Monreal J, Bailey P, et al. Increased adrenocorticotropin suppression following dexamethasone administration in sexually abused adolescents with posttraumatic stress disorder. *Psychoneuroendocrinology.* 2004;29:1281-1289.

80. Elzinga BM, Schmahl CG, Vermetten E, van Dyck R, Bremner JD. Higher cortisol levels following exposure to traumatic reminders in abuse-related PTSD. *Neuropsychopharmacology.* 2003;28:1656-1665.

81. Aubrun A, Grady J, Cultural Logic. Moving the public beyond familiar understandings of early childhood development: findings from talkback testing of simplifying models [FrameWorks Institute Web site]. November 2003. Available at: http://www.frameworksinstitute.org/assets/files/PDF/cl_shonkoff_sm_report.pdf. Accessed February 27, 2009.

82. Cohen JA, Deblinger E, Mannarino AP, Steer R. A multisite, randomized controlled clinical trial for children with sexual abuse–related PTSD symptoms. *J Am Acad Child Adolesc Psychiatry.* 2004;43:393-402.

83. Deblinger E, Heflin A. *Treating sexually abused children and their non-offending parents.* Thousand Oaks, CA: Sage Publications; 1986.

84. Deblinger E, Stauffer LB, Steer RA. Comparative efficacies of supportive and cognitive behavioral group therapies for young children who have been sexually abused and their nonoffending mothers. *Child Maltreat.* 2001;6:332-343.

85. Kolko D, Swenson C. *Assessing and treating physically abused children and their families.* Thousand Oaks, CA: Sage Publications; 2002.

86. Lieberman AF. Child-parent psychotherapy: a relationship-based approach to the treatment of mental health disorders in infancy and childhood. In: Sameroff AJ, McDonough SC, Rosenblum KL, eds. *Treating parent-infant relationship problems: strategies for intervention.* New York: Guilford Press; 2004:97-122.

87. Stuber ML, Schneider S, Kassam-Adams N, Kazak AE, Saxe G. The medical traumatic stress toolkit. *CNS Spectr.* 2006;11:137-142.

88. Phillips SD, Allred CA. Organizational management: what service providers are doing while researchers are disseminating interventions. *J Behav Health Serv Res.* 2006;33:156-175.

Chapter 22

THE PATH TO PREVENTION

Carol A. Plummer, PhD
Vincent Palusci, MD, MS, FAAP

The costs of sexual abuse are great in human terms (psychological, physical, developmental) but also have an economic price tag. The Department of Justice has estimated that child sexual abuse costs $23 billion per year in the United States, including medical expenses of over $1 billion. To understand the financial impact of sexual abuse in the US, it is helpful to look at the facts:

While it is difficult to precisely estimate the total costs for sexual abuse and assault for children under age 18 years, the total direct cost for all child abuse and neglect was estimated at over $33 billion in 2007, with an additional $70 billion in indirect costs.* Data from the US National Child Abuse and Neglect Data System for 2007 indicated that there were an estimated 794 000 children who were victims of maltreatment, 7.6 percent of whom were sexually abused. This is thought to be an underestimate as it only reflects children meeting criteria for CPS substantiation or indication. A separate survey of sexual assault administered as part of the National Incidence Studies of Missing, Abducted, Runaway and Thrownaway Children estimated that there were 285 400 cases of rape and other sexual assault among children in 1999.† Data from adults in 2001 suggest that the costs of sexual abuse/assault are $100 000 per episode, with 90% being indirect.‡ Using a conservative estimate of 100 000 children per year being sexually abused, the total lifetime cost is therefore estimated to be $10 billion.

Health care professionals have unique reasons for wanting to prevent child sexual abuse—to prevent pain of their patients, to spare future health problems, and because it is congruent with the goals of the health care profession regarding health and safety promotion. However, the details of why, how, when, and where health care professionals can promote prevention may seem murky or ill-defined, especially as violence against children remains one of the least well-documented crimes.[1] This chapter provides both the rationale for prevention and some concrete ideas about how prevention can become a part of not only what health care professionals support in the community, but also what can they do in the day-to-day care of their patients.

THE PROBLEM OF CHILD SEXUAL ABUSE AND THE IMPORTANCE OF PREVENTION

In the past several decades, awareness of sexual abuse and its connection to other social and health problems has skyrocketed. Self-report surveys conclude that at least 1 in 5 females and 1 in 10 males in the United States are sexually abused before the age of 18 years.[2,3] Incidence rates show that as many as one in 1000 children are sexually abused in

---

* *Wang CT, Holton J. Total Estimated Costs of Child Abuse and Neglect in the United States. Prevent Child Abuse America Web site. http://www.preventchildabuse.org/about_us/media_releases/pcaa_pew_economic_impact_study_final.pdf. Published September 2007. Accessed July 29, 2010.*
† *Finkelhor D, Hammer H, Sedlak AJ. NISMART: Sexually Assaulted Children: National Estimates and Characteristics. Washington, DC: US Dept of Justice; 2008.*
‡ *Clark KA, Biddle AK, Martin SL. A cost-benefit analysis of the Violence Against Women Act of 1994. Violence Against Women. 2002;8(4):417-428.*

the United States every year, but these rates are considered low because most abuse never gets reported to authorities.[4] In fact, a large part of the problem is being unable to identify when or where sexual abuse has occurred because there are often active cover-ups by the shamed child victims, denial by alleged offenders, and, at least initially, disbelief by caregivers. Statistics clearly show that a majority of offenders are known to or are even relatives of the sexual abuse victims, further contributing to the secrecy and underreporting.[5]

In addition, more facts about the old problem of sexually exploited runaway youth and the new problems of so-called cyberstalking or Internet use to facilitate child sexual exploitation are being discovered. The sexual abuse of children through sex tourism, nationally and internationally, as well as production of and use of child pornography, is also being increasingly publicized. Abuse at childcare centers, by religious leaders, or stings of nationwide perpetrator rings are also regular news items. It is becoming clearer that sexual abuse and exploitation are strongly linked, and it is increasingly evident that both occur worldwide.[6] While the façade of sexual abuse may change somewhat, the vastness of its reach and the depth of its outcomes are undeniably great.

Although no one symptom can "rule out" or "rule in" sexual abuse, with the possible exception of pregnancy or sexually transmitted infections, certain symptoms or behaviors at least raise concerns that beg for additional inquiry. The sexual abuse of children has long been linked to a variety of mental health and behavioral problems. Relationship difficulties, depression, suicidal tendencies, and eating disorders are related to a history of child sexual abuse.[7-9] In fact, juvenile delinquency and future criminal behavior have also been strongly linked to a history of childhood abuse.[10] Some children are more resilient than others after sexual abuse experiences, and not all are immediately symptomatic, yet a significant number report emotional reactions or distress.[11,12] Several victim variables, such as relationship to the perpetrator, age, duration, prior victimization, and use of force are also sometimes predictive of reactions the child may have to the abusive experience. In addition, some children may exhibit short-term effects and others may show long-term effects of the sexual abuse.

Many health care professionals are still unaware of increasing evidence that child sexual abuse predicts not only emotional and mental health problems, but also future physical health ailments. A large retrospective study linked child sexual abuse with diabetes, heart disease, somatization, drug abuse, and other psychosomatic illnesses.[13] The distress resulting from childhood adversity often results in physical health problems that have long-term effects on those victimized as children. Although the former US Surgeon General has declared child sexual abuse "a serious public health challenge," a unified plan to address this problem and prevent sexual abuse has not yet been prioritized in this country.[14] This lack of a well-defined prevention plan has contributed to weak public involvement in prevention, resulting in the perpetuation of the problem.

DEFINING PREVENTION

Prevention of child sexual abuse is, of course, recommended by all those who are familiar with the problems associated with sexual abuse and its sequelae. Because intervention with and treatment for sexual abuse is both difficult and expensive, efforts aimed at preventing abuse are promoted by agencies, governmental officials, and individual practitioners. Unfortunately, beyond a blanket endorsement of the concept of prevention, there are many different ideas about what the term actually means or what activities are considered "prevention." Definitions for prevention may vary slightly, yet 3 categories of prevention are generally noted: primary, secondary, and tertiary. The most commonly used definitions of the levels of prevention categorize them in the following way:

— **Primary:** Efforts aimed at the general population for the purpose of keeping abuse from happening to the target victims.

— **Secondary:** Efforts aimed at a particularly high-risk group to keep abuse from happening to them given that the risk to this group is elevated.

— **Tertiary:** Efforts aimed at preventing abuse from happening again to those who have already been victimized. This level of prevention may include treatment of the patient and perpetrator for the original abuse.

The Centers for Disease Control and Prevention (CDC) has recently relabeled the 3 levels of prevention in a new way, emphasizing that abuse operates in a context and requires an entire spectrum of necessary prevention strategies over time.[15] These efforts are explicitly based on Bronfenbrenner's ecological model, which promotes intervening at the individual, relationship, community, and societal levels.[16] Approaches inferred from these new labels emphasize a shift away from risk reduction as the predominant prevention approach and toward promotion of positive social changes. Some argue that prior definitions may limit the prevention strategies by focusing primarily on the potential individual targets of abuse and how to intervene with them, rather than the environmental and societal context that supports and even condones abusive acts. These newer definitions of prevention focus on WHEN the prevention effort occurs:

— **Primary:** This is taking action *before* abuse has occurred to prevent it from happening.

— **Secondary:** This level of prevention is intervening right *after* abuse has occurred.

— **Tertiary:** Tertiary prevention is seen as that which takes the long view and *works over time to change conditions* in the environment that promotes or supports abusiveness.

Physicians and other health care professionals are invited to become more active in prevention efforts as part of this definitional shift. The National Sexual Violence Resource Center[17] has recently published information about how to involve a broader constituency in prevention through using the "Spectrum of Prevention." Prevention is explicitly not the responsibility of any one agency, one profession, or one intervention, but it is being framed as the responsibility of all to create a society less conducive to child sexual abuse. In this spectrum, individual skill development, community and provider education, coalition building, organizational change, and policy innovations are all components of the prevention solution.

RISK AND PROTECTIVE FACTORS

Through the use of an ecological model to examine child sexual abuse, both risk and protective factors can be examined on the individual level, the relationship/family level, the community level, and the broader societal level. Prevention includes activities that diminish risk and bolster protective factors. Prevention, then, requires that those of us involved recognize not only what we are against, or what we want to avoid, but also what we are for and want to promote. Examining risk factors can inform us about which individuals might have the greatest vulnerabilities. Likewise, recognizing personal, family, or community strengths and supporting them is another approach to preventing negative life outcomes.

On an individual level, risks of child sexual abuse include being a female child and being under the age of 11 years.[18,19] More females are reported as child sexual abuse victims, but most experts also believe there are a substantial number of male victims who are not reported because of societal double standards, pressure on males to not express "weakness" or admit vulnerabilities, and increased embarrassment if the abuse is same-gender.[20] Although the mean age of children being sexually abused is generally reported to be between 9 and 11 years old,[21-23] other studies report that more than half of those sexually victimized are younger than age 7 years.[4,24] Undeniably, the vulnerability of younger children is heightened for several additional reasons other than offender age preference: difficulty in adults understanding communication of the very young child, difficulty for the child in verbalizing or otherwise communicating what has happened, heightened dependence upon adults, and a higher likelihood of these children being tricked or successfully threatened.

Relationship dynamics and family characteristics may also influence the likelihood of abuse. Presence of a stepfather in the home, living with parents who have a conflictual relationship or substance abuse problems, and living apart from one's natural parents are all variables that increase risk of sexual abuse.[2] There is some evidence that low socioeconomic status may increase the possibility of sexual abuse, perhaps in part because of neediness, lack of supervision, or increased familial stress levels.[4] Studies of ethnicity and rural/urban differences have been inconclusive. What is definitive is that sexual abuse exists in high numbers in all groups: racial, ethnic, socioeconomic, and religious.

On a community, or even societal, level, some factors may increase vulnerability to sexual abuse: having a weak friendship network, lack of employment opportunities, lack of institutional support from police and the judicial system, general tolerance of sexual assault within the community, settings that support sexual violence, weak community sanctions against sexual violence perpetrators, and being isolated from the broader community.[25] Other societal factors include poverty, societal norms that support sexual violence, societal practices that support male superiority and sexual entitlement, attitudes that maintain women's inferiority and sexual submissiveness, weak laws and policies related to gender equity, and high tolerance levels toward crime and other forms of violence.[25]

Perhaps in part because of different levels of supervision, freedom, self-reliance, and social roles of males and females, community risks can be categorized with regard to gender. Males are abused more often by nonrelatives than are females,[23] and females are more likely to be sexually abused by family members[26]—but both are likely to know the perpetrator.[27]

SOME KEY POINTS TO UNDERSTAND ABOUT SEXUAL ABUSE OF CHILDREN

Prior to discussing details of prevention efforts, including the role of health care professionals in prevention, a few key points need to be stressed. This list highlights what is known about sexual abuse and provides guidance in our responses to that problem. These points about child sexual abuse help to frame the work by providing a common understanding of the dynamics of child sexual abuse, which should guide our prevention and intervention efforts.

DISCOVERY OF CHILD SEXUAL ABUSE MORE OF A PROCESS THAN AN EVENT

Not all children who have experienced sexual abuse will be clearly identified, or perhaps even identified at all, prior to coming to your office for medical services. Although some cases of sexual abuse are immediately apparent, owing to the presence of sexually transmitted infections or acute physical injury, the vast majority of child sexual abuse is discovered through a child's own accidental or purposeful disclosure of abuse. Children often grapple with whether to tell, whom to tell, and when to disclose so as to minimize negative outcomes to themselves or their families. These children may be faced with adults who are unprepared to respond appropriately because of lack of information, fears, or adults' own emotional reaction. Even when adults listen, they may respond in ways that upset the child or contribute to a retraction of the report or they may misinterpret the message, either exaggerating or minimizing the situation.[28,29]

A goal of secondary prevention is to minimize harm after sexual abuse is discovered and thereby reduce the risk of further victimization. When children are officially questioned, much effort is put into reducing the number of times and increasing the sensitivity in interviewing children to help them tell their stories accurately and without retraumatization. However, at any point in the investigative process, a true report can be changed by a child victim to stop removal from the home, foster care placement, court proceedings, and so on. It is important for health care professionals to recognize that they may need to provide care and intervention at an initial report or, for a variety of reasons, long after the first or most recent incident of abuse. In fact, they may not be informed until the abuse has resumed or been ongoing for a period of years. Awareness of this issue also means knowing the possibility of children being tricked or forced into behaviors or situations that are nearly unbelievable to us, including sexual activities with other children, animals, maternal caregivers, teachers, and religious leaders; child pornography; and being prostituted (even by their own parents). Full disclosure of such events may only be revealed over months or even years.

Children React in a Wide Variety of Ways After Victimization

Some children victimized by sexual abuse will be primarily relieved once the sexual abuse has stopped. Other children will experience ongoing posttraumatic stress disorder; some will not want to discuss it; and others will need to vent their experience and emotions. It is impossible to "diagnose" the accuracy of a child's report or predict any long-term medical or psychological needs based on the immediate presentation of symptoms, especially because many children are actually asymptomatic.[30] While children may react favorably to specialized evaluation techniques such as videocolposcopy during a physical examination, such responses do not allow one to interpret the accuracy of their victimization history and need for long-term mental health treatment.[31]

Parents Are Central for Both Successful Prevention and Intervention

Parents will react differently than their children and than one another and are critical to healing after abuse. Assessment of and attention to parents may be a critical component of successful intervention. Parents may need a referral for mental health care or crisis support. Health care professionals can play a central role in informing parents regarding the necessity and techniques for talking to their children, supervising behaviors, and selecting care providers in order to prevent the sexual abuse of their children. Furthermore, if there are questions or abuse allegations, physicians and other health care professionals may be asked for, or want to offer, referral services for parents.

Some Children Are More Vulnerable to Child Sexual Abuse

Prevention is important before abuse ever occurs, but also from the perspective of risks to those who have been previously abused or those with special needs. Children with physical disabilities, cognitive impairments, or developmental delays are all at a greatly elevated risk of being sexually abused.[32-35] For that reason, parents and caregivers of these children need to be especially informed of the need for safety for these vulnerable categories of children.

Studies also have shown that children who have already experienced sexual abuse are at increased risk of experiencing additional sexual abuse.[36-38] These children also are at an increased risk of experiencing other types of interpersonal violence, both as children and later as adults.[19,39]

HISTORY OF CHILD SEXUAL ABUSE PREVENTION EFFORTS

EDUCATIONAL EFFORTS TARGETING CHILDREN

Since the late 1970s, when efforts first were made to prevent child sexual abuse in the United States, educational methods have been the main approach. Programs have been designed to help children understand what abuse is, to instruct them on ways to avoid potentially dangerous situations, and to inform them of what to do if grooming (ie, gradually acclimating a child to activities that will ultimately lead to sexual abuse) or actual abuse takes place. This child-education component was initially mandated in 1979 by federal authorities at the National Center on Child Abuse and Neglect (NCCAN) when deciding to fund child sexual abuse prevention programs.[40] Approaches to preventing sexual abuse were designed differently than those aimed to address neglect or physical abuse. Sexual abuse had been shrouded in secrecy and silence for so long, and in most cases only the perpetrator and the child were aware of it. Perpetrators were perceived to have few incentives to report themselves and limited motivation to willingly stop the behavior. In addition, many children didn't even know what this behavior (sexual abuse) was, had no knowledge of where or how they could seek help, or what to do if they were approached in a potentially dangerous situation. For these reasons, educating children was seen as one necessary step in child sexual abuse prevention's initial efforts.

Educational programs for children often focused on victimization prevention. Many aimed to alter children's level of knowledge, skills, and resources regarding potential sexual abuse. For example, factual information was given to make children more aware of abuse, as well as to address attitudes that may have contributed to self-blame. Many programs addressed lies that perpetrators may tell to confuse children or keep them quiet and isolated with their abuse secret. These messages challenged ideas presented by some offenders (eg, "you shouldn't have worn that outfit," "your mother will be mad at you if you tell," "this is how uncles always show love to their nieces"). Most programs addressed myths about sexual abuse (eg, that offenders were mostly strangers, that it was the victim's fault, that sexual abuse only happened to girls or in "bad" neighborhoods). Programs also endorsed and emphasized communication with trusted adults. Some of this was to build support networks for consulting with trusted adults regarding all kinds of problems or confusion. Building communication was a strategy to help prevent abuse by involving adults when luring of the child had begun but had not yet led to abuse. Other programs focused solely on the need for children to report abuse and to keep telling until someone believed and helped them.

Other programs for children, albeit in smaller numbers, also focused on educating children about related topics. These included bullying prevention, respect for others, protecting your own child when you become a parent, and even "offender prevention." Offender prevention pertains to programs that actually try to alter behaviors and attitudes in those youth who may be considering sexually abusive acts, and these programs may emphasize morals, laws, or social norms. Many of these programs were developed later in the 1980s and 1990s and were integrated into already existing child abuse prevention programming.

Child education programs aimed at prevention developed quickly over the next decade, resulting in millions of children receiving a wide variety of programs: from weak to strong, comprehensive to one-shot deals, risk reduction to reporting directions, assertiveness training to avoidance-oriented, antisex to discussing a "continuum" of touching experiences.[41] Fortunately, these early efforts showed promise and had the ability to reach children, doing so with broad adult approval.[42,43] Unfortunately, the quality of programs vacillated from very useful to potentially harmful or confusing.[44,45]

EDUCATIONAL EFFORTS TARGETING ADULTS

Several groups of adults were particularly targeted in the earliest years of sexual abuse prevention programming. These included parents, teachers, mental health professionals who treated children and victims, and the general public. A plethora of newspaper articles, books, movies, and talk shows about the sexual abuse of children saturated the public in the early to mid-1980s. While awareness of the problem undoubtedly increased, efforts may have helped create a "backlash" that challenged claims of the astronomical rates of abuse, the extent of damage to victims and families, and even the veracity of specific victim statements. An overreaction to concerns about sexual abuse has been termed "moral panic" by some writers[46] and may have resulted in overzealous pursuits of those perceived to be offenders in large childcare center cases or bizarre stories being publicized about ritual abuse, baby-killing, and other unusual child sexual abuse claims.[47]

Even nonsensationalized public awareness efforts had their weaknesses in the earliest years of the awareness of sexual abuse. For example, most programs were aimed at the generic public, meaning that they were primarily focused on images and approaches that would appeal to white, middle-class Americans. Few programs were in other languages, focused on messages to subcultures, or had a distinct audience in mind.

Programs for parents initially accompanied almost every child-oriented educational effort. This was partly because parents had never before heard of talking with children about sexual abuse and had grave concerns about what would be said and how it would be communicated. Educational programs for parents were not just about gaining entry to work with children, but often became that, even though prevention advocates also attempted to engage parents as partners in prevention. Once parents realized the programs appeared to be safety-oriented, did not differ from their personal values, and had some developmental appropriateness (or claimed to), they gave consent for their children to attend programs. They also stopped coming to parent education meetings themselves, either expecting that the experts would do a great job or believing that they knew what they needed to know after the media blitz or from a prior meeting they had attended.

CONCERNS ABOUT SEXUAL ABUSE PREVENTION EFFORTS

Prevention programs, and especially those geared toward children, are not without critics. Early criticism focused on the fear that children would make false allegations, "practice" sex, be traumatized by the topic, or be incapable of understanding concepts. As is the case in arguments against sex education, some felt that parents should educate their children about sexual abuse. Others countered that when incest was the problem, relying on parents alone to reach children with sexual abuse prevention messages meant that these children would be at great risk and never get prevention messages from parents.

Most critics today do not advocate completely dismantling child education, but they encourage expanding the emphasis to decrease placing the sole responsibility on the shoulders of children or their own protection. Although there is no empirical evidence that any program actually promotes children taking full responsibility to prevent sexual abuse, there is no doubt that some programs have underemphasized their parent education, public awareness, and advocacy efforts to focus on child education. Numerous efforts were neglected while children, parents, certain professionals, and the public was given awareness information. These areas include a broader focus on community ownership of the problem, organizational responses, long-term changes in social norms, and rigorous efforts to see if offending behaviors could be stopped so there were fewer offenders, to name a few.

Bolen[27] suggests that potential offenders should be targeted by providing school-based programs (for youth) that promote healthy relationship patterns, rather than a "victim-based paradigm," because there is such a diversity of approaches taken by offenders. Unfortunately, though the idea of outreach to offenders is gaining in popularity and has promise, no solid empirical evidence exists yet to show whether this will produce change in the rates of sexual abuse or whether new or potential offenders are amenable to change.

The sex offender registry, initially driven by concerns about missing and exploited children, has been considered a prevention strategy by some. Efforts to learn where offenders are, to monitor their movement, and to limit their access to children have been expanding over the past decade. Those in the child sexual abuse prevention movement, though initially strongly supportive of the idea, have often withdrawn support for this direction, deeming it a poor substitute for other prevention efforts. First, it reinforces the idea that most offenders are those dangerous stranger pedophiles. Second, it may reduce other prevention efforts by diverting funds away from primary prevention programs and give parents a false sense of security, reducing their perception of the need for them to be involved in other prevention efforts. Third, it inequitably has penalized the young, the poor, minorities, and the mentally challenged. For example, professionals recognize the dangers of labeling youth with sexual behavior problems as "offenders" and the unfortunate outcome of dating relationships resulting in persons placed on the registry when in peer consensual liaisons. Finally, many of these offenders are maltreated children all grown up—and extremely punitive measures may make some people feel some release for their anger but not really solve the overall problem. In fact, leaving no room for offender rehabilitation and reentry into society may even exacerbate the long-term problem.

The biggest questions of how best to prevent sexual abuse, how to reduce rates over time, and eventually eliminate sexual abuse remain unanswered. However, there are numerous signs that prior efforts have been useful and new methods still need to be further explored and researched. Study after study characterizes the merits of past prevention efforts with regard to learning and skill acquisition for children and adults as a result of policy change, education, or media campaigns. Until recently, no study actually showed that participation in a prevention program resulted in reduced rates of sexual abuse for participants, with only anecdotal reports on successes and actions taken to stay safe as evidence.[48,49] A recent study, however, showed that college women (n = 825) who had participated in a child sexual abuse prevention program as children were significantly less likely to experience subsequent sexual abuse than those who had not completed such a program.[50] In addition, although some argue that sexual abuse has not decreased as a result of sexual abuse prevention efforts,[27] actual rates of sexual abuse do seem to be decreasing and one proposed explanation is that sexual abuse prevention efforts may be at least part of the reason.[51]

PREVENTION TODAY: TRENDS AND FUTURE DIRECTIONS

SETTING STANDARDS

The variability in past prevention programming aimed toward children has resulted in many efforts to find more effective prevention programs. One current trend in child-focused sexual abuse education programs is toward "best practices" for ensuring quality. The Association for Sexual Abuse Prevention, a program of the National Children's Alliance, has recently instituted a "Prevention Institute" to promote high-quality programming. Another example is Prevent Child Abuse Iowa, which provides a list of expected practices for their funded programs that specifies topics to address, skills to develop, structure of sessions, school and family involvement expectations, ways to handle disclosures, and evaluation guidelines.[52]

Similarly, the New Jersey Task Force on Child Abuse and Neglect has created a booklet titled, "Standards for Prevention Programs: Building Success through Family Support," based on research findings about effective programs.[53] Included in their list of factors used to evaluate programs are conceptual standards (ie, the content and approaches to imparting information to the target group), practice standards, and administrative standards. Recommendations for programs include being family centered, community-based, and culturally competent, and using a strengths-based approach. Other suggestions include being easily accessible, being linked to informal and formal supports, and having a long-range plan and ongoing evaluations. These efforts are promising and may help to build the highest quality into programs that currently vary greatly in their level of comprehensiveness. Evidence-based interventions will be useful, but standardizing programs across settings and cultures may not entirely work. At the same time that high standards must be set, there must remain room for creativity and the use of feedback from diverse community settings to respond to their unique needs and situations. Also, to be fair, some programs may be hampered in their opportunity to be truly comprehensive, to reach broader audiences, and to use creative methods because of lack of funds, a problem that has been identified by many prevention program leaders.[54] Demands for quality will probably need to be combined with demands for adequate funding for prevention so that truly valuable programs can even exist.

MEANINGFUL PARENT INVOLVEMENT

As discussed earlier, parents have generally been included in sexual abuse education programs. The earliest child sexual abuse prevention programs included strong parent education components, but in subsequent years, parent attendance has dwindled, shifting the focus even more to children.[55-57]

Parents are in the best position to prevent sexual abuse, because it can begin at a very young age (before children have contact with any professionals) and because parents know how to talk to their own children, children are more likely to believe their parents, parents know what their children need to know, and children will understand from the conversation that parents are approachable.[58,59] Promising outcomes in parent education on sexual abuse include substantial parental support for in-school programs[56] and the finding that programs may increase the confidence of parents to talk with their children about sexual abuse.[60]

At the same time, survey results have indicated that parents may mistakenly believe their own children are well supervised and able to avoid danger, and as such they do not want to frighten them unnecessarily.[58] Some results of parent education have been encouraging, yet new methods of engaging parents meaningfully, with information they truly need, must still be creatively developed. Reppucci et al[57] found that parents are enthusiastic about parent programs "but in different formats, at different times and in different environments than the current typical PTO one evening, one-time meeting."

Some prevention advocates are currently developing programs that better meet parents' needs. These include a topical focus on Internet safety or common lures for teens at malls, areas of new concern for parents and for which parents are offered information they truly believe they require. Programs may need to reach out to parents in new formats: take-home videos, videos played in waiting rooms of doctors' offices, meetings held over lunch in employment settings, and the incorporation of sexual abuse prevention messages into general pamphlets about the health care of children.

BROADEN THE TARGETS OF PREVENTION MESSAGES

Awareness programs need to include education of professionals, the general public, and even perpetrators or potential perpetrators. A survey of 87 sexual abuse prevention programs showed that one quarter of these programs had included some adolescent offender prevention messages or approaches in their overall education.[54] Rates of offender prevention efforts should be improved. One approach developed by Dr. Gene Abel teaches parents to watch for sexual behavior problems in their children so patterns of dysfunction can be identified and interrupted earlier.[61] This program uses data about current offenders—including how they developed without effective interventions—to prevent young people who are at some risk of developing sexual problems from doing so. In large part, it engages parents to help prevent their own children from developing sexual problems by recognizing concerning signs early and taking them to sex-specific therapists, rather than fearfully retreating into denial and ignoring these concerns.

Bystanders also are being encouraged to be more proactive, rather than silently ignoring internal concerns that a professional colleague, relative, or neighbor is displaying concerning behavior toward children. A booklet by Stop It Now details an approach that can be taken to ask questions of, and show concern for, a friend, colleague, or loved one who you are concerned may have interest in sexual contact with children (or who may have acted inappropriately toward them).[62] Approaching a potential perpetrator may alert them to a friend's awareness and force reconsideration of certain preabusive or abusive behavior. However, care must also be taken that this is done advisedly; in some cases, discussing concerns with an offender may only make the abuse go deeper underground or may inappropriately reassure the concerned party that nothing is occurring. This method, and others, needs to be undertaken with awareness of the dynamics of sexual abuse and the potential for harm, as well as good, coming from our prevention innovations. One thing is certain: sexual abuse prevention will need to involve many types of people and many diverse approaches if we are to alter the family and community context where sexual abuse occurs.

SUPPORT QUALITY EDUCATION OF CHILDREN

School-based educational programs that teach children what abuse is and how to avoid and report it have merit.[49,63] Those studies with the most compelling findings revealed that age of the child, number of sessions, participant involvement, and the use of behavioral skills training to be significant moderator variables. Dozens of studies show that children can and do learn information, change attitudes, and can even gain skills from quality prevention education that is child-focused.[49,64] Despite this, communities should be wary of relying on children to be solely or primarily responsible for their own safety and protection. All communities must do more than simply educate children about sexuality or abuse.

Health care professionals are also well aware that good sex education programs, including messages about positive sexuality and good choices, are sorely lacking. To provide quality sexual abuse prevention, it is necessary to have a model for healthy sexual development and behavior to provide to children and to their parents.

CREATE DIVERSE APPROACHES FOR DIVERSE COMMUNITIES

Different forms of abuse in distinctive communities and cultures will require unique types of prevention strategies. For example, as abuse of children in schools is addressed, administrators may need to establish stronger policies on student-to-student sexual harassment, working to change norms on allowable on-campus behavior. Teachers may need to address attitudes of sexual entitlement, provide sex education, and demand training on how to respond when sexual abuse is suspected or disclosed. Recent high-profile cases in which teachers, both male and female, have sexually exploited young students have also expanded our awareness that schools need to do more to screen teachers, set appropriate student/teacher relationship standards, and train bystanders to take action when it appears a teacher colleague is acting inappropriately.

Education of a whole range of groups, including health care professionals, is necessary to help in the prevention of child sexual abuse. Some groups are effectively addressing child sexual abuse as a public health problem and are attempting to change the willingness of adults to report abuse based on public awareness efforts. For example, Stop It Now found that there was an increase of willingness to report abuse after they conducted a multiyear public education campaign on the importance of reporting.[62]

Some communities have chosen to focus on offender prevention. Currently, efforts aimed at offenders and potential offenders are being explored: billboards and telephone hotlines aimed at current offenders, education programs for parents of children with sexual behavior problems that could lead to offending, and socialization skills training for youth focused on making abusive behavior unacceptable. Hotlines have been used by friends or family of suspected offenders, and they encourage concerned adults to take appropriate action. Importantly, each of these approaches needs to be designed, evaluated, and updated based on specific local cultural values to maximize relevance and community endorsement and ownership.

One innovative community-based approach was developed by a group called "Generation Five." In addition to providing community-specific consultation and capacity building to make programs emerge from and be relevant to the participants, Generation Five encourages taking a look at the long view as we try to change society to eradicate child sexual abuse. They anticipate it will take five generations to totally rid society of sexual abuse and prescribe tasks for each generation as we work for long-term outcomes (http://www.generationfive.org).

THE INTERNET AND MEDIA MUST BE ADDRESSED

The expanded use of the Internet by young people and by sexual offenders has placed children at additional risk of being lured into sexual contact. Although the public is broadly aware of this risk, school-based child education programs have only recently incorporated strong Internet-safety programs into their sexual abuse prevention curricula. Further, still fewer parents are monitoring their children's use, nor do they believe that their own child is personally at risk of such exploitation. In this area, in particular, strong parent engagement and concrete training are necessary to minimize the risk to children in terms of Internet predators.

The World Wide Web is an invaluable teaching tool, but it can also enable exposure to unsavory topics or materials, as well as provide an avenue for luring children into sexually abusive situations. It is unlikely that prevention advocates or parents will force a discontinuation of children's use of the Internet because of its problems or because of the difficulties in monitoring its use. However, one promising approach is that children and youth are being targeted with information on how to be "Netsmartz," (http://www.netsmartz.org/index.aspx) with interactive Internet games, school programs, and print material that instruct them on safe practices, both online and in their broader lives.

ORGANIZATIONAL INTERVENTIONS

Another type of prevention receiving attention is aimed at changing organizations to maximize safety for children. Nationally known speaker and consultant on the prevention of child sexual exploitation and sexual violence Cordelia Anderson[65] has highlighted the work of groups as diverse as the Boy Scouts of America, the National Alliance of Youth Sports, the Chicago Children's Museum, and the Greater Twin Cities Youth Symphonies, with all having done work to prevent child sexual abuse. Actions taken by these groups include developing organizational policies, installing security hardware, creating training mandates, instituting supervision and hiring requirements, making public statements about their commitment to child safety, and adopting proactive risk management plans. Even consideration of facility design to minimize one-on-one opportunities between unsavory adults and vulnerable children has resulted in cameras or mirrors in youth facilities or doors left off stalls where younger children may need assistance while toileting.

All organizations can develop policies and procedures that acknowledge that child sexual abuse occurs, in and outside of child-serving agencies. Youth-serving organizations have an implicit responsibility to their clientele. However, even organizations that do not solely or primarily focus on children can, and should, be involved in the same prevention process. For example, doctors' offices, clinics, hospitals, community mental health centers, and other health care facilities that serve children could also enhance children's safety and decrease their own liability by taking similar actions.

WHY AND HOW SHOULD HEALTH PROFESSIONALS BE INVOLVED IN PREVENTION EFFORTS?

There are several reasons why health professionals, particularly pediatricians, should be involved with prevention efforts. Most health professionals already understand and appreciate the linkages among prevention, intervention, and treatment. It is equally critical that health care personnel embrace the importance of professionals having a role in prevention beyond merely treating and reporting suspicious injuries. Ray Helfer, a physician who spearheaded the creation of the Children's Trust Funds to promote prevention, suggested decades ago that health professionals should be an important part of a multifaceted approach with concurrent maneuvers to prevent violence. The approaches listed include community commitment, mass media messages, training for new parents, early childhood development programs for all preschoolers, interpersonal skills programs for all school-aged children, and adult education programs for those caring for children.[66]

Health care professionals are sometimes reluctant to intervene in potential cases of abuse. There are several reasons for this: lack of knowledge, fear of offending the patient (or caregiver), time pressures, discomfort of the patient with questions, fear of loss of control of the provider/patient relationship, and attitudes about accountability. Hamberger and Patel[67] have found these hesitancies in cases of domestic violence, and many of the same factors are relevant in cases of child sexual abuse. Examining barriers to optimal service provision is important for every health care professional.

It is vital for health care professionals to be knowledgeable regarding current issues of sexually abused patients. If the child is treated medically, the physician's lack of knowledge about abuse may impede discussion regarding sexual abuse with the child, and therefore, subsequent intervention. Frequently, this interaction has replicated the child's experience of family denial or minimization.[68] For example, touch is often experienced as invasive, intrusive, and noxious. Persistent revictimization themes may emerge during medical treatment. The patient may even feel that the medical experience triggers associations with childhood abuse. In addition, because of the patient's difficulty with trust or inability to remember, abuse issues may only be revealed to the provider over time.

Health professionals have unique relationships with families and special opportunities to intervene to prevent child sexual abuse. Dubowitz[69] has suggested that it is important that physicians be able to ask sensitive questions, gather information, and use astute observation and careful assessment skills if they are to be successful in these endeavors. Johnson[70] has provided a simple checklist for comprehensive screening. Keys to effectiveness are professional comfort with hearing sensitive issues, an ability to teach children about sensitive issues, familiarity with normal genital anatomy and routine child and parent concerns, an ability to diagnose and treat suspected maltreatment, and knowledge of the child welfare system.

Physicians specializing in forensic examinations and emergency department physicians charged with evaluating alleged abuse should be attuned to the need for thorough assessments. Physical examinations should include discussions with the patient and his or her family as part of the process. Physicians, nurse practitioners, and nurses can also assist in communicating messages that may prevent additional abuse.[59] Anticipatory guidance is provided to parents and families by health care professionals about a variety of topics during childhood. However, pediatricians also reported they need additional training and support to make anticipatory guidance regarding abuse prevention more effective.[71]

These messages can be in the form of pamphlets, video education, or interpersonal discussions that communicate safety information to victims, parents, and caregivers. Prevention messages may be critical if no medical evidence is found, if a child victim changes his or her story, or if action by child protective services or prosecutors is not possible because of the lack of medical evidence.

Lack of medical evidence,[72] victim-recantation,[73,74] and general lack of evidence for legal action[2,75] are, in fact, very common. Health care professionals need to communicate to families that medical evidence is often not present (depending on the type of abuse), that coming in for help was the right thing to do, and that resources are available if other concerns arise.[24] Given that maternal support is important for a child's recovery and that maternal adjustment is predictive of the child's adjustment, attention to the needs of the maternal caregiver is critical.[76,77] Mothers need to not only believe that health care providers care about the child victim, but that their needs and feelings are also of interest. Professional support of mothers during early discovery and disclosure has been shown to have a positive relationship to maternal emotional stability.[44] Thus, supporting a mother with empathy and patience during this crisis may be one of the best ways to support the child victim. The mother, particularly in cases of incest, will need to be understood before she can take guidance or challenges, and her strength will determine the ability of a child or children to remain in a home. In cases in which nonoffending fathers are actively involved after the sexual abuse, it is likely that support for them is equally important; however, few studies have examined the role of fathers in child adjustment after abuse.[78]

Screening for family and community violence should be included in routine health visits, even though some pediatricians need skills to better identify and manage injuries caused by such violence.[79] Collecting information about possible abuse experiences on intake forms is another way to learn about and create opportunities to address certain problems. Some physicians may be skeptical that patients would reveal information about a history of sexual abuse on health forms, though patients are more forthcoming if asked than if never asked.[80] In addition, by mentioning "unmentionable" topics, those providing health care show that they are aware of these issues and probably are knowledgeable about how to be helpful. The American Academy of Pediatrics is currently developing and assessing the effectiveness of a violence prevention program called "Connected Kids: Safe, Strong, Secure."[81] This program includes a guide for office clinicians, provides 21 parent/patient information brochures and supporting training materials, and encourages implementing a strengths-based approach for clinicians to provide anticipatory guidance, in order to help parents raise resilient children.

TEN STEPS HEALTH CARE PROFESSIONALS CAN TAKE TO PREVENT CHILD SEXUAL ABUSE

In addition to the prevention opportunities in the health care setting, health care professionals can also involve themselves in communitywide efforts to change the societal conditions that promote or allow sexual abuse of children. The following steps provide possible avenues for the prevention of abuse that broaden collaboration and enlarge health care professionals' role in the prevention of sexual abuse. This list is not exhaustive, but it provides examples for consideration.

1. ***Child Education:*** Health care professionals can endorse and support quality comprehensive child-focused education, using their professional status to reassure parents and communities. They can also serve on an advisory board for a local child abuse prevention agency, thereby assisting in networking alliances between prevention programs and the treatment field. Physicians and nurses can play a key role in promoting both healthy sexuality and sexual abuse education.

2. ***Parent Involvement:*** Health care professionals can provide parents with ideas of how to speak with their own children about sexuality and sexual abuse, providing materials or consultation. They can promote issues of Internet safety, supervision, selecting safe babysitters, and choosing a quality childcare program. Posters in waiting rooms, take-home brochures, and lists of Web addresses readily available for referrals for parents' use can be used to further provide outreach. Additional resources on child abuse prevention programs that exist in and around the community and referrals to area agencies for additional information or assistance can also be vital prevention interventions.

   When parents learn that their child has been sexually abused, it is essential for the health care professional to communicate to nonabusive parents that they are likely to feel distress and that counseling for their own reactions, in addition to treatment for their victimized child, is normative and advisable, at least short-term.[82] Care must be taken not to communicate blame toward parents who are not the abusers, leaving clinical interventions to those who provide counseling. At the same time, health care professionals need to make a commitment to reporting suspected abuse and following up when necessary, to promote children's safety.

3. ***Community Awareness:*** Health care professionals can offer to provide radio or TV public service announcements to build awareness of child sexual abuse as a public health issue and an issue that is related to physical health. Health care professionals

need to promote awareness of the links between childhood trauma and future health problems, and they have the credibility to do so. They can participate in Child Abuse Prevention Month, promoting activities from their practices and in their offices; they can also donate money to the Children's Trust Fund in their state.

4. ***Bystander Involvement:*** In personal or professional capacities, health care professionals should be willing to become involved when they are concerned about a child's safety and should seek supervision or consultation when necessary. Despite great demands on their time, health care professionals must be willing to make appropriate referrals to child protective services based on reasonable suspicions, rather than waiting to report abuse when they are certain. Child protective services investigates suspicions and has the authority, expertise, and responsibility for that job.

5. ***Early Sexual Behavior Problem Identification:*** Caregivers often consult with medical authorities about sexual or social behavior problems with their children, who may be exhibiting sexually reactive symptoms of being abused or early sexual deviancy. Behavioral problems are often nonspecific, but physicians can guide parents to seek additional assistance rather than ignoring these problems, while guarding against parental overreaction to self-exploration or age-appropriate sexual curiosity.[24,83] Consider having materials and referral sources on hand for sexual behavior problems. Even parents who won't verbally address their concerns may pick up a pamphlet.

6. ***Offender Prevention:*** Support efforts to reach out to those with problematic sexual feelings or desires and make certain that referrals are made to therapists knowledgeable about the assessment and treatment of sexual deviance. Be alert to early signs of sexual problems in youth so that patterns of deviant behavior do not become established through lack of responsiveness.

7. ***Policy and Organizational Prevention Efforts:*** Be willing to make changes in policy, hiring, supervision, and training in your own office or organization to put proven risk-reducing procedures in place. This can include establishing clinical practice guidelines to address these issues in the office, hospital, and clinic. For example, new initiatives might include routine staff trainings conducted for updates on family violence issues, and intake protocols for patients that ask about past or present traumatic events.

8. ***Improved Clinical Care and Education:*** Pediatricians should recognize risk factors for violence when providing clinic care and be able to diagnose and treat violence-related problems at all stages of child development. Pediatricians need to identify, for example, issues with mental illness, substance abuse, and stress in family constellations, as well as inappropriate supervision; family violence and exposure to media violence; access to firearms; and gang involvement and other signs of poor self-esteem, school failure, and depression.[81] Pediatricians should also support early bonding and attachment and educate parents on normal age-appropriate behaviors for children of all ages. Pediatricians can educate parents about parenting skills, limit-setting, and protective factors to be nurtured in children to help prevent a variety of injuries. Consistent discipline practices and body safety techniques should be emphasized. Pediatricians can also provide information about what constitutes safe, appropriate dating and relationships, as well as information on safe sex practices. During adolescence, this can mean supporting parents to foster independence in teens and teaching children about adult roles and responsibilities. During an examination, health care professionals can teach children about sexuality and preventing victimization. Statements such as

"I can examine you because I am a doctor and your parent is here" are helpful in reducing anxiety and providing key information. Also, with so many parents anxious about the possibility of abuse, encouraging open communication in families is important. Parents should be encouraged to tell their children to let them know if something bothers them.

9. ***Treatment and Referral:*** Pediatricians need to know what they can handle through office counseling and when they need to refer families for help. They must also be cognizant of the resources available in their community to address these risks. This will require knowledge of the child welfare, emergency shelter, and substance abuse treatment systems and how to make referrals to appropriate therapists and mental health professionals. Health care professionals need to understand when to make reports, the reporting laws, and how the reporting process works for sexual abuse in their jurisdiction.

10. ***Advocacy:*** Pediatricians should use their given status in the community to advocate for the needs of individual families and for the broader needs of children in society. This may include working on public policy. This can best be achieved by working in conjunction with nonmedical organizations that address the needs of children in different arenas. Pediatricians can also work with medical schools and pediatric training programs to provide opportunities for students to learn these techniques and to assist in research evaluating the effectiveness and implementation of child abuse prevention programs.

CONCLUSION

It is an exciting time for those working to prevent child sexual abuse. There is already a wealth of information on what programs are doing and where they are making a difference. At the same time, with decades of experience, it is now apparent that gaps exist in prevention efforts. A level of awareness has been reached so that stronger efforts can proceed to prevent child sexual abuse by addressing individual, family, community, and societal changes. Programs must involve the cultures and communities they serve and be geared toward a specific message to specific populations. Although child-focused programs have grown and provided some protection, involvement of a much wider range of targets and approaches is necessary. In particular, quality programs that involve key adults, including health care professionals, need support and financial backing. Involving the public, bystanders, organizations, parents, offender providers, social change advocates, the media, teachers, policymakers, and health care professionals will be important to ongoing and expanded success of child sexual abuse prevention efforts. Pediatricians and others caring for children have a special position in relation to society and the family and have a multitude of steps they can take to reduce and prevent child sexual abuse.

REFERENCES

1. Miller TR, Cohen MA, Wiersema B. *Victim costs and consequences: a new look* [National Institute of Justice report]. January 1996. Available at: http://www.ncjrs.gov/pdffiles/victcost.pdf. Accessed August 15, 2006.

2. Finkelhor D. Current information on the scope and nature of child sexual abuse. *Future Child.* 1994;4:31-53.

3. World Health Organization. *Gender and health in disasters.* July 2002. Available at: www.who.int/gender/other_health/en/genderdisasters.pdf. Accessed August 13, 2006.

4. United States Department of Health and Human Services. Child Maltreatment 2007. Available at: http://www.acf.hhs.gov/programs/cb/pubs/cm07/. Accessed June 29, 2009.

5. Barnett O, Miller-Perrin CL, Perrin RD. *Family violence across the lifespan.* Thousand Oaks, CA: Sage Publications; 1996.

6. Finkelhor D, Mitchell KJ, Wolak J. Online victimization: what youth tell us. In: Cooper SW, Estes RJ, Giardino AP, Kellogg ND, Vieth VI, eds. *Medical, legal, and social science aspects of child sexual exploitation: a comprehensive review of pornography, prostitution, and Internet crimes.* Vol 1. St Louis, MO: GW Medical Publishing, Inc; 2005:437-467.

7. Berliner L, Elliott DM. Sexual abuse of children. In: Myers JEB, Berliner L, Briere J, Hendrix TC, Jenny C, Reid TA, eds. *The APSAC handbook on child maltreatment.* Thousand Oaks, CA: Sage Publications;2002;55-78.

8. Tyler KA. Social and emotional outcomes of childhood sexual abuse: a review of recent research. *Aggression Violent Behav.* 2002;7:567-589.

9. Dube SR, Anda RF, Whitfield CL, Brown DW, Felitti VJ, Dong M, et al. Long-term consequences of childhood sexual abuse by gender of victim. *Am J Prevent Med.* 2005;28:430-438.

10. Goodkind S, Ng I, Sarri RC. The impact of sexual abuse in the lives of young women involved or at risk of involvement with the juvenile justice system. *Violence Against Women.* 2006;12:456-477.

11. Whiffen VE, MacIntosh HB. Mediators of the link between childhood sexual abuse and emotional distress: a critical review. *Trauma Violence Abuse.* 2005;6: 24-39.

12. Feerick MM, Snow KL. The relationships between childhood sexual abuse, social anxiety, and symptoms of Posttraumatic Stress Disorder in women. *J Fam Violence.* 2005;20(6):409-419.

13. Felitti VJ, Anda RF, Nordenberg D, Williamson DF, Spitz AM, Edwards V, et al. Relationship of childhood abuse and household dysfunction to many of the leading causes of death in adults. The Adverse Childhood Experiences (ACE) Study. *Am J Prev Med.* 1998;14:245-258.

14. Satcher D. The surgeon general's call to action to promote sexual health and responsible sexual behavior. July 9, 2001. Available at: http:// www.surgeon general.gov/library/sexualhealth/call.pdf. Accessed August 12, 2006.

15. Grunbaum JA, Kann L, Kinchen S, Ross J, Hawkins J, Lowry R. Youth risk behavior surveillance—United States, 2003 [published corrections appear in MMWR Morb Mortal Wkly Rep. 2004;53:536 and MMWR Morb Mortal Wkly Rep. 2005;54:608]. MMWR Surveill Summ. 2004;53:1-96.

16. Bronfenbrenner U. Toward an experimental ecology of human development. *Am Psychol.* 1977;32:513-531.

17. National Sexual Violence Resource Center. *A National Resource Directory & Handbook Preventing Child Sexual Abuse.* 2006. Available at: http:// www.nsvrc.org/publications/directories/csa_directory/index.html. Accessed August 18, 2006.

18. Snyder HN. Sexual assault of young children as reported to law enforcement: victim, incident, and offender characteristics. [US Department of Justice, Office of Justice Programs, Bureau of Justice Statistics Web site]. July 2000. Available at: http://www.ojp.usdoj.gov/bjs/pub/pdf/saycrle.pdf. Accessed August 15, 2006.

19. Mullen PE, Martin JL, Anderson JC, Romans SE, Herbison GP. Childhood sexual abuse and mental health in adult life. *Br J Psychiatry*. 1993;163:721-732.

20. Rew L, Esparza D. Barriers to disclosure among sexually abused male children: implications for nursing practice. *J Child Adolesc Psychiatr Ment Health Nurs*. 1990;3:120-127.

21. Gomes-Schwartz B, Horowitz JM, Cardarelli AP. *Child sexual abuse: the initial effects*. Newbury Park, CA: Sage Publications; 1990.

22. Anderson J, Martin J, Mullen P, Romans S, Herbison P. Prevalence of childhood sexual abuse experiences in a community sample of women. *J Am Acad Child Adolesc Psychiatry*. 1993;32:911-920.

23. Finkelhor D, Hotaling G, Lewis IA, Smith C. Sexual abuse in a national survey of adult men and women: prevalence, characteristics, and risk factors. *Child Abuse Negl*. 1990;14:19-28.

24. Palusci VJ, Cox EO, Cyrus TA, Heartwell SW, Vandervort FE, Pott ES. Medical assessment and legal outcome in child sexual abuse. *Arch Pediatr Adolesc Med*. 1999;153:388-392.

25. National Center for Injury Prevention and Control. *Understanding sexual violence: fact sheet*. 2007. Available at: http://www.cdc.gov/ncipc/pub-res/images/SV%20 Factsheet.pdf. Accessed April 7, 2009.

26. Romans S, Martin J, Anderson J, O'Shea M, Mullen P. Factors that mediate between childhood sexual abuse and adult psychological outcome. *Psychol Med*. 1995;25:127-142.

27. Bolen RM. Child sexual abuse: Prevention or promotion? *Social Work*. 2003; 48:174-185.

28. Jensen TK, Gulbrandsen W, Mossige S, Reichelt S, Tjersland OA. Reporting possible sexual abuse: a qualitative study on children's perspectives and the context for disclosure. *Child Abuse Negl*. 2005;29:1395-1413.

29. Staller KM, Nelson-Gardell D. "A burden in your heart": lessons of disclosure from female preadolescent and adolescent survivors of sexual abuse. *Child Abuse Negl*. 2005;29:1415-1432.

30. Kelly P, Koh J, Thompson JM. Diagnostic findings in alleged sexual abuse: symptoms have no predictive value. *J Paediatr Child Health*. 2006;42:112-117.

31. Palusci VJ, Cyrus TA. Reaction to videocolposcopy in the assessment of child sexual abuse. *Child Abuse Negl*. 2001;25:1535-1546.

32. Mandell DS, Walrath C, Manteuffel B, Sgro G, Pinto-Martin J. The prevalence and correlates of abuse among children with autism served in comprehensive community-based mental health settings. *Child Abuse Negl*. 2005;29:1359-1372.

33. Andrews AB, Veronen LJ. Sexual assault and people with disabilities. Special issue: sexuality and disabilities: a guide for human service practitioners. *J Soc Work Hum Sex*. 1993;8:137-159.

34. Nosek MA. Sexual abuse of women with physical disabilities. In: Krotoski DM, Nosek MA, Turk MA, eds. *Women with physical disabilities: achieving and maintaining health and well-being.* Baltimore: Paul H. Brookes Publishing Co, Inc; 1996:153-173.

35. Kelly L. Pornography and child sexual abuse. In: Itzin C, ed. *Pornography: women, violence and civil liberties.* Oxford, England: Oxford University Press; 1992.

36. Briere J, Runtz M. Differential adult symptomatology associated with three types of child abuse histories. *Child Abuse Negl.* 1990;14:357-364.

37. Fergusson DM, Horwood LJ, Lynskey MT. Attentional difficulties in middle childhood and psychosocial outcomes in young adulthood. *J Child Psychol Psychiatry.* 1997;6:633-644.

38. Fleming J, Mullen P, Bammer G. A study of potential risk factors for sexual abuse in childhood. *Child Abuse Negl.* 1997;21:49-58.

39. National Resource Center on Child Sexual Abuse. *The Incidence and Prevalence of Child Sexual Abuse.* Huntsville, AL: NRCCSA; 1994.

40. Plummer CA. The history of child sexual abuse prevention: a practitioner's perspective. *J Child Sex Abuse.* 1999;7:77-95.

41. McCurdy K, Daro D. Child maltreatment: a national survey of reports and fatalities. *J Interpersonal Viol.* 1994;9(1):75-94.

42. Miller-Perrin CL, Wurtele SK. The child sexual abuse prevention movement: a critical analysis of primary and secondary approaches. *Clin Psychol Rev.* 1988; 8:313-329.

43. Finkelhor D, Asdigian N, Dziuba-Leatherman J. The effectiveness of victimization prevention instruction: an evaluation of children's responses to actual threats and assaults. *Child Abuse Negl.* 1995;19:141-153.

44. Plummer CA. Child sexual abuse prevention is appropriate and successful. In: Gelles R, Loseke D, Cavanaugh MM, eds. *Current controversies in family violence.* Newbury Park, CA: Sage Publications; 2004:257-270.

45. Reppucci ND, Haugaard JJ, Antonishak J. Is there empirical evidence to support the effectiveness of child sexual abuse prevention programs? In Gelles R, Loseke D, Cavanaugh MM, eds. *Current controversies in family violence.* Newbury Park, CA: Sage Publications; 2004;271-284.

46. Edwards SM, Lohman JSS. The impact of "moral panic" on professional behavior in cases of child sex abuse: an international perspective. *J Child Sex Abuse.* 1994;3:103-126.

47. Schreiber N. Interviewing techniques in sexual abuse cases—a comparison of a daycare abuse case with normal abuse cases. *Swiss J Psychol.* 2000;59:196-206.

48. Davis K, Gidycz C. Child sexual abuse prevention programs: a meta-analysis. *J Clin Child Psychol.* 2000;29:257-265.

49. Rispens J, Aleman A, Goudena P. Prevention of child sexual victimization: a meta-analysis of school programs. *Child Abuse Negl.* 1997;21:975-987.

50. Gibson L, Leitenberg H. Child sexual abuse prevention programs: do they decrease the occurrence of child sexual abuse? *Child Abuse Negl.* 2000;24:1115-1125.

51. Finkelhor D, Jones LM. Explanations for the decline in child sexual abuse cases. *OJJDP:* Juvenile Justice Bulletin. 2004. Available at: http://www.ncjrs.gov/pdffiles1/ojjdp/199298.pdf. Accessed June 29, 2009.

52. Prevent Child Abuse Iowa. *Together for Prevention* [newsletter]. Summer/Fall 2005. Available at: http://www.pcaiowa.org/documents/newsletter/PCAIA-SuF05.pdf. Accessed August 10, 2006.

53. New Jersey Task Force on Child Abuse and Neglect. Standards for Prevention Programs: Building Success through Family Support. 2003. Retrieved August 18, 2006 from http://www.familysupportamerica.org/downloads/FinalNJDoc11-14-03.pdf.

54. Plummer CA. Prevention of child sexual abuse: a survey of 87 programs. *Violence Vict.* 2001;16:575-588.

55. Berrick JD. Parental involvement in child abuse prevention training: what do they learn? *Child Abuse Negl.* 1988;12:543-553.

56. Elrod JM, Rubin RH. Parental involvement in sexual abuse prevention education. *Child Abuse Negl.* 1993;17:527-538.

57. Reppucci ND, Jones LM, Cook SL. Involving parents in child sexual abuse prevention programs. *J Child Fam Stud.* 1994;3:137-142.

58. Finkelhor D. *Child sexual abuse: new research and theory.* New York: The Free Press; 1984.

59. Wurtele SK. Comprehensiveness and collaboration: key ingredients of an effective public health approach to preventing child sexual abuse. *Sex Abuse.* 1999;11:323-325.

60. Wilson CG, Golub S. Sexual abuse prevention programs for preschool children: what do parents prefer? *Psychol Rep.* 1993;73:812-814.

61. Abel G, Harlow N. *Stop child molestation.* Philadelphia: Xlibris Corporation; 2001.

62. Stop It Now. Let's talk: speaking up to prevent child sexual abuse. 2006. Available at: http://www.stopitnow.com/sites/stopitnow.rivervalleywebhosting.com/files/webfm/green/LetsTalk.pdf. Accessed April 7, 2009.

63. Finkelhor D, Strapko N. Sexual abuse prevention education: a review of evaluation studies. In: Willis D, Holden EW, Rosenberg M, eds. *Prevention of child maltreatment.* New York: Wiley & Sons; 1992:150-167.

64. MacMillan HL, MacMillan JH, Offord DR, Griffith L, MacMillan A. Primary prevention of child physical abuse and neglect: a critical review. Part I. *J Child Psychol Psychiatry.* 1994;35:835-856.

65. Anderson C. *Sexual abuse prevention with organizations.* Paper presented at: Imagine: The National Conference on Sexual Abuse Prevention; August 2005; Huntsville, AL.

66. Helfer RE. A review of the literature on the prevention of child abuse and neglect. *Child Abuse Negl.* 1982;6:251-261.

67. Hamberger L, Patel D. Why health care professionals are reluctant to intervene in cases of ongoing domestic abuse. In: Kendall-Tackett K, ed. *Health consequences of abuse in the family: a clinical guide for evidence-based practice.* Washington, DC: American Psychological Association; 2004;63-80.

68. Trepper T, Barrett MJ. *Systemic treatment of incest: a therapeutic handbook.* New York: Brunner/Mazel; 1989.

69. Dubowitz H. Preventing child neglect and physical abuse: a role for pediatricians. *Pediatr Rev.* 2002;23:191-196.

70. Johnson CF. *Actions Pediatricians Can Take to Prevent Child Maltreatment: A Checklist.* 1998.

71. Sege RD, Hatmaker-Flanigan E, De Vos E, Levin-Goodman R, Spivak H. Anticipatory guidance and violence prevention: results from family and pediatrician focus groups. *Pediatrics.* 2006;117:455-463.

72. Bays J, Chadwick D. Medical diagnosis of the sexually abused child. *Child Abuse Negl.* 1993;17:91-110.

73. Rieser M. Recantation in child sexual abuse cases. *Child Welfare.* 1991;70:611-621.

74. Sorenson T, Snow B. How children tell: the process of disclosure in child sexual assault. *Child Welfare.* 1991;70:3-15.

75. Myers JB. *The backlash: child protection under fire.* Thousand Oaks, CA: Sage Publications; 1994.

76. Everson MD, Hunter WM, Runyon DK, Edelsohn GA, Coulter ML. Maternal support following disclosure of incest. *Am J Orthopsychiatry.* 1989;59:197-207.

77. Goodman R. A Modified Version of the Rutter Parent Questionnaire Including Extra Items on Children's Strengths: A Research Note. *J Child Psychol Psychiatry.* November 1994;35(8):1483-1494.

78. Dubowitz H, Black MM, Cox CE, Kerr MA, Litrownik AJ, Radhakrishna A, et al. Father involvement and children's functioning at age 6 years: a multisite study. *Child Maltreat.* 2001;6:300-309.

79. Trowbridge MJ, Sege RD, Olson L, O'Connor K, Flaherty E, Spivak H. Intentional injury management and prevention in pediatric practice: results from 1998 and 2003 American Academy of Pediatrics Periodic Surveys. *Pediatrics.* 2005;116:996-1000.

80. Diaz A, Manigat M. The healthcare provider's role in the disclosure of sexual abuse: the medical interview as a gateway to disclosure. *Child Health Care.* 2000; 28:141-149.

81. American Academy of Pediatrics. Connected kids: safe, strong, secure. *A new violence prevention program from the American Academy of Pediatrics.* Elk Grove Village, IL: AAP; 2005.

82. Plummer CA. Non-abusive mothers of sexually abused children: The role of rumination in maternal outcomes. *J Child Sex Abuse.* 2006;15:103-122.

83. Crisci G. *Youth sexually abusing youth.* Paper presented at Imagine: National Conference on Child Sexual Abuse Prevention, Florence, AL; Aug 2006.

INDEX

A

ABO group antigens based testing, 234
ABP. *See* American Board of Pediatrics
Abuse prevention, 375–395
    adult educational efforts, 381
    age of victims and likelihood of abuse, 378
    bystander involvement in, 389
    child education, 381–382, 384–385, 388
    child victim's reaction to abuse, 379
    clinical care and education improvement,
        389–390
    community awareness involvement in, 388–389
    criticism of current prevention efforts, 381–382
    current trends and future directions, 383–386
    defining, 376–377
    diversity-based approaches, 385
    early sexual behavior problem identification, 389
    of exploitation of children, 300–301, 306–308,
        306f–307f, 313–315
    familial mental and behavioral problems as
        indicators, 376
    future health problems of victims, 376
    health professional involvement in, 386–388,
        390
    history of prevention efforts, 380–381
    identification of abuse cases, 378–379
    importance of, 375–376
    incidence rates of child abuse, 375–376, 382
    individual vulnerability, 379–380
    Internet and media safety programs, 385–386
    organizational interventions, 386, 389
    parental involvement in, 379, 383–384,
        387–388
    prevention messages, 384
    risk of abuse and protective factors, 377–378
    school-based education programs, 384–385
    societal factors leading to abuse, 378
    and special needs children, 379–380
    support for parents and extended family,
        387–388
    treatment and referral, 390
    youth offender prevention, 380, 382, 389
    See also Reframing our perspective of child abuse

Abuser
    confessions of abuse, 223–224, 239
    danger to intimate partner presented by, 67–68,
        90–91
    demographics of, 291
    protection of the, 63–64
    protection of the victim from, 61, 63, 90–91
    relationship to victim, 59
    sex offender registries, 382
    youth as sexual abuse offenders, 293, 380, 382
    See also Prosecution of sexual abuse
Accreditation Council for Graduate Medical
        Education, 263
ACEs. *See* Adverse Childhood Experiences
Acute sexual assault. *See* Forensic evidence; Medical
        examination and evaluation
Adolescents, 85–102
    emotional issues
        anxiety and emotional health of, 77, 90–93,
            96–100, 100t
        behavioral symptoms and detection of
            abuse, 88
        cognitive development issues in, 85
        confidentiality and consent issues, 85–86,
            217
        disclosure of abuse, 87
        interviewing, 213–214
        long term healing management, 98–100
        perception of sexual abuse of, 87
        self-blame in, 87
        trust and safety issues of, 90–91
    legal issues
        evidence collection, 216–221
        jurisdictional interpretations of sexual
            abuse, 86
        mandatory sex offender registration and,
            293
    physical issues
        anal trauma evidence in, 226–227
        anogenital examination techniques,
            215–216
        development of bacterial vaginosis, 203
        drug- and alcohol-facilitated sexual assault
            of, 87, 98, 221, 223–224

B

C

I

J

L